Common Complications in Endodontics

Priyanka Jain
Editor

Common Complications in Endodontics

Prevention and Management

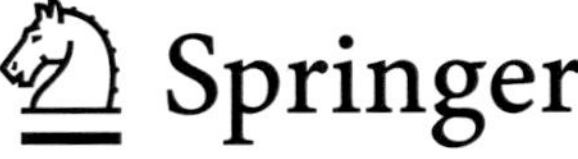

Editor
Priyanka Jain
Department of Endodontics
Apex Medical Clinics
Dubai
United Arab Emirates

ISBN 978-3-319-86979-7 ISBN 978-3-319-60997-3 (eBook)
https://doi.org/10.1007/978-3-319-60997-3

Softcover reprint of the hardcover 1st edition 2017

Printed on acid-free paper

This Springer imprint is published by Springer Nature
The registered company is Springer International Publishing AG
The registered company address is: Gewerbestrasse 11, 6330 Cham, Switzerland

Foreword

It is a pleasure for me to write the Foreword to the first edition of *Complications in Endodontics: Prevention and Management.*

This is a fine collaboration of internationally renowned authors that summarizes every clinical aspect of how to avoid procedural errors that might occur and how to correct these errors if they should occur.

The twenty-first-century style of this textbook reflects the most current ways of imparting information and acquiring knowledge in this digital era.

The multitude of well-documented case presentations, including outstanding photographs, illustrations, and radiographs, helps to reinforce, in a step-by-step approach, the concepts discussed in each chapter.

The flawless continuity between the following chapters and the coordination of topics is a real tribute to the authors and editors to inform and educate the clinician.

The clinically based "how to" style in which each of these chapters is written will be a great help for the clinician. The superb organization and comprehensive nature of *Complications in Endodontics: Prevention and Management* makes it a valuable addition for all clinician's libraries.

Stephen Cohen, M.A., D.D.S., F.I.C.D., F.A.C.D.
Diplomate, American Board of Endodontics
San Francisco
CA, USA

Preface

The common problems clinicians encounter during practice continue to stem from the areas of diagnosis and cleaning and shaping techniques. Successful endodontics requires a thorough diagnosis, a complete knowledge of the anatomy of the canal systems being treated along with their complete debridement, and careful shaping techniques, thus providing for complete obturation and a coronal seal provided by a final permanent restoration. Assessment of the risks associated with any treatment procedure is aimed to prevent, identify, and manage any potential complication. A clinician should always be prepared to manage any undesirable results.

Complications can occur during many dental procedures. The clinician responds by either correcting the problem during treatment or, ideally, preventing the problem from occurring in the first place.

A decision on how or whether to treat or not cannot be made without a proper diagnosis. Endodontic treatment is not a diagnosis but is a treatment plan arrived at after a thorough and careful assessment. A radiolucency on a radiograph alone cannot provide a diagnosis. Separate pulpal and periapical diagnoses must be reached. Careful examination along with a detailed history is of prime importance. It must be kept in mind that the findings can change between appointments.

The importance of correct radiographic interpretation cannot be emphasized enough. It is a common understanding that both large and small lesions and anatomical entities can be routinely missed in radiographic interpretation both by the operator and the limitations of the technology when encountering differences in anatomic variation. Digital imaging of dental structures has become a common diagnostic modality in the last decade in dental offices around the world. New radiographic imaging systems have recently become available for use in the dental field and have completely transformed the way we diagnose and treat problems. Among these are cone beam computed tomography (CBCT), which allows for precise and accurate visualization and evaluation of teeth and their surrounding structures. CBCT has become an essential diagnostic tool in the modern endodontic practice. But we need to carefully evaluate the potential risk and maximize the benefit to the patient.

Although an emphasis is placed in the literature on instrumentation and obturation techniques, we cannot forget that a basic aspect of providing care is doing the treatment painlessly. True anesthesia failures (i.e., primary, secondary, and adjunct forms of anesthesia delivered skillfully that fail to anesthetize the pulp) are rare occurrences. Adequate anesthesia can be achieved despite initial failure through patience, skillful delivery of the anesthetic, and understanding of the original cause of failure. Factors that contribute to anesthesia failure are discussed, and recommendations to overcome them are proposed and discussed in Chap. 3.

Paresthesia due to over-obturation as well as other neural complications must be considered as a serious problem. These injuries require a thoughtful strategy for prevention during endodontic procedures as well as a careful systematic approach toward its management, should the endodontic procedure result in such injury.

The next section talks about the various mishaps encountered during the procedural phase of endodontic therapy. Procedural errors may be defined as improper action or inaction of the practitioner either before or after the procedure. These may not have any effect or may, in some cases, result in a complication.

The cause of perforations during access is mainly due to lack of axial inclination and failure to hold the bur parallel to the tooth. Inadequate access can also lead to misdirection and unnecessary gouging. Prevention is the key to success and includes a thorough understanding of the tooth morphology, having multiple radiographs to reference, and patience.

In endodontic treatment separated rotary Ni-Ti files are a common procedural problem. Through understanding that the main causes of file breakage are cyclic fatigue and torsional stress, a dentist can best prevent this occurrence by using hand files before rotary files, creating a straight-line access into a canal, and pre-flaring the coronal portion before using rotary files in the apical third of the canal. A case does not necessarily fail if the separated file cannot be removed. The prognosis in these cases can still be favorable, if care is taken to reduce the concentration of canal debris with hand instrumentation and chemical irrigation prior to rotary file insertion.

Wouldn't it be nice and simple if all canals were straight? Since they aren't, we must understand how curved canal cleaning and shaping can be achieved without creating ledges. The most common canals that are "prone to ledging are small, curved, and long." Prevention of ledging can be minimized with accurate preoperative and working radiographs, copious irrigation, pre-curved files, and incremental instrumentation. The prognosis of teeth that have ledges in them varies and surgical endodontics may be needed.

The next chapter discusses the obturation complications. These are best prevented by giving proper attention to the working length and attaining a smooth and even taper and flare during the cleaning and shaping process.

In the dental literature, several mishaps during root canal irrigation have been described, from damage to the patient's clothing, splashing of the irrigant into the patient's or operator's eye, to injection through the apical foramen or air emphysema and allergic reactions to the irrigant. Forcibly injecting sodium hypochlorite (or other types of irrigants) into the radicular tissues can cause tissue damage, paresthesia, muscle weakness, and extreme discomfort. The author discusses various management measures should such a complication occur in Chap. 7. Measures that can prevent and/or minimize such accidents, which can occur during the course of endodontic therapy, are also discussed.

Chapter 8 describes the way to maximize disinfection and avoid reinfection via case preselection, antimicrobial strategy, and reinfection prevention. Occasionally, a nonsurgical root canal procedure alone cannot save the tooth and a surgical approach may be needed. Surgical endodontics and the common risks/complications such as wound healing impairment, infection, and bleeding are discussed under this chapter.

An endo-perio lesion can have a varied pathogenesis ranging from simple to a relatively complex one. Having proper knowledge of these disease processes is essential in coming to the correct diagnosis. It is important to remember that the recognition of pulp vitality is essential for a differential diagnosis and for the selection of primary measures for treatment of inflammatory lesions in the marginal and apical periodontium.

Endodontic needs of today's and tomorrow's growing older adult population present increasing challenges for clinicians. Biologic and anatomic differences in the dental pulpal tissues between older and younger patients must be carefully understood and considered in treatment planning and performance for appropriate endodontic procedures. These differences generally do not contraindicate treatment, which, when performed correctly, will be successful in the elderly patient.

When the endodontic procedure is carried out in patients with systemic illness or who are under medical management, it is important to avoid the potential medical emergencies. Hence, clinicians must be aware of common diseases and drugs that have an impact in endodontic treatment and the management options in such cases. The last chapter aims to highlight the most commonly occurring clinical conditions that require special endodontic attention.

This book presents up-to-date recommendations for the prevention, diagnosis, and management of complications in endodontic procedures, based on the best available scientific evidence. It is ideal for both endodontists and general dentists, as the text combines the precision of quality endodontic care with achievable and pain-free outcomes for the patient. Each chapter has been carefully written from a clinical viewpoint to help the clinician and accompanied by an extensive bibliography, allowing the reader to explore the topic further, should they desire.

The aim is to provide the readers with in-depth knowledge and tools to incorporate an evidence-based approach to prevent, identify, and manage complications that occur during the endodontic procedure. Every attempt has been made to discuss the common procedural complications in depth and detail. The text presents the material in a reader-friendly manner with helpful flowcharts, tables, and figures.

Enjoy the book and we welcome your feedback at any time.

Dubai, UAE Priyanka Jain

Acknowledgments

This book is for all my teachers, colleagues, and friends in the field of endodontics. It took close to 18 months in conceiving and executing this project. A book of this caliber and scope cannot be accomplished by a single person. It is the result of a great multiauthor dedication and effort. I have several people to thank, for without their help, guidance, perseverance, and patience, this book would not have seen the light of the day. They are the true heart and spirit of the book.

Therefore, my sincere gratitude to Carla Cabral dos Santos Accioly Lins, Flavia Maria de Moraes Ramos Perez, Andrea dos Anjos Pontual de Andrade Lima, and Maria Luiza dos Anjos Pontual, authors of the chapter on radiographic interpretation; Alexander J Moule, Unni Krishnan, and Tara Renton, authors of the chapter on complications of local anesthesia; Ray Bradford Johnson for his expertise on access-related complications; Sami Chogle, Obadah Attar, and Tun-Yi Hsu for the chapter on instrument-related complications; Gianluca Plotino, Nicola Maria Grande, and Mauro Venturi for their work on obturation-related complications; Zuhair Alkatib and Rashi el Abed, authors for the chapter on complications due to medicaments; Federico for his expertise on strategies to reduce the risk of reinfection in endodontics; Igor Tsesis, Eyal Rosen, Tamar Blazer, and Shlomo Elbahary for their work on complications during surgical endodontics; Prof. Omer for his chapters on endo-perio relationship and geriatric patient; and finally Catherine Wynne for contributing to the chapter on endodontic considerations in systemically compromised patients.

I would also like to thank Mr. Kumar Krishna Mohan, for his help with the images and illustrations.

I would also like to extend my thanks to Dr. Reem, Dr. Dana, Dr. Aga and Dr. Hessa for their help with cases.

Sincere thanks to Dr. Stephen Cohen for once again providing the Foreword. He has always been my inspiration and I was very grateful when he agreed to write the Foreword.

I would also like to thank Dr. Sverre Klemp for his faith in me and giving me this opportunity to write the book. My sincere thanks to Ms. Abha Krishnan, Springer, and their team for their professional expertise in making this book a reality.

Most importantly, thanks to my husband Gaurav and my children, Navya and Armaan, and all my family members who put up with all my apprehensions and late working hours.

And finally and most important of all, I thank them who are responsible for whatever I am today—my parents.

Contents

Part I

Diagnosis

Clinical Diagnosis and Treatment Planning

1

Priyanka Jain

1.1 Introduction

Establishing an accurate diagnosis (both pulpal and periapical) is the most important step in determining the appropriate treatment [1, 2]. If an incorrect diagnosis/assessment of the clinical findings is made, improper management may result often leading to confusion, for example, performing endodontic treatment when it is not needed or providing some other treatment when root canal treatment is indicated. Tooth pain is usually considered the worst and least tolerable kind of pain. It usually originates in dentine, pulp, or periapical tissue and is thus considered of endodontic origin. Therefore, 90% of all patients with orofacial pain require a thorough endodontic assessment and diagnosis, and 60% of them may require endodontic treatment. A proper diagnosis is only possible following the subjective description of complaints by the patient coupled with objective clinical findings. Identification of a coronal or radicular fracture is also important. Although this is not specifically a pulpal or periradicular diagnosis, but it is important to note that fractures may change the proposed treatment plan. Temporomandibular joint (TMJ) dysfunctions may also present as dental pain, so we should keep in mind the clinical presentation of patients with those symptoms as well.

Following a definitive diagnosis of the need for root canal treatment, the treatment planning stage should be straightforward. The goal of endodontic treatment is to preserve the tooth as a functional unit within a functioning dentition. Therefore, the endodontic treatment must be integrated into a comprehensive treatment plan that includes both restorative and periodontal management.

This chapter will talk about the various endodontic diagnosis and describe each condition typical of clinical and radiographic characteristics supported by clinical

P. Jain, M.Sc., M.D.S., B.D.S.
Specialist Endodontist, Dubai Health Authority, Dubai, UAE

Part Time Faculty (Endodontics)- College of Dental Medicine, University of Sharjah, Dubai, UAE
e-mail: tracyjain@hotmail.com

P. Jain (ed.), *Common Complications in Endodontics*,
https://doi.org/10.1007/978-3-319-60997-3_1

cases. But we as clinicians have to recognize the fact that diseases of the pulp and periapical tissues are dynamic and their signs and symptoms may vary between patients. A simple and practical system which uses terms related to clinical findings is essential and will help clinicians understand the progressive nature of pulpal and periapical disease, directing them to the most appropriate treatment approach for each condition. The proposed endodontic treatment should be part of an agreed, comprehensive treatment plan that includes the patient's participation in the treatment decisions. The author will also discuss the various treatment planning considerations to be kept in mind. Pulpal obliteration and its management are also discussed in brief.

In 2008, the American Association of Endodontists proposed universal recommendations regarding endodontic diagnoses and developed a standardized definition of key diagnostic terms that will be generally accepted by endodontists, educators, test construction experts, third parties, generalists and other specialists, and students [3]. This will help in the interpretation of results and determine the radiographic criteria and clinical criteria needed to validate these.

1.2 Examination

Endodontic diagnosis cannot be made from a single complaint. The clinician must gather all the data presented to him to be able to make a probable diagnosis (Table 1.1).

1.2.1 History of Chief Complaint

The initial step for an exact endodontic diagnosis involves taking the patient's past and present medical history and any current medication. The relationship between the medical conditions and endodontic treatment are discussed later in the book. The medical case history is followed by a dental history, with particular emphasis on the current history. This should be clearly structured and suggestive questions must always be avoided.

Table 1.1 Examination procedures required to make an endodontic diagnosis

Medical/Dental history	Past/recent treatment, drugs
Chief complaint (if any)	How long, symptoms, duration of pain, location, onset, stimuli, relief, referred, medications
Clinical exam	Facial symmetry, sinus tract, soft tissue, periodontal status (probing, mobility), caries, restorations (defective, newly placed?)
Clinical testing:	
Pulp tests	Cold, electric pulp test, heat
Periapical tests	Percussion, palpation, tooth sloth (biting)
Radiographic analysis	New periapicals (at least 2), bitewing, cone beam computed tomography
Additional tests	Transillumination, selective anesthesia, test cavity

Possible questions for a detailed dental history:

1. Reason for consultation of dentist?
   If the patient indicates pain as a reason, a differentiated history of pain is required.
   (a) When did the pain start?
   (b) Kind of pain: spontaneous, constant, intermittent, continuously worsening, or improving periodically?
   (c) Does the pain radiate?
   (d) Can you localize it?
   (e) Pain during the night? Is it worse in the morning?
   (f) Any aggravating or relieving factors like heat/cold?
   (g) How long does it last?
   (h) Quality of the pain: dragging, stabbing, and throbbing?
2. Is there any swelling, and if so, where?
3. Is there a sensitivity to temperature? If so, describe the nature of it.
4. Has there been a need to take pain medication for this tooth? Does it help in controlling the pain?
5. Has there been any sinus problem lately?
6. Is the tooth sensitive to chewing or pressure?
7. Have you had any recent dental work?

It is important to recreate the patient's chief complaint during the clinical examination. This reduces the chance that you will miss an important piece of evidence. Also note that antibiotics and pain medications can make the diagnostic process more challenging and less reliable.

The clinical and radiographic examinations must be always combined with a thorough periodontal evaluation and clinical testing (pulp and periapical tests) before arriving at a preliminary diagnosis. In case the findings are inconclusive and a definitive pulpal and periapical diagnoses cannot be made, it is better that treatment should not be rendered at this stage. The patient may have to wait and be reassessed at a later date.

Endodontic diagnosis is composed of two parts: pulpal diagnosis and the periapical diagnosis. Pulpal diagnosis indicates the status of the pulp (nerve and connective tissue inside the tooth) and can be accomplished by using thermal and electric pulp tests. The periapical diagnosis indicates the status of the periapex (tissues around the root of the tooth) and, according to the *American Association of Endodontists*, is based upon pain and swelling. Diagnostic terminology used in this chapter is approved by the American Association of Endodontists and the American Board of Endodontics [4–6].

For clarification, the acute classifications refer to recent symptomatology. The chronic classifications refer to a situation that is long standing and can be viewed on a radiograph. Suppurative periradicular periodontitis is used when a sinus tract or drainage area is present. An acute periradicular abscess occurs when there is acute swelling, pus formation, tenderness, and eventual swelling with or without radiographic pathology.

1.2.2 Pulpal Diagnosis [7–12]

1.2.2.1 Normal Pulp

In this case, the pulp is symptom-free and usually responsive to pulp testing normally. A "clinically" normal pulp results in a mild or transient response to thermal and cold testing, lasting for few seconds after the stimulus is removed. The response should always be compared with adjacent and contralateral teeth.

1.2.2.2 Reversible Pulpitis

This is based upon both subjective and objective findings indicating that the pulp will return to normal following appropriate management of the cause. Pain is experienced when a stimulus such as cold or sweet is applied but goes away quickly (within a couple of seconds) following the removal of the stimulus. Etiological factors may include exposed dentin (dentinal sensitivity), caries, or deep restorations. There are no significant radiographic changes in the periapical area of the affected tooth. Pain elicited is not spontaneous but is usually hypersensitive. After the management of the etiology, the tooth requires further evaluation to determine whether the "reversible pulpitis" has returned to a normal status. Symptoms of dentinal sensitivity mimic those of a reversible pulpitis.

1.2.2.3 Symptomatic Irreversible Pulpitis (SIP)

This scenario is based on subjective and objective findings that the vital inflamed pulp is incapable of healing (returning to normal status) and that root canal treatment is indicated. Characteristics may include sharp pain upon thermal stimulus which lingers (often 30 seconds or longer after stimulus removal), spontaneous pain (unprovoked pain), and referred pain. At times, the pain may be accentuated by postural changes such as lying down or bending over, and over-the-counter analgesics are typically ineffective. Common factors include deep caries, extensive restorations, or fractures exposing the pulpal tissues. Such teeth may be difficult to diagnose because the inflammation has not yet reached the periapical tissues, thus resulting in no pain or discomfort to percussion. In such cases, detailed dental history and careful examination in conjunction with thermal testing are the primary tools for assessing pulpal status (Fig. 1.1).

1.2.2.4 Asymptomatic Irreversible Pulpitis

This is a clinical diagnosis also based on subjective and objective findings and root canal treatment is indicated. These cases have no clinical symptoms and usually respond normally to thermal testing but may have deep caries that would likely result in exposure during removal.

1.2.2.5 Pulp Necrosis

This is a clinical diagnostic category indicating death of the dental pulp, necessitating root canal treatment. The pulp is nonresponsive to pulp testing and is asymptomatic. Pulp necrosis by itself does not cause apical periodontitis (pain to percussion or any radiographic changes) unless the canal is infected. Some teeth may be nonresponsive to pulp testing due of calcification, or recent history of trauma. Therefore, vitality testing must be comparative in nature with the adjacent teeth (Fig. 1.2).

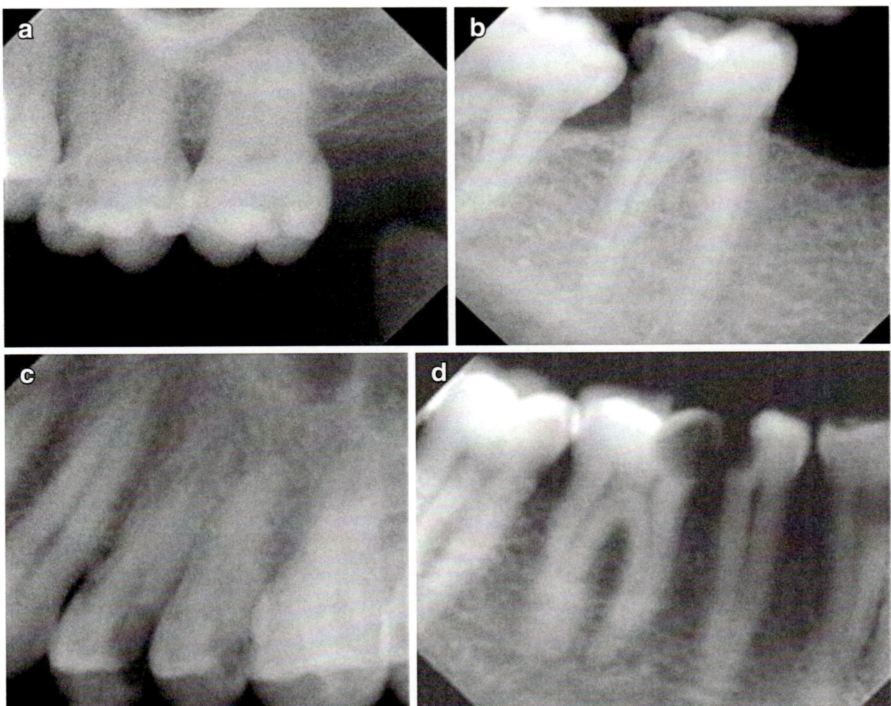

Fig. 1.1 (**a**, **b**) Symptomatic irreversible pulpitis. (**c**) Irreversible pulpitis on tooth 24, 25. (**d**) Irreversible pulpitis and widening of PDL on tooth 45, 46

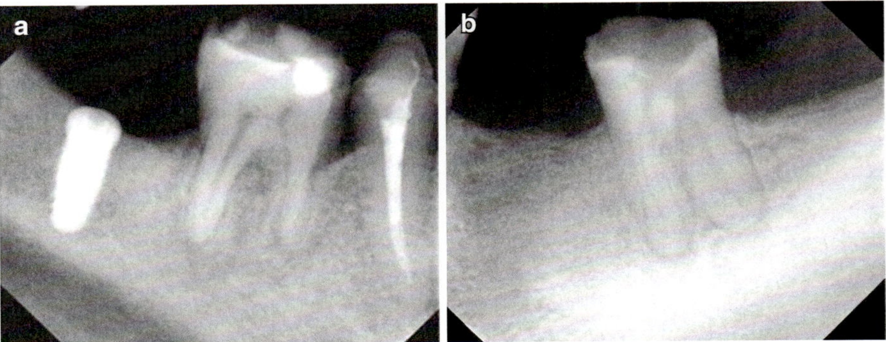

Fig. 1.2 (**a**) Partial pulp necrosis with root resorption (tooth 46). (**b**) Pulpal necrosis with uncertain periapical status

If the pulp necrosis is asymptomatic, there:

1. May or may not be an observable radiographic lesion. If there is no observable lesion radiographically, caution is advised. If the tooth requires a new crown and there is evidence that the pulp is necrotic, it is optimal to perform endodontic

therapy before placing the crown. If the tooth was once symptomatic with clear signs of irreversible pulpitis (especially spontaneous pain) and later became asymptomatic with or without a lesion, the tooth should be treated.
2. May be a lack of response to thermal pulp testing.

1.2.3 Apical Diagnoses [7–12]

1.2.3.1 Normal Apical Tissues

In teeth which are not sensitive to percussion or palpation during testing and radiographically, the lamina dura surrounding the root is intact with the periodontal ligament space as uniform. As with pulp testing, comparative testing for percussion and palpation should always begin with normal teeth as a baseline for the patient.

1.2.3.2 Symptomatic Apical Periodontitis (SAP)

This represents inflammation, usually of the apical periodontium. Clinical symptoms include a painful response to biting and/or percussion or palpation. This may or may not be accompanied by radiographic changes (i.e., depending upon the stage of the disease, there may be normal width of the periodontal ligament or there may be a periapical radiolucency). Severe pain to percussion and/or palpation is highly indicative of a degenerating pulp, and root canal treatment is needed (Table 1.2) (Fig. 1.3a, b).

1.2.3.3 Asymptomatic Apical Periodontitis

In this case, inflammation of the apical periodontium is of pulpal origin. It manifests as an apical radiolucency and does not present clinical symptoms (no pain on percussion or palpation) (Fig. 1.4a–c).

1.2.3.4 Chronic Apical Abscess

This is an inflammatory reaction to pulpal infection and necrosis characterized by gradual onset, little or no discomfort, and an intermittent discharge of pus through an associated sinus tract. Radiographically, there are signs of a radiolucency.

1.2.3.5 Acute Apical Abscess (AAA)

This is necrosis characterized by rapid onset, spontaneous pain, and extreme tenderness of the tooth to pressure, pus formation, and swelling of associated tissues. There may be no radiographic changes, and the patient often experiences malaise, fever, and lymphadenopathy (Fig. 1.5).

Table 1.2 Clinical findings used to differentiate between SIP and SAP

Criteria	Symptomatic irreversible pulpitis (SIP)	Symptomatic apical periodontitis (SAP)
Sensitivity to cold (carbon dioxide snow)	+	–
Radiographically widened ligament space	±	+
Swelling or sinus tract	–	–
Periapical radiolucency	–	±

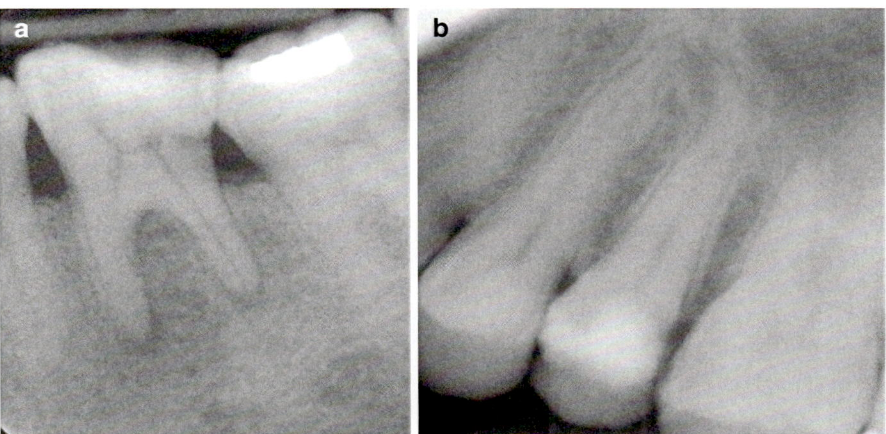

Fig. 1.3 (**a**, **b**) Pulpal necrosis symptomatic apical periodontitis

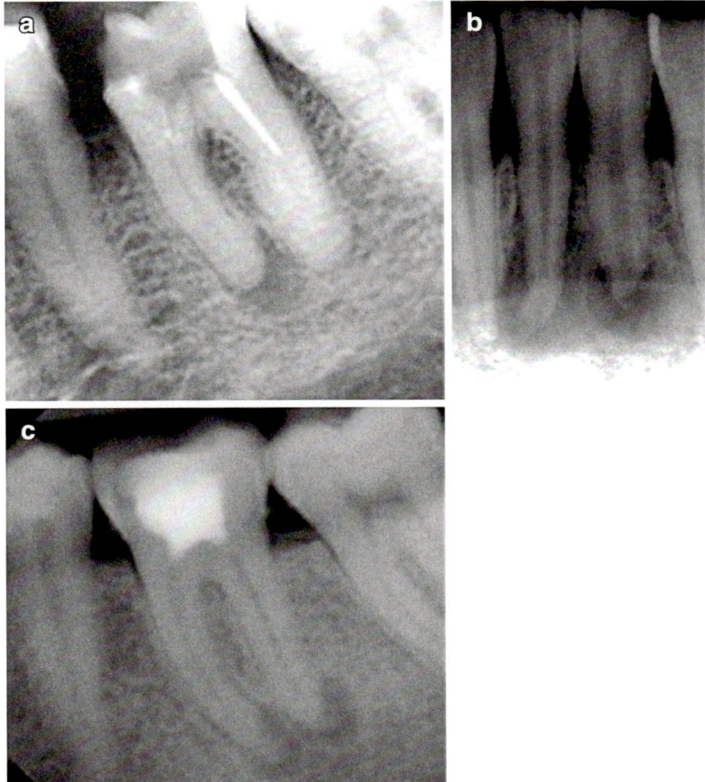

Fig. 1.4 (**a**) Posttreatment asymptomatic apical periodontitis on lower left first molar. (**b**) History of trauma 15 years ago—pulp necrosis with asymptomatic apical periodontitis with grade 2 mobility and pocket depth of 8 mm. (**c**) Asymptomatic apical periodontitis and root resorption

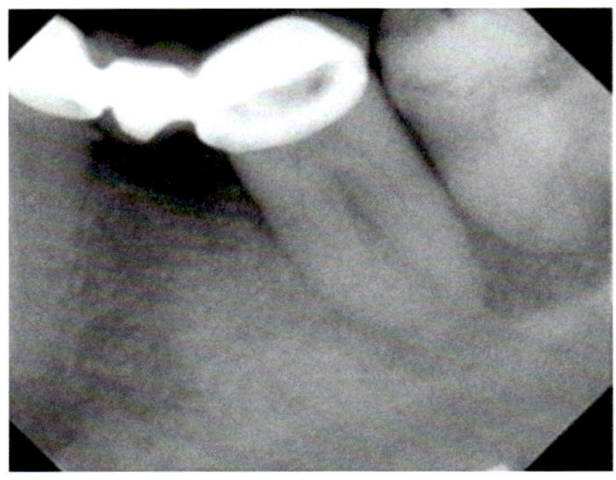

Fig. 1.5 Pulp necrosis with acute apical abscess

1.2.4 Condensing Osteitis

This is a diffuse radiopaque lesion representing a localized bony reaction to a low-grade inflammatory stimulus usually seen at the apex of the tooth.

Symptomatic clinical conditions such as symptomatic irreversible pulpitis (SIP), symptomatic apical periodontitis (SAP), and acute apical abscess (AAA) can be extremely painful [13, 14]. Unfortunately, the current diagnostic nomenclature of the American Association of Endodontists (AAE; [15]) does not differentiate between teeth that cause significant enough pain to require the patient to seek emergency care from those that merely show an increased reaction to diagnostic tests [16].

Due to the obvious clinical symptom of edema (swelling) associated with the diagnosis of AAA, this diagnosis poses no challenge. In contrast, clear-cut symptoms have not been identified to differentiate between SAP and SIP. While SIP is merely painful, SAP is the beginning of the spread of infection with a possibility of untoward systemic consequences [17]. The emergency treatment for SIP and SAP differs [18, 19]. With SIP, simply removing the coronal pulp is sufficient for relief [20], while with SAP the disinfection of the entire root canal system is needed.

1.3 Clinical Evaluation

The clinical evaluation consists of several tests including but not limited to palpation, percussion, periodontal probing, thermal/electrical testing, biting and release (Tables 1.3 and 1.4). For a comparative result to help in establishing a diagnosis, all tests should be performed on the tooth in question and the contralateral/adjacent teeth as well.

1.3.1 Palpation, Percussion, and Periodontal Probing

The first step in the examination is to do a visual evaluation by looking at the patient straight on to check if there is any visible swelling or asymmetry. Both extraoral and

Table 1.3 Pulpal diagnosis

Clinical classification	Signs and symptoms	Diagnostic tests	Endodontic treatment needed or not
Reversible pulpitis	*Pain*—no history of pain, pain is non-spontaneous *Radiographically*—no radiographic evidence of internal resorption or periapical change	*EPT*—response is normal and within range *Thermal tests*—moderate to sharp response to thermal, sweet; response subsides when stimulus is removed *Percussion and Palpation*—negative, no response	**NOT** needed
Irreversible pulpitis (with or without apical pathosis) *Etiology* Deep caries and/or restorations, exposed dentin (attrition, abrasion, and erosion), traumatic injuries, orthodontic forces	*Pain* • May have acute or chronic symptoms, • Pain may be spontaneous/continuous; previous repeated episodes of pain, • Pain with mastication (on biting) *Radiology* • Radiographic evidence may reveal normal pulp, narrow pulp chamber, "calcified" canals, or condensing osteitis • An enlarged PDL may also be present	*EPT* Tooth may test within normal limits, but response may be markedly different from control; rapid/delayed onset, may be persistent, and may be of severe intensity *Thermal test* A key factor in making a diagnosis. Sharp, exaggerated, painful response to thermal stimulus; pain lingers after stimulus is removed *Percussion test* May or may not be positive *Palpation* May or may not be positive	**IS** needed
Necrotic pulp (with or without apical pathosis) *Etiology* Deep caries and/or restorations, exposed dentin (attrition, abrasion, and erosion), traumatic injuries, orthodontic forces	*Pain* • May have acute or chronic symptoms • Pain may be spontaneous/continuous; previous repeated episodes of pain, often dull and throbbing • Pain on biting *Radiology* • May be normal • Enlarged PDL maybe evident • Periapical or lateral lesions maybe evident	*EPT* No response/may have false positives *Thermal test* No response *Palpation/percussion test* May or may not be positive	**IS** needed

Table 1.4 Periapical diagnosis

Clinical classification	Signs and symptoms	Diagnostic tests	Endodontic treatment needed or not
Acute apical periodontitis *Etiology* Irreversible pulpitis, traumatic injuries, Periodontal disease, orthodontic forces, restoration in hyperocclusion	*Pain* Sharp, intermittent pain of pulpal origin (moderate to severe intensity), aggravating factors are usually present	*EPT and thermal tests* may be normal, or similar to irreversible pulpitis or pulpal necrosis *Palpation/percussion* Moderate to severe pain *Radiology* Usually thickening of PDL, may have periapical or lateral radiolucency	**MAY** need endodontic treatment
Chronic apical periodontitis (etiology—same as above)	*Pain* • Slight intensity to no pain, pain may be absent or constant • Periapical pain can be spontaneous. • Pain is dull throbbing • Pain can occur with mastication	*EPT and thermal tests* may be normal, or similar to irreversible pulpitis or pulpal necrosis *Percussion* Moderate to none *Palpation* Moderate to none. May be swelling *Radiology* Periapical or lateral radiolucency	**MAY** need endodontic treatment
Chronic suppurative apical periodontitis *Etiology* Irreversible pulpitis, traumatic injuries, periodontal disease, orthodontic forces, restoration in hyperocclusion	*Pain* • Usually no pain present • A draining sinus tract or other evidence of suppuration is evident	*EPT and thermal tests* may be normal, or similar to irreversible pulpitis or pulpal necrosis *Percussion* None to slight pain *Palpation* Slightly tender *Radiology* Periapical or lateral radiolucency	**IS** needed
Acute alveolar abscess (acute apical abscess) *Etiology* The result of coronal apical progression of pulpal necrosis into the periapical tissues	*Pain* • Severe pain which is constant and spontaneous • Pain is pulsing and throbbing • Pain can occur with mastication	*Pulp tests* No response *Percussion* Moderate to severe *Palpation* Moderate to severe, swelling probable *Radiology* PDL thickening, periapical or lateral radiolucency	**IS** needed

A pulpal diagnosis is required for a definitive determination intraoral digital palpation should be performed, including palpating the lymph nodes on the affected side. Make sure to palpate the buccal and lingual/palatal surfaces of the affected tooth and ask the patient if the areas are sensitive.

Percussion testing is a short and indirect mechanical irritation of the tooth or the periodontium in order to obtain information about the condition of pulp or periodontium from the patient's reaction. It is a very reliable means for diagnosing irreversible pulpitis or apical periodontitis. Percussion should be performed carefully, especially in patients who have the chief complaint of biting, chewing, or pressure sensitivity. A finger, "Tooth Slooth," or the blunt end of any plastic instrument may be used to elicit symptoms. Start gently and increase the intensity slowly. Testing the adjacent teeth first is a good way to gauge the patient's reaction. If he responds strongly with a healthy tooth, be extra gentle when testing the tooth in question.

Periodontal probing is important, especially in diagnosis of suspected root fractures or combined periodontic-endodontic problems. Always examine the gingiva for inflammation and exudate. Documentation of all relevant periodontal findings such as pocket probing depth, probing for furcation involvement, and tooth mobility should be done.

If a sinus tract is present, always trace it by inserting the tip of a small gutta-percha point into the sinus tract and taking a radiograph with the point in place. It acts like an arrow directing you to the root of the problem.

1.3.2 Sensitivity Testing

Sensitivity testing is required prior to any kind of root canal treatment and the result must be documented. The pulpal diagnosis is obtained by using thermal or electrical tests. Thermal tests may be hot or cold, depending on the chief complaint. Sensitivity testing will only determine the ability of pulpal tissue for nervous conduction but will not give any information on the vascular supply of the pulp. *Therefore, the tests used are referred to as sensitivity tests and not vitality tests.* As stated before, any thermal or electrical sensitivity testing should always be compared with the adjacent teeth or its counterpart in the other quadrant.

1.3.2.1 Thermal Tests

Cold Test

The pulpal diagnosis is obtained by using thermal or electrical tests. Thermal tests may be hot or cold, depending on the chief complaint.

There are several ways to reproduce the sensation of cold. These include a skin refrigerant (such as Endo Ice®), ice pellets, or a CO_2 stick. The simplest thermal test is the cold test which is performed using ethyl chloride spray (Fig. 1.6), dichlorodifluoromethane (CC12F2—Frigen®, Freon®, Arcton®), a propane-butane mixture, or carbon dioxide snow. A cold test is usually a very reliable means for diagnosis of a pulpless (devitalized) tooth (the reason for majority of negative cold tests is pulpal

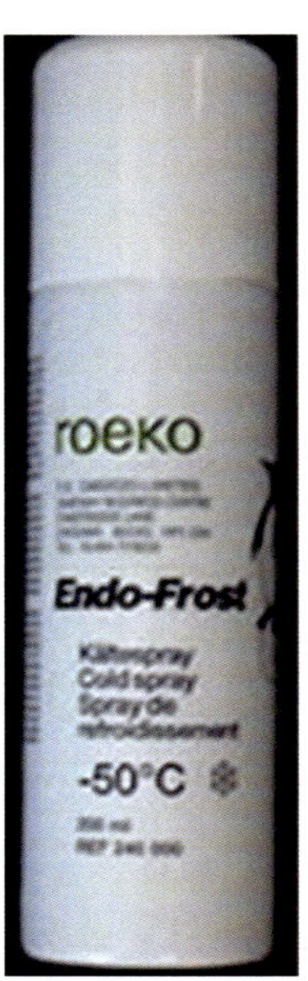

Fig. 1.6 Refrigerant spray for cold vitality testing

necrosis), but a lack of response to a cold test does not always necessarily mean a pulpal necrosis. In this case, additional electrical sensitivity testing is required. Reversible pulpitis can also be diagnosed using the cold test.

Heat Test

Heat test can be very helpful to establish a provisional diagnosis of suppurative pulpitis. This kind of pulpitis reacts with a clear sensation of pain even at slight temperature increase of only 2–3 °C. The most effective way to heat test the teeth is to isolate each tooth using a rubber dam and flood the area with water with similar temperature to that of a warm or hot beverage. Warn the patient that there will be some pressure/sensation. Heat testing should never be performed with a melted stick of wax or an electrically or flame-heated instrument. This type of heat is difficult to control and may cause pulpal damage in healthy teeth. As soon as the patient feels any type of sensation, remove the stimulus and ask him to report his feelings: Is the sensation painful? Does it linger? Is this what he feels when he drinks or eats something hot or cold?

Suppurative pulpitis, however, will cause a feeling of pain described by the patient. Heat test must never be used for routine testing—in order to obtain any reaction from healthy pulp, the temperature within the pulp cavity would have to be raised such that this would result in denaturation of pulpal tissue protein.

Electrical Sensitivity Test

The electrical pulp test is helpful when natural tooth structure is available and the results of the thermal tests are inconclusive. It is not suitable, however, for the control of teeth with metallic or ceramic crowns or dental bridges and is not reliable

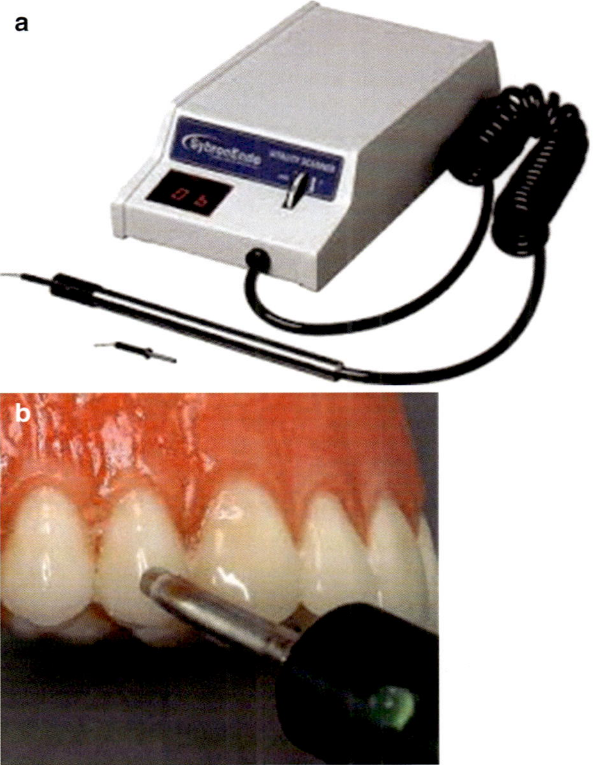

Fig. 1.7 Electric pulp testing

when placed too close to the gingiva. Electrical pulp testing devices should not be used on patients with cardiac pacemakers. Ideally, the area should be isolated and the tooth dry. Conducting medium, such as topical anesthetic or toothpaste, should be used. Testing a normal tooth first is good to give the patient a baseline of what the test feels like, even if it is not an adjacent tooth (Fig. 1.7a, b).

Although the results are given numerically, usually from a scale of 1 to 80, it is impossible to know how "alive" the tooth is. A response before the scale is at its maximum means that there is some vital tissue inside the tooth; no response at the maximum number means that there is not.

1.3.3 Biting and Release

This test is useful for the diagnosis of a coronal fracture. It is best to have a Tooth Slooth for testing cusps individually. When using the Slooth, ask the patient to bite down on his teeth together and open quickly. Instruct him to note if the pain is upon biting or release. Pain upon release from biting with the absence of any other symptoms and normal responses to the other diagnostic tests is frequently correlated to a coronal fracture. This is usually effectively treated with a full-coverage restoration.

1.4 Radiographic Evaluation and Diagnosis

Radiological diagnosis is a valuable additional method in clinical examination. It will not inform about the condition of the pulp or different types of pulpitis but can give various other bits of information such as carious lesions not identified in clinical examination, root resorption, internal resorption, width of the periodontal ligament space, condition of the periapical tissue, and root fractures. Radiological diagnosis of the affected tooth is important prior to any root canal treatment.

The clinical evaluation is the most important part of the diagnostic process because there is often a lack of radiographic pathology associated with an endodontic problem. To view radiographic bone destruction, there must be erosion of one of the cortical plates. There can be extensive loss of cancellous bone without any radiographic pathology.

1.5 Treatment Planning and Considerations

Endodontic diagnosis can be challenging. Understanding both the pulpal and periradicular diagnoses and how to obtain them is crucial. Although it can be frustrating for the patient and the provider, sometimes no treatment until the symptoms localize is the best option.

An ideal treatment plan should address the chief complaints of the patient, provide long-lasting and cost-effective treatment, and at the same time meet the patient's expectations. Treatment should always be patient centered and based on scientific and clinical evidence and should preserve the biological environment while maintaining comfort and function. The selection of cases for endodontic therapy should take into consideration the prognosis of the endodontic, restorative, and periodontal procedures [21, 22]. Although certain teeth are endodontically treatable, the amount of tooth structure remaining may not be readily restorable, and a durable coronal restoration is not achievable [23]. The periodontal condition of the tooth must be assessed prior to endodontic therapy because optimal periodontal health is critical to the long-term success of teeth that are endodontically treated [24]. At the same time, it is essential to consider the patient's needs, attitude, and willingness to accept treatment [25].

Factors which help in deciding whether the tooth concerned has a good or poor prognosis include:

1. Strategic value of the tooth
2. Periodontal factors
3. Patient factors (systemic and oral health)
4. Restorability of the tooth

The clinician should also take into account the patient's medical condition and motivation to maintain oral health [26]. The above considerations will aid the dentist in determining whether a tooth can be preserved via endodontic therapy or whether it is in the best interests of the patient to consider extraction and possibly a prosthetic replacement [27]. Both the dentist and patient must agree on the definitive plan. The dentist should consider whether he or she possesses the necessary skills and knowledge to perform endodontic treatment for this particular tooth to a high standard. The components of the treatment planning are summarized in Flow chart 1.1.

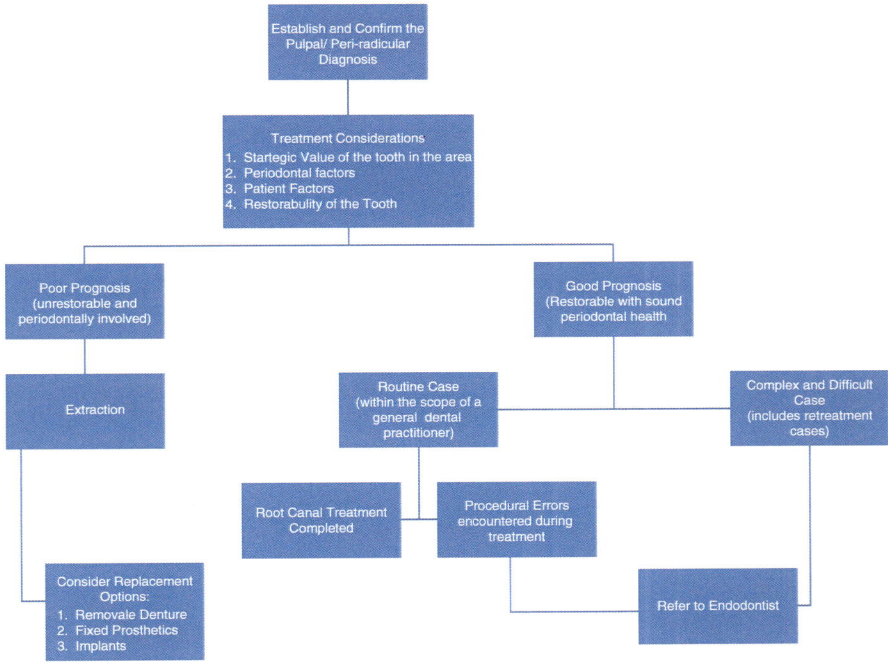

1.5.1 Strategic Value of the Tooth

The primary concern is the long-term preservation of a healthy functional dentition. The dentist should consider the strategic value of the tooth to be endodontically treated in relation to the overall function of the dentition. For example, a second or third molar is generally considered to be of little strategic value, unless it is required to support a prosthesis. This is because a denture is more stable if it has a posterior abutment tooth to retain and support it [28].

Other strategic considerations may include the structural integrity, remaining sound tooth structure, morphology and dimensions of the root, the level of surrounding bone, amount of periodontal support, and whether the tooth is in the esthetic zone [27]. Endodontic treatment is contraindicated when there is limited remaining tooth structure, and the definitive crown will not be able to engage at least 1.5–2.0 mm of tooth structure with a cervical ferrule [29, 30]. Retaining a tooth with a poor long-term prognosis via endodontic treatment, particularly a cracked tooth, can lead to substantial bone loss by the time the tooth is eventually removed. The resulting bone defect can substantially affect the esthetic result.

Endodontic treatment is associated with procedural accidents occasionally. These mishaps can occur during access preparation, cleaning and shaping, and obturation (discussed later in the book), as well as during preparation of the post space [31]. Some of these errors can have a negative effect on the outcomes and subsequent prognosis of endodontic treatment [32–34].

A number of adjunctive procedures affect the comparison of complicated and/or high-risk endodontic treatment with tooth extraction and placement of an implant and a crown. For instance, retaining some teeth via endodontic therapy may require treatment for periodontal disease, crown lengthening through surgery or orthodontic extrusion, a core buildup or a post and core, or a crown. Each of these procedures adds complexity to the treatment plan and can present additional complications and risks. It also increases the overall cost of treatment and makes it more difficult for patients to comprehend and accept a treatment plan.

1.5.2 Periodontal Factors

The health of the periodontium needs to be assessed because in a compromised dentition, the long-term prognosis for retaining a single tooth may be poor [35]. Approximately one-third of endodontically treated teeth requiring extraction are lost because of periodontal problems [36]. Periodontal management of patients is important to the long-term success of any treatment plan.

1.5.3 Patient Factors

The dentist should be aware and prepared that some patients will opt to have an extraction of a tooth on the grounds of time involved in treatment, fear of treatment, or the financial cost [28]. A patient's previous positive or negative experiences with either treatment may also affect his or her decision as to which treatment modality should be pursued.

Although medical conditions (e.g., diabetes or habitual tobacco smoking) may complicate or delay healing, but in general, medical reasons are not a contraindication to root canal therapy. Endodontic considerations in patients with underlying medical condition are discussed later in the book. However, conditions which limit a patient's ability to lie supine (e.g., spinal arthritis), to open the mouth wide for a prolonged period (e.g., rheumatoid arthritis), or to have anxiety disorders [35] may make endodontic treatment more difficult but not impossible. Things to consider before starting a root canal treatment are [28].

- Is endodontic treatment in the patient's best interest?
- What are the patient's expectations?
- Will the patient be able to afford the treatment planned?

1.5.4 Restorability of the Tooth in the Arch

Extraction of the tooth is a viable treatment if endodontic therapy is not applicable or where successful completion of the treatment plan is impossible because of periodontal or restorative concerns [24]. The tooth in question must be assessed for any restorative challenges before the start of the treatment that would compromise the restorability following root canal treatment.

The prognosis for endodontic treatment of the tooth or teeth in question must take into account the treatment planning. Although we, as dentists, would like to give the patient as accurate a prognosis as possible before the start of an endodontic treatment, a less than ideal technical standard provided or procedural errors and/or an inadequate coronal restoration will lead to a reduced prognosis for the tooth.

1.5.5 Other Considerations

1.5.5.1 When to Refer and When to Perform Endodontic Retreatment

Dentists should be able to assess when the difficulty of the treatment exceeds their skill and be able to refer the patient to an endodontist as necessary [27]. Sometimes, the technical difficulty of the case dictates that the patient be referred to a specialist for treatment and management [26]. Other factors that may complicate and increase the difficulty of an endodontic case include [23]:

- Calcifications
- Inability to isolate the tooth with a rubber dam
- Resorptive defects
- Extra roots and canals
- Retreatment cases
- Presence of a post
- Ledges and perforations

Referring the patient before commencement of endodontic treatment is better than after the problem has been created because the error will compromise the prognosis of the tooth [26]. Retreatment is acceptable only after an acceptable observation period with no signs of radiographic improvement. In some cases where the extra-radicular infection is the source of ongoing disease, apical surgery is considered the treatment of choice [37]. Dentists must be aware of their level of clinical skill, knowledge, and experience.

The treatment plan should be divided into various stages such as

- Initial relief of pain, e.g., emergency pulp extirpation
- Corrective treatments, e.g., complete root canal treatment and restorative treatment
- Maintenance, e.g., measures to prevent the disease recurrence [35].

Treatment plans can also be divided into "simple" and "complex." A plan may be considered simple if only one tooth is involved and the overall status of the dentition is acceptable [26]. A complex treatment plan is required for patients who have not attended for some time or where there is a need for a major reassessment of the entire dentition. In such a case, it is important to manage the acute pain and swelling associated with a tooth that requires root canal treatment before offering a definitive treatment plan.

1.5.5.2 Post-endodontic Restoration

The choice of the final coronal restoration will influence the outcome of endodontic treatment. It should provide adequate coverage to protect the endodontically treated tooth against fracture [26]. Other potential problems associated with the final restoration playing a role in the breakdown of root canal treatment include a permanent restoration with marginal breakdown, or bacterial penetration due to restorative procedures such as post space preparation [38].

Research has suggested that both root canal filling and the coronal restoration serve as a barrier against fluid and bacterial penetration into the periapical area [39]. In reality, there are no available materials or obturation techniques that can confidently assure an impervious seal of the complex root canal system [40]. Fractures of endodontically treated teeth could lead to infection of the root canal system or extraction of the tooth.

The difficulty of a case should be balanced with the skill and experience of the dentist in deciding whether to manage the case in general practice or to refer the patient to an endodontist [26]. The overall treatment planning in endodontics should be in agreement with the overall dental management of the patient.

1.6 Pulp Canal Obliteration

Pulp canal obliteration, also known as calcific metamorphosis, is defined as a pulpal response to trauma that is characterized by the loss of root canal space due to the deposition of hard tissue along the root canal walls and the pulp space proper [5] (Fig. 1.8). It is also referred to as dystrophic calcification, diffuse calcification, and calcific degeneration. Calcified canals may pose diagnostic challenge. In spite of improved magnification methods like the dental operating microscope, it may still be difficult to locate and negotiate them. In the process, excessive tooth structure may be removed, and the tooth or a root may be at risk of untoward sequelae of perforation. The new imaging technologies such as cone beam computed

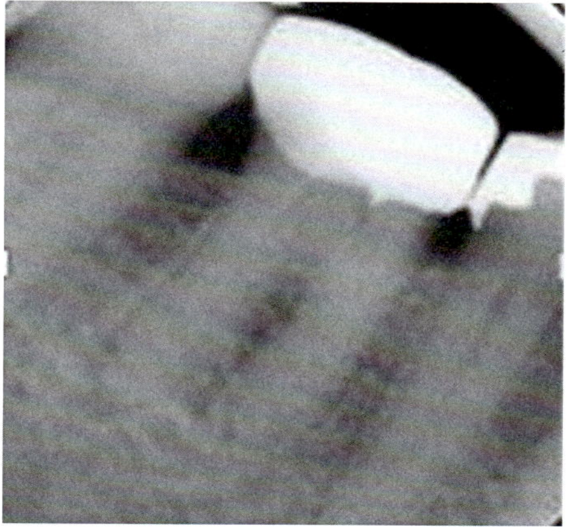

Fig. 1.8 Pulp canal obliteration

tomography (CBCT) are very useful and can help to ascertain if the root canal lumen is present in a tooth that appears calcified on periapical radiograph and if the tooth is amenable to conventional endodontic treatment [41].

Teeth with calcification provide an endodontic treatment challenge. Traumatized teeth frequently develop partial or total pulpal obliteration characterized evidently by loss of the pulp space radiographically and a yellow discoloration of the clinical crown. Since only a small percentage of such teeth develop pulp necrosis with radiographic signs of apical periodontitis, it is difficult to decide whether to treat these teeth immediately upon detection of the pulpal obliteration or to wait until signs and symptoms of pulp and/or apical periodontitis occur.

1.6.1 Clinical Picture

The calcification of the pulp chamber results in a darker hue than the adjacent and the loss of translucency due to a greater thickness of dentin under the enamel. Some teeth also have a gray/yellowish appearance of the crown of the tooth [42]. The affected teeth do not always react to sensibility tests, and generally there is no sensitivity to percussion [43]. Pulp necrosis is most frequently a complication with ranges varying from 1% to 16% [44, 45].

Research shows that tooth discoloration has no diagnostic value. Not all teeth with radiographic signs of pulpal obliteration undergo a color change [46]. Furthermore, more than two-thirds of teeth with pulpal obliteration are asymptomatic. These teeth are often an incidental finding following clinical or radiographic investigations. As the pulp calcification becomes more pronounced, there is a progressive decrease in the response to thermal and electrical pulp testing. But, partially obliterated teeth can give positive results; hence, in the presence of pulpal obliteration, it is generally accepted that sensibility tests are unreliable [46].

1.6.2 Radiographic Appearance

The radiographic appearance is partial or total obliteration of the pulp canal space with a normal periodontal ligament space and intact lamina dura. A thickening of the periodontal ligament space or periapical radiolucency may sometimes be observed with or without subjective symptoms. Complete radiographic obliteration of the root canal space does not necessarily mean the absence of the pulp or canal space; in the majority of these cases, there is a pulp canal space with pulpal tissue.

1.6.3 Management

Most authors believe that endodontic treatment should only be initiated following the development of periapical disease radiographically. Research shows that pulpal necrosis and periapical disease are not a common complication of pulpal obliteration. Teeth demonstrating pulpal obliteration but no periapical disease should be managed conservatively through clinical observation and periodic radiographic examination. They should only be treated if an area of rarefaction or clinical symptoms develop. Teeth with pulpal obliteration requiring root canal treatment fall into the high difficulty category of the American Association of Endodontists Case Assessment criteria [47].

It is essential to remember that the pulp chamber is always located in the center of the tooth at the level of the CEJ [44, 48] and, also, that the CEJ is the most consistent repeatable landmark for locating the pulp chamber [48].

Thus, if the access preparation remains well centered, aligned to the long axis of the tooth, and limited initially to the level of the CEJ, the root canal system is normally easy to locate. Selden (1989) emphasized on the role of the dental operating microscope in treating calcified canals and improving the treatment outcome [49]. Modified burs and ultrasonic tips have been designed for performing the deep troughing required to locate and enter calcified pulp chambers and canals. Dyes such as methylene blue may assist in locating the canal system under the microscope. Sodium hypochlorite may also prove to be useful in the identification of a calcified canal using the "bubble" or "champagne" test. The test involving placing 5% sodium hypochlorite into the pulp chamber over a calcified canal containing remnants of pulp tissue will result in a stream of bubbles emerging from the oxygenation of the tissue. This can be seen under the microscope and used to identify the canal orifice [50].

It is essential to take radiographic images at different angles to maintain the alignment and direction. Combining orthoradial and angulated radiographs provides an impression of a three-dimensional anatomical space. If both centered and angulated radiograph images show the file in the same position relative to the root canal or centered in the long axis of the root, then the scouter instrument can be safely apically advanced. Conversely, if a deviation is noted, the file position must be corrected.

The endodontic treatment performed under these circumstances poses the risk complications such as instrument fracture and perforating the root, which can seriously affect the long-term prognosis of the tooth.

Ideally, smaller-sized instruments are required for initial pathfinding; however, these files lack the rigidity required to transverse restricted spaces and often fracture when used with vertical watch-winding forces. One method is to alternate between size 8 and 10 K-files with a gentle watch-winding motion with minimal vertical pressure with regular replacement of the instruments before fatigue occurs. However, a variety of "pathfinding" instruments are available with this objective in mind. Instruments with reduced flute, such as a Canal Pathfinder (JS Dental, Ridgefield. Conn.) or instruments with greater shaft strength such as the Pathfinder CS (Kerr Manufacturing Co.), may be used as they are more likely to penetrate even highly calcified canals.

Chelating agents such as EDTA are of limited value except as a lubricant or to assist instrumentation after the canal has been negotiated [44, 51]. A "crown-down" approach is highly recommended as it improves tactile sensation and ensures better apical penetration [44]. As a general rule, the calcification process as seen in pulpal obliteration occurs in a corono-apical direction, so once the initial canal has been captured, an instrument tends to progress more easily as it advances toward the canal terminus.

Treatment recommendations are given in Flow chart 1.2.

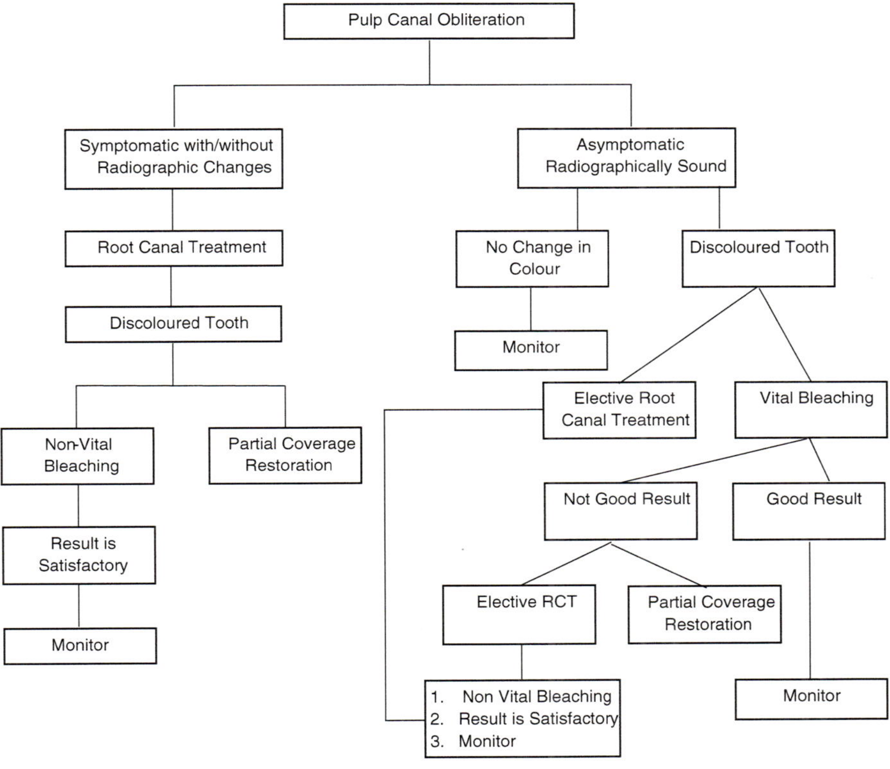

Conclusion

To conclude, when a patient presents to the dental office with a complaint of a toothache, it is important to do appropriate investigations with sensibility testing. If testing results are inconclusive or don't add up, consider either seeing the patient on a different day to repeat testing or refer for a second opinion. No treatment should be rendered without a diagnosis. The diagnosis will dictate which, if any, treatment needs to be done.

The dentist must determine whether the needs are best served by providing endodontic treatment or advising extraction. The overall treatment planning in endodontics should always be in agreement with the overall dental management of the patient.

References

1. Berman LH, Hartwell GR. Diagnosis. In: Cohen S, Hargreaves KM, editors. Pathways of the pulp. 11th ed. St. Louis: Mosby/Elsevier; 2011. p. 2–39.
2. Schweitzer JL. The endodontic diagnostic puzzle. Gen Dent. 2009;57(6):560–7.
3. Glickman GN. AAE consensus conference on diagnostic terminology: background and perspectives. J Endod. 2009;35:1619.
4. AAE Consensus Conference. Recommended diagnostic terminology. J Endod. 2009;35:1634.
5. American Association of Endodontists. Glossary of endodontic terms. 8. 2012. AAE Chicago.
6. Glickman GN, Bakland LK, Fouad AF, Hargreaves KM, Schwartz SA. Diagnostic terminology: report of an online survey. J Endod. 2009;35:1625.
7. Jafarzadeh H, Abbott PV. Review of pulp sensibility tests. Part 1: general information and thermal tests. Int Endod J. 2010;43:738–62.
8. Jafarzadeh H, Abbott PV. Review of pulp sensibility tests. Part II: electric pulp tests and test cavities. Int Endod J. 2010;43:945–58.
9. Newton CW, Hoen MM, Goodis HE, Johnson BR, McClanahan SB. Identify and determine the metrics, hierarchy, and predictive value of all the parameters and/or methods used during endodontic diagnosis. J Endod. 2009;35:1635.
10. Levin LG, Law AS, Holland GR, Abbot PV, Roda RS. Identify and define all diagnostic terms for pulpal health and disease states. J Endod. 2009;35:1645.
11. Gutmann JL, Baumgartner JC, Gluskin AH, Hartwell GR, Walton RE. Identify and define all diagnostic terms for periapical/periradicular health and disease states. J Endod. 2009;35:1658.
12. Rosenberg PA, Schindler WG, Krell KV, Hicks ML, Davis SB. Identify the endodontic treatment modalities. J Endod. 2009;35:1675.
13. Sindet-Pedersen S, Petersen JK, Gotzsche PC. Incidence of pain conditions in dental practice in a Danish county. Community Dent Oral Epidemiol. 1985;13:244–6.
14. McCarthy PJ, McClanahan S, Hodges J, Bowles WR. Frequency of localization of the painful tooth by patients presenting for an endodontic emergency. J Endod. 2010;36(5):801.
15. American Association of Endodontists. AAE consensus conference recommended diagnostic terminology. J Endod. 2009;35:1634.
16. Iqbal M, Kim S, Yoon F. An investigation into differential diagnosis of pulp and periapical pain: a PennEndo database study. J Endod. 2007;33:548–51.
17. Zero DT, Zandona AF, Vail MM, Spolnik KJ. Dental caries and pulpal disease. Dent Clin N Am. 2011;55:29–46.
18. Carrotte P. Endodontics: part 3. Treatment of endodontic emergencies. Br Dent J. 2004;197:299–305.
19. Nalliah RP, Allareddy V, Elangovan S, Karimbux N, Lee MK, Gajendrareddy P, et al. Hospital emergency department visits attributed to pulpal and periapical disease in the United States in 2006. J Endod. 2011;37:6–9.
20. Asgary S, Eghbal MJ. The effect of pulpotomy using a calcium-enriched mixture cement versus one-visit root canal therapy on postoperative pain relief in irreversible pulpitis: a randomized clinical trial. Odontology. 2010;98:126–33.
21. Friedman S, Mor C. The success of endodontic therapy—healing and functionality. J Calif Dent Assoc. 2004;32:493–503.
22. Montgomery S, Ferguson CD. Endodontics. Diagnostic, treatment planning, and prognostic considerations. Dent Clin N Am. 1986;30:533–48.
23. Rosenberg P. Case selection and treatment planning. In: Cohen S, Burns R, editors. Pathways of the pulp. 8th ed. St Louis: Mosby; 2002. p. 91–102.
24. Wagnild GW, Mueller K. Restoration of the endodontically treated tooth. In: Cohen S, Burns R, editors. Pathways of the pulp. 8th ed. St Louis: Mosby; 2002. p. 765–95.
25. Marshall FJ. Planning endodontic treatment. Dent Clin N Am. 1979;23:495–518.
26. Messer HH. Clinical judgement and decision making in endodontics. Aust Endod J. 1999;25:124–32.

27. Pothukuchi K. Case assessment and treatment planning: what governs your decision to treat, refer or replace a tooth that potentially requires endodontic treatment? Aust Endod J. 2006;32:79–84.
28. Kidd EAM, Smith BGN. Making clinical decisions. In: Kidd EAM, Smith BGN, editors. Pickard's manual of operative dentistry. Oxford: Oxford University Press; 1998. p. 28–49.
29. Libman WJ, Nicholls JI. Load fatigue of teeth restored with cast posts and cores and complete crowns. Int J Prosthodont. 1995;8(2):155–61.
30. Tan PL, Aquilino SA, Gratton DG, et al. In vitro fracture resistance of endodontically treated central incisors with varying ferrule heights and configurations. J Prosthet Dent. 2005;93:331–6.
31. Torabinejad M, Lemon RR. Procedural accidents. In: Walton R, Torabinjad M, editors. Principles and practice of endodontics. 3rd ed. Philadelphia: Saunders; 2002. p. 310–30.
32. Ingle JI, Simon JH, Machtou P, Bogaerts P. Outcome of endodontic treatment and re-treatment. In: Ingle JI, Bakland LK, editors. Endodontics. 5th ed. London: Decker; 2002. p. 748–57.
33. Kvinnsland I, Oswald RJ, Halse A, Gronningsaeter AG. A clinical and roentgenological study of 55 cases of root perforation. Int Endod J. 1989;22(2):75–84.
34. Farzaneh M, Abitbol S, Friedman S. Treatment outcome in endodontics: the Toronto study. Phases I and II—orthograde retreatment. J Endod. 2004;30:627–33.
35. Stewart T. Diagnosis and treatment planning are essential prior to commencing endodontic treatment: discuss this statement as it relates to clinical endodontic management. Aust Endod J. 2005;31:29–34.
36. Vire D. Failure of endodontically treated teeth. J Endod. 1991;17:338–42.
37. Friedman S. Considerations and concepts of case selection in the management of post-treatment endodontic disease (treatment failure). Endod Top. 2002;1:54–78.
38. Heling I, Gorfil C, Slutzky H, Kopolovic K, Zalkind M, Slutzky-Goldberg I. Endodontic failure caused by inadequate restorative procedures: review and treatment recommendations. J Prosthet Dent. 2002;87:674–8.
39. Kirkevang LL, Hörsted Bindslev P. Technical aspects of treatment in relation to treatment outcome. Endod Top. 2002;2:89–102.
40. Gutmann JL. Clinical, radiographic, and histologic perspectives on success and failure in endodontics. Dent Clin N Am. 1992;36:379–92.
41. American Association of Endodontists; American Academy of Oral and Maxillofacial Radiology. Use of cone-beam computed tomography in endodontics joint position statement of the American Association of Endodontists and the American Academy of oral and maxillofacial radiology. Oral Surg Oral Med Oral Pathol Oral Radiol Endod. 2011;111:234–7.
42. Patersson SS, Mitchell DF. Calciic metamorphosis of the dental pulp. Oral Surg Oral Med Oral Pathol. 1965;20(1):94–101.
43. Oginni AO, Adekoya-Sofowora CA, Kolawole KA. Evaluation of radiographs, clinical signs and symptoms associated with pulp canal obliteration: an aid to treatment decision. Dent Traumatol. 2009;25(6):620–5.
44. Amir FA, Gutmann JL, Witherspoon DE. Calciic metamorphosis: a challenge in endodontic diagnosis and treatment. Quintessence Int. 2001;32(6):447–55.
45. Tavares WLF, Lopes RCP, Menezes GB, Henriques LCF. Ribeiro- Sobrinho AP. Non-surgical treatment of pulp canal obliteration using contemporary endodontic techniques: case series. Dental Press Endod. 2012;2(1):52–8.
46. McCabe PS, Dummer PM. Pulp canal obliteration: an endodontic diagnosis and treatment challenge. Int Endod J. 2012;45:177–97.
47. American Association of Endodontics. Case difficulty assessment form and guidelines B. Chicago: American Association of Endodontists; 2006.
48. Krasner P, Rankow HJ. Anatomy of the pulp chamber floor. J Endod. 2004;30:5–16.
49. Selden HS. The role of the dental operating microscope in improved non surgical treatment of calcified canals. Oral Surg Oral Med Oral Pathol. 1989;68:93–8.
50. Johnson BR. Endodontic access. Gen Dent. 2009;57:570–7.
51. Ngeow WC, Thong YL. Gaining access through a calcified pulp chamber: a clinical challenge. Int Endod J. 1998;31:367–71.

2 Importance of Radiographic Interpretation

Carla Cabral dos Santos Accioly Lins,
Flavia Maria de Moraes Ramos Perez,
Andrea Dos Anjos Pontual de Andrade Lima,
and Maria Luiza dos Anjos Pontual

2.1 Introduction

Radiographic examination is an indispensable adjunct in endodontics, especially for diagnosis, treatment, and follow-up after endodontic therapy. Currently, periapical radiography is the first choice of imaging method in endodontics clinical practice and a valuable tool to diagnose and to follow up patients (Fig. 2.1). Furthermore, the practice of radiography is traditionally used in various stages of root canal therapy, such as for determination of work length. Digital intraoral radiography systems are being used increasingly for these purposes, with having similar accuracy as film radiography [1–3]. Currently, a variety of digital intraoral systems are commercially available.

2.2 Digital Radiography

Digital intraoral receptors have several advantages compared to conventional film-based imaging, for example, the lower dose per exposure, the ability to perform image quality enhancements, task-specific image processing, an almost instantaneous availability of images, and a greater reduction in working time. An additional environmental advantage is the elimination of processing chemicals [4].

C.C. dos Santos Accioly Lins (✉)
Department of Anatomy, Centre for Biological Sciences, Federal University of Pernambuco, Recife, PE, Brazil
e-mail: cabralcarla1@hotmail.com

F.M. de Moraes Ramos Perez • A.D.A.P. de Andrade Lima • M.L. dos Anjos Pontual
Oral Radiology Area, Department of Clinical and Preventive Dentistry, School of Dentistry, Federal University of Pernambuco (UFPE), Recife, Pernambuco, Brazil
e-mail: Flavia.ramosperez@ufpe.br; Pontual.andrea@gmail.com; mlpontual@gmail.com

P. Jain (ed.), *Common Complications in Endodontics*,
https://doi.org/10.1007/978-3-319-60997-3_2

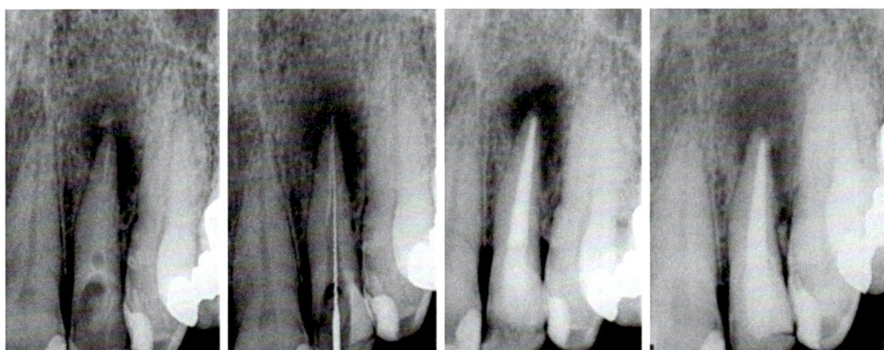

Fig. 2.1 Periapical radiographic images obtained by intraoral solid-state sensors, used for diagnosis, odontometry, and follow-up

Table 2.1 Some commonly used terms

Pixel	It is the foundation block of digital imaging and is the smallest complete sample of an image. It is a unit of digital resolution
Bit depth	This indicates the shades of gray used to define each pixel. It is commonly measured as "number of bits"
Spatial resolution	This refers to the ability of the imaging modality to differentiate two objects

Digital images are fundamentally composed of numeric information that can be differentiated from each other based on two characteristics: pixel spatial distribution and gray values attributed to them. The pixel size and the bit depth are important features, which determine the spatial and contrast resolutions for the acquisition of digital radiographs (Table 2.1). Presently, the pixel size is about 19–50 μm in intraoral digital radiographic systems, similar to conventional films, which allows a theoretical maximum spatial resolution of about 25 line pairs per mm [4, 5]. High image resolution appears to improve the accuracy for the diagnosis of root fractures and the determination of file lengths [6, 7].

With respect to the contrast resolution, image acquisition software offers various bit depths, allowing 8, 10, 12, and 16 bits, the last generating images with 65,536 different shades of gray per pixel. It is important to note that the higher the bit depth, the greater the contrast resolution will be. Thus, it enables a more detailed visualization of subtle differences which may increase the diagnostic accuracy, such as for the determination of file lengths, in which high contrast resolution is recommended [6, 8]. Regarding the detection of subtle radiographic density differences, 12-bit image or higher is needed for accurate determination of endodontic file position [8]. However, it is important to remember that the human is capable to perceive a limited number of shades of gray.

2.3 Digital Image Acquisition and Receptors

Digital image acquisition can be performed by two distinct ways: (1) indirect acquisition by means of digitizing films using flatbed scanners with a transparency adapter, slide scanners, or digital cameras to convert an existing analog radiograph into a digital image and (2) direct acquisition. In direct acquisition, the conventional film could be replaced by a solid-state sensor with/without a cord (charged coupled devices or complementary metal-oxide semiconductors) or by a photostimulable storage phosphor (PSP) plate.

Intraoral solid-state sensors (CCD and CMOS) are composed by silicon chips wrapped in a rectangular, rigid, 5–10.5 mm thick plastic pack [9]. Most intraoral solid-state sensors are connected to the computer by a cable, and the image is displayed almost immediately on a computer monitor after exposure [9, 10]. Usually, the cable is 0.40–3 m long, which can be extended on some digital systems. There are few direct digital systems that use wireless technologies for data transmission. Wireless digital systems can either use common radiofrequency waves or Bluetooth data transmission [9]. Intraoral solid-state sensor systems could be efficient aids in endodontic procedures, in which an additional image effortlessly can be acquired from a different angle with the sensor in the same position. This might make these sensors the elected digital receptor in endodontic practice [10].

The intraoral solid-state sensor's disadvantages include (1) smaller active areas of image receptors when compared to films and phosphor plate—which limits the visualized structures and increases the number of radiographic exams needed; (2) the reduced dynamic scale resulting in overexposed images and requiring several repeats; and (3) solid-state image receptors which are rigid and thicker than others, causing discomfort to the patient and difficulty in the placement of the sensor for intraoral radiographs for posterior teeth. The cable used to connect the sensor to the computer also brings discomfort to the patient.

PSP plate systems use plates covered with phosphor crystals. A wide variety of intraoral imaging plate's sizes are available, with dimensions compatible to conventional film sizes 0, 1, 2, 3, and 4. The PSP plates are as comfortable as radiography film [10]. The substantial dose reduction compared with film is one of the advantages of PSP plates, and no repeats are required when overexposing phosphor plates [11]. The main disadvantage of PSP-based digital systems is the need of phosphor plate continual reposition, since they can present image artifacts as small or big scratches and stains with a related deterioration of image quality as time progresses and by usage. Handling the plates with gloves and wiping the soiled plates with a soft cloth should increase the reusability of plates. Vigorous rubbing is not recommended as it produces scratches on the plates [12].

In contrast with the conventional film, an intraoral digital radiographic receptor is projected to be used for several patients. However, they should not be sterilized by the methods commonly available in dental practice. Thus, the most viable method to prevent the transfer of microorganisms to the digital receptor is to use barrier envelopes as the plastic covers. When phosphor storage plates are used, the use of a second plastic barrier is recommended to minimize contamination by microorganisms from the oral microbiota. Also, the barrier should then be disinfected before the plate is removed from the barrier and placed in the scanner [12].

2.4 Limitations of Bidimensional Radiography

As mentioned previously, the periapical radiographs are currently used for management of endodontic problems, from diagnosis until follow-up assessment. Although these images present high detail and the image receptors show high spatial resolution, some limitations are evident, such as the compression of three-dimensional anatomy (Fig. 2.2), geometry distortion, and anatomical noise, which may impair the diagnosis. Additionally, it must be emphasized that all radiographs taken during diagnosis, treatment, posttreatment, and follow-up should be standardized with respect to alignment between the X-ray beam, tooth, and the receptor, avoiding under- or overestimation of the disease and the healing process [13].

2.5 Cone Beam Computed Tomography in Endodontics

Cone beam computed tomography (CBCT) is a diagnostic imaging modality that provides an accurate three-dimensional image of dento-maxillofacial structures. This imaging technology has been growing rapidly in recent years in the field of dentistry, replacing medical computed tomography (CT), due to its superior image

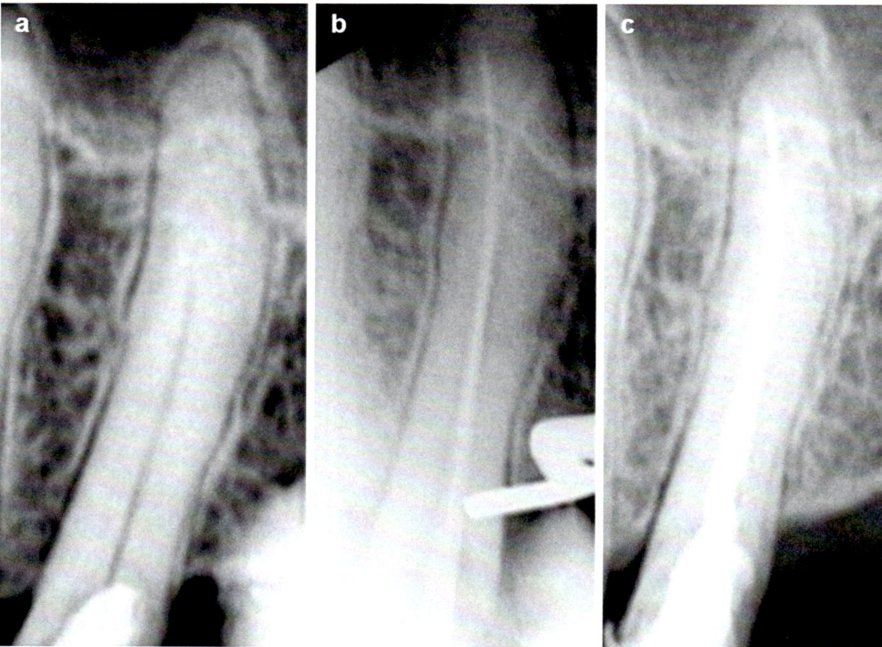

Fig. 2.2 Limitation of the periapical radiograph. (**a**) Nonvisualization of the root canal bifurcation on the third apical of the orthoradial incidence. (**b**) A variation of the horizontal angulation. (**c**) The presence of the filling material allowed its precise identification

quality of dental hard tissue and bone, in addition to low radiation dose. While CT images present anisotropic voxels, CBCT data are isotropic, which allows geometrically accurate measurements [13, 14]. Other advantages include faster scan time and low economic cost. The main disadvantage of CBCT is its inability to assess soft tissue lesions.

Several CBCT systems are available, with different parameters of exposure, scan volume, spatial resolution, and image quality. Among them, the size of the *field of view* (FOV) can vary from 3 × 4 cm (limited) to up to 20 cm (large) and the voxel size from 0.076 to 0.4 mm. Some equipments were developed specifically to scan limited volumes, such as a particular tooth, and it's desired that the optimal resolution does not exceed 0.2 mm for endodontic evaluations [14]. In general, the smaller the scan volume, the smaller the radiation dose and higher is the spatial resolution [14], which is essential for endodontic purposes. The choice for dose-reduced protocols should be preferable, considering the *ALARA* (*as low as reasonably achievable*) principle, whenever possible.

The criteria for referring patients to CBCT endodontics exams should be prudently selected, due to the higher radiation dose employed, in comparison with two-dimensional dental radiographs. Three-dimensional images are not recommended as a usual method for diagnosis [15]. A request for CBCT images should consider the impact both on the diagnosis and on its ability to change the treatment planning. Thus, after a careful clinical examination, only complex diagnosis tasks must be referred [16].

There are many indications of CBCT in endodontics, such as canal morphology evaluation, periapical lesions, dental trauma, identification of broken instrument, extent of extruded root canal material, root resorptions, vertical root fracture, non-healing root canals, etc., among others. Each case should be individually assessed, keeping in mind the radiation risk and the high economic cost involved in CBCT exams.

2.5.1 Canal Morphology

The success of an endodontic treatment depends on the precise identification of root canal morphology. Periapical radiography is the usual diagnostic tool to evaluate the morphology of the root canals. Intentional variation in X-ray beam angulation may provide additional information not readily available from the orthoradial images. The horizontal beam angulation for number identification and morphology of the root canals depends on the separation and divergence between the canals, and a horizontal beam angulation between 20 and 40° is recommended. Although radiography may reveal the characteristics, it is unlikely to show the complexities of the canal's anatomy.

Three-dimensional imaging allows a better identification of accessory canals, root curvatures, and root canal anomalies in teeth with complex morphology when intraoral conventional radiograph fails to demonstrate the real anatomy (Fig. 2.3). A superior performance is notable, especially in multi-rooted teeth and in the

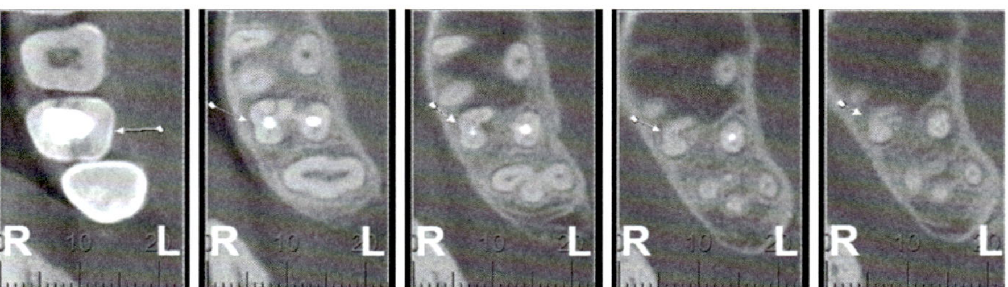

Fig. 2.3 Axial views. Right maxillary second molar with buccal root in "C" with the absence of endodontic material, verified after a CBCT exam to investigate possible cause of apical lesion

identification of second mesiobuccal canal in upper first molars [17]. However, CBCT should be avoided as a standard method for the screening of root canal anatomy.

2.5.2 Periapical Pathosis

The periapical inflammatory lesion is one of the most common diseases affecting the jaws. The diagnosis is performed based on clinical signs and symptoms and complemented by radiographic exams.

Frequently, the graduation of the periapical lesion is underestimated by periapical radiography. However, it usually shows healthy periapical conditions. To increase the possibility of a correct diagnosis, the patient could be submitted to an intraoral radiographic examination using different projections.

As stated earlier, high-resolution CBCT images allow earlier diagnosis with better accuracy than periapical radiographs [18, 19], especially in small lesions. When evaluating the impact of three-dimensional imaging on planning decisions, considering the size of lesion, some evidences point out no differences between periapical radiographs and volumetric acquisitions [20], whereas for preoperative assessment, additional informations provided by CBCT directly influence the treatment plan in approximately 62% compared to periapical conventional radiographs [18]. In fact, limited high-resolution CBCT scans should be indicated in selected cases, particularly in those with positive clinical signs and symptoms and negative finding in bidimensional radiographs [16] (Figs. 2.4 and 2.5).

2.5.3 Root Resorption

Pathological root resorption is characterized by a loss of mineralized tissue, involving dentin and/or cementum, and can be idiopathic or caused by dental trauma, pulp infections, bone lesions, orthodontic movements, and impacted teeth, among others. According to the teeth surface involved, root resorption can be classified as internal or external (Figs. 2.6 and 2.7). An early and precise diagnosis is mandatory because it is an irreversible process, which presents rapid progression [21]. Periapical

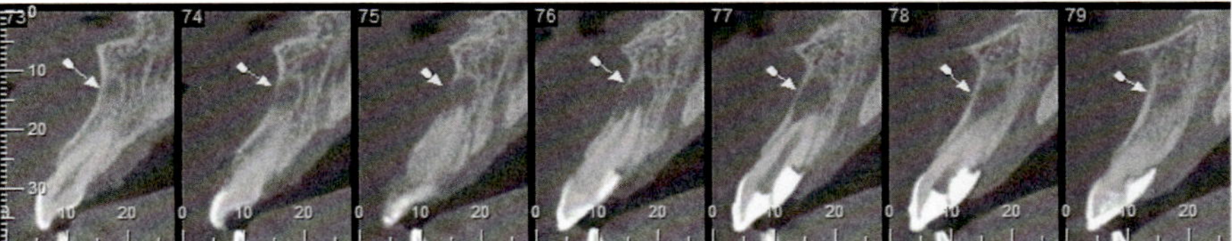

Fig. 2.4 Hypodense image, unilocular, of defined and corticalized limits suggests granuloma or radicular cyst and radicular resorption on the apical region

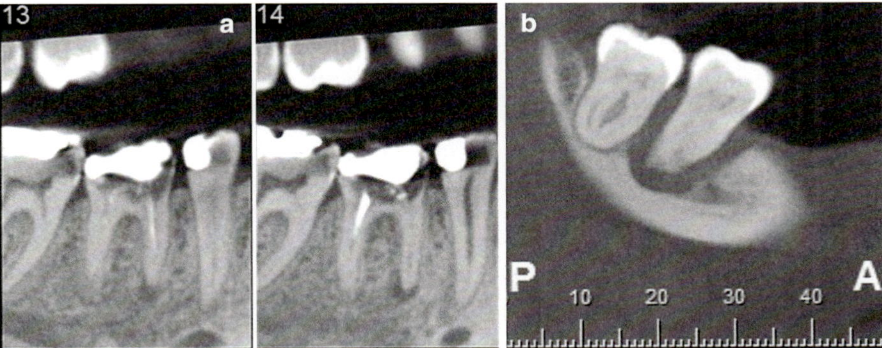

Fig. 2.5 Sagittal reconstructions, showing apical and endo-perio lesions on right mandibular first molar (**a**) and left mandibular second molar (**b**-arrow), respectively

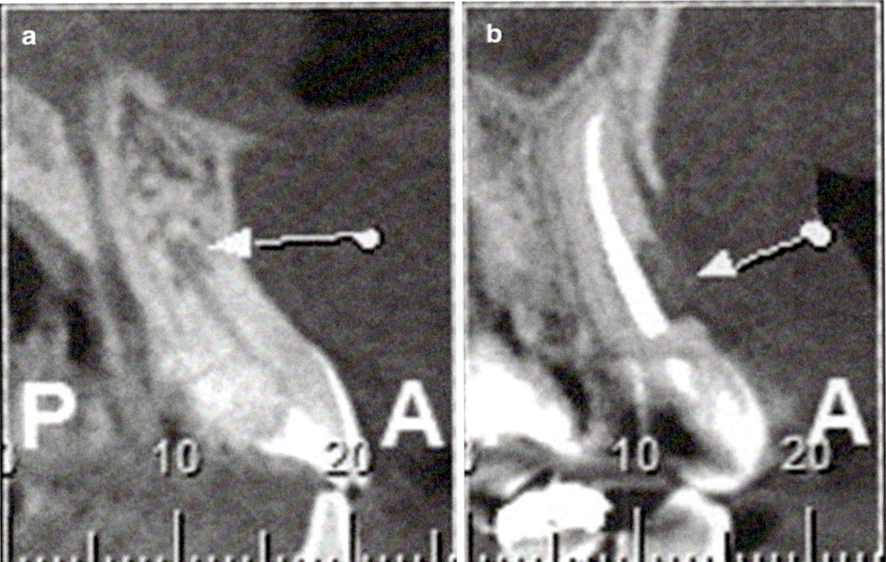

Fig. 2.6 Sagittal view of the CBCT exam shows internal and external resorption on the roots of the left maxillary central incisor (**a**) and left maxillary canine (**b**), respectively

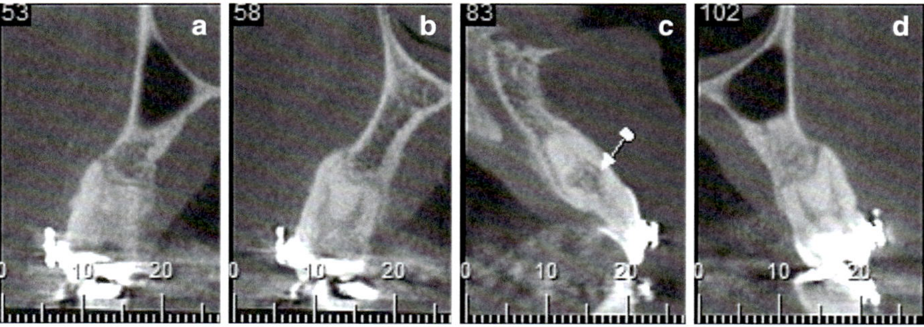

Fig. 2.7 CBCT. Sagittal views External root resorption on right maxillary second premolar (**a**) right maxillary first premolar (**b**) and left maxillary first premolar (**d**) teeth Internal root resorption on left maxillary central incisor tooth (**c**) in a patient, during orthodontic treatment

radiographs and CBCT are diagnostic tools commonly used for root resorption assessment. Each case should be individually evaluated based on the professional clinical experience and the stage the tissue is demineralized in.

There are some evidences that a periapical radiograph is not sufficiently accurate, especially in small lesions and in those located in buccal and lingual root surfaces [22]. On the other hand, CBCT presents high sensitivity and superior accuracy in diagnosing. Its capability to alter the management or prognosis of the tooth is one of the main reasons for referring patients [16]. As recommended for all endodontic complications, a three-dimensional scanner with high resolution and limited volume must be employed.

2.5.4 Vertical Root Fractures

The precise identification of root fractures is a major challenge for dentists, mainly in cases of lack of signals and symptoms, such as pain, swelling, fistula, and osseous resorptions surrounding teeth. For diagnosing such problems using periapical radiographs, it is necessary that central X-ray beam passes parallel to the fracture line. Otherwise, it will not be visible, especially if there is no fragment displacement. Radiographs taken using parallax technique may help for correct visualization.

On the other hand, high-resolution scanners offer images with high accuracy when compared with periapical radiographs [23]. The presence of root fillings and metallic posts presents a negative impact on diagnosis, reducing significantly the correct identification, due to high incidence of beam-hardening artifact formation [23–25] (Figs. 2.8 and 2.9).

2.6 Artifacts in CBCT

Knowledge about artifacts is important in day-to-day clinical practice. Artifact can be defined as a distortion or error in the reconstructed data that is not present in the object investigated [26, 27]. Artifacts cause the degradation of the quality of CBCT

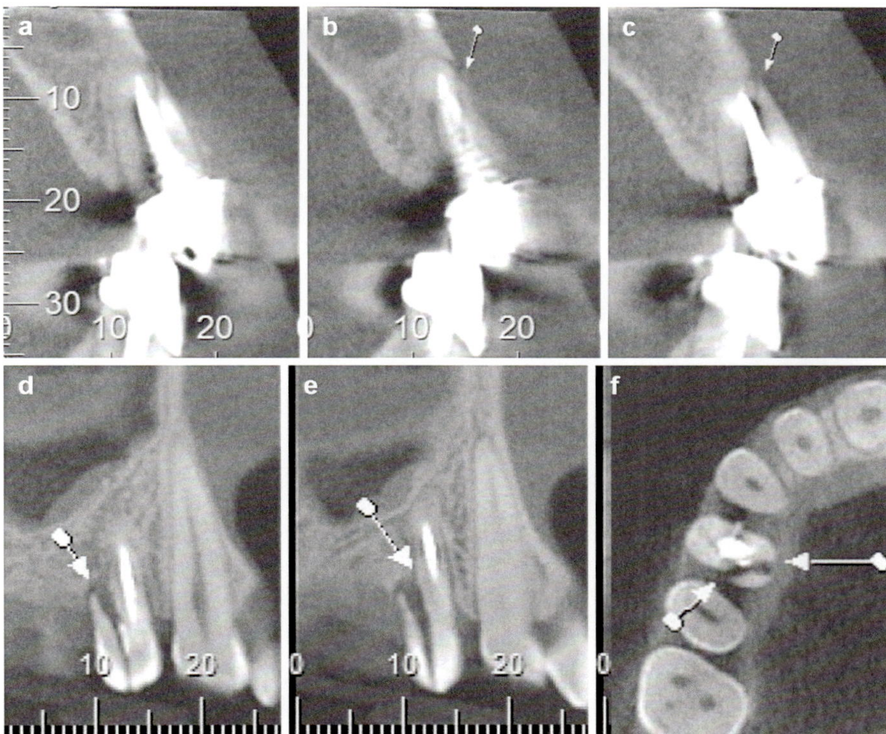

Fig. 2.8 CBCT images. (**a–c**) Oblique root fracture in left maxillary canine. (**d–f**) Vertical fracture of the crown and root of right maxillary first premolar, with fragment separation

images. Consequently, it may obscure or simulate pathology like root fractures, making them diagnostically unusable.

Interestingly enough, there seems to be a misconception among dental professionals that artifacts are reduced in CBCT volumes when compared with classic CT. It may be attributed to the cone beam geometry or lower energetic spectra that these artifacts appear differently in the CBCT data.

Based on their etiology, the artifacts can be categorized into several groups. There are many different types, including noise, scatter, cupping, ring, and streaks. The knowledge of these different types and the understanding of their causative factors are important to avoid diagnostic errors and to improve the image quality.

The most common is the beam-hardening artifacts [26]. They are often visible in CBCT images of teeth filled with dense material such as gutta-percha and metallic posts and are also observed when implants, metal crowns, and other restorations are present [26, 28]. The polychromatic X-rays lower the energy of CBCT and suffer significant absorption when passing through these materials [29]. Beam hardening also causes different artifact patterns such as cupping artifact, hypodense halo, and dark streaks. They are more numerous in axial than in the coronal sections [29].

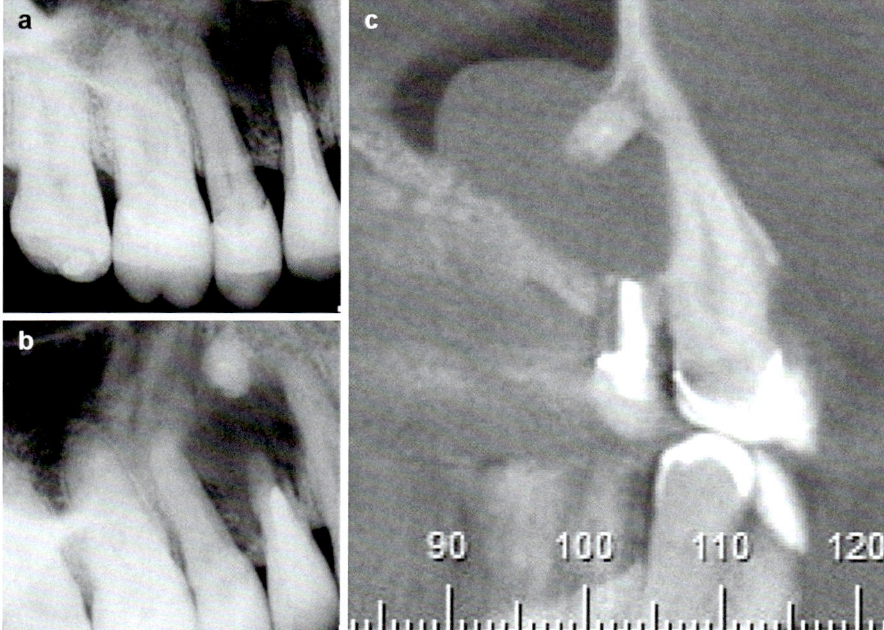

Fig. 2.9 (**a**) Radiographic periapical digital image for the diagnosis for visualization of right maxillary first premolar. (**b**) Variation in horizontal angulation to locate displaced radicular fragment. (**c**) CBCT. Sagittal views show radicular fragment of the palatal root, superiorly, displaced on the hypodense lesion

Additionally, other artifacts can also occur due to the patient motion, the image capture, and reconstruction process (Fig. 2.10).

2.6.1 Hypodense Halo

Hypodense halo is the name given to the dark area adjacent to gutta-percha caused by corrupted data also due to beam hardening. It represents 35% of CBCT images of roots with gutta-percha and root canal sealers [26].

2.6.2 Streak Artifacts

The streak artifacts can also be caused by the beam-hardening phenomenon and by those photons that are diffracted from their original path after interaction with matter [26, 27]. They correspond to 16% of CBCT images of roots with gutta-percha and root canal sealers [26] and are more visible in the axial views. In the reconstruction of image, they are seen as dark streaks. Thus, it reduces soft tissue contrast, and it also affects the density values of all other tissues.

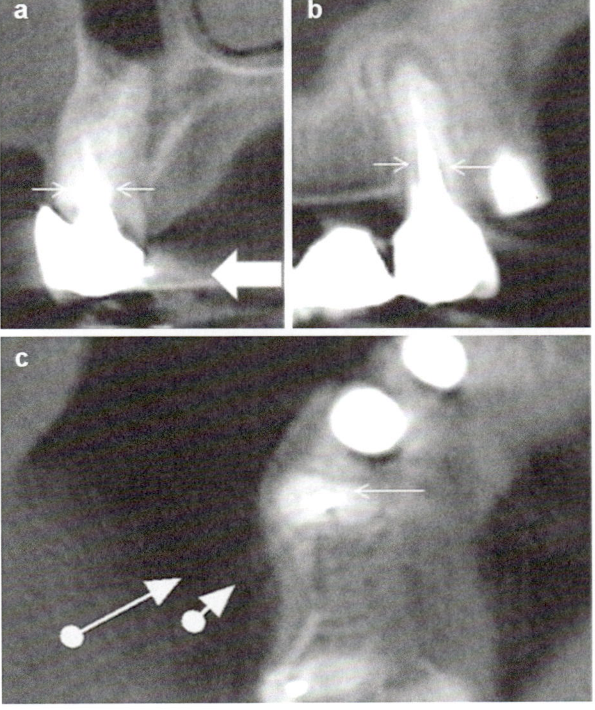

Fig. 2.10 (**a**) Coronal reconstruction, the small arrow points to the cupping artifact and the big arrow points to streaks. (**b**) Sagittal reconstruction, the arrow points to the hypodense halo. (**c**) Axial reconstruction, the small arrow points to cupping and the bigger arrows point to streak artifacts

2.6.3 Cupping Effect Artifact

The cupping effect artifact is demonstrated when a uniform cylindrical object is imaged. X-rays passing through the center portion of a uniform aluminum cylindrical phantom are hardened more than those passing through the edges because they are passing through more material. As the beam becomes harder, the rate at which it is attenuated decreases. The gray levels decrease in value in the center of the phantom owing to the increase in transmitted intensity to the sensor from the presence of beam hardening and scatter radiation occurring during image acquisition. Therefore, the resultant attenuation profile differs from the ideal profile that would be obtained without beam hardening and displays a characteristic cupped shape artifact.

In endodontics, cupping artifact in the CBCT images of roots with gutta-percha and root canal sealers corresponds to 70% of artifacts [26].

2.7 Root Fracture Detection in Endodontically Treated Teeth

The correct identification of vertical root fractures (VRF) in endodontically treated teeth is one of the most challenging tasks in dentistry. Despite CBCT having higher accuracy for detection of root fractures than periapical radiographs, the presence of metal artifacts caused by high-density material, such as gutta-percha and metallic posts, impairs the diagnosis. In these situations, it is possible to observe an obscuration of anatomical structure, reducing the contrast between adjacent objects, thus leading to false-positive diagnosis.

An increase in contrast-to-noise ratio is needed to improve the diagnosis. This could be obtained by using a smaller field of view (FOV), which is routinely employed for endodontic purposes. A smaller FOV results in an enhanced contrast-to-noise ratio, allowing better visibility of the external surfaces of the teeth. Additionally, a modification of the patient's head position or separate dental arches to avoid scanning of the areas susceptible to beam hardening (i.e., metal restorations, metal posts, and dental implants) are also good alternatives. A lower *mA* should also be preferably used for detection of VRFs in teeth with intracanal posts [30]. To overcome this unwanted artifact phenomenon, some CBCT manufactures have incorporated software in their systems to reduce their appearance in the image [26, 30]. In addition, post-processing image filters can also help to correct raw data in areas of low photon count, identify portions of the raw projection data where there is a disproportionate loss in X-ray signal, and apply a local 3D filter with smoothing effect.

Therefore, CBCT provides valuable information. However, it is important to interpret the images accurately and recognize artifacts to avoid false-positive diagnosis. Whenever is possible, the professional can use resources to improve image quality for diagnosis and to an endodontic treatment of excellence.

Conclusion

Imaging technology is important in the diagnosis of endodontic pathosis, canal morphology, assessing root and alveolar fractures, identification of the pathosis of non-endodontic origin, and presurgical assessment before root-end surgery. CBCT has increased accuracy, higher resolution and also eliminates the superimposition of the surrounding structures, providing clinically relevant information. But at the same time, CBCT has limited availability and requires significant capital investment. As accurate diagnostic information leads to better clinical outcomes, CBCT might prove to be an invaluable tool in the modern dental practice.

References

1. Mentes A, Gencoglu N. Canal length evaluation of curved canals by direct digital or conventional radiography. Oral Surg Oral Med Oral Pathol Oral Radiol Endod. 2002;93:88–91.
2. Raghav N, Reddy SS, Giridhar AG, Murthy S, Yashodha Devi BK, Santana N, et al. Comparison of the efficacy of conventional radiography, digital radiography, and ultrasound in diagnosing periapical lesions. Oral Surg Oral Med Oral Pathol Oral Radiol Endod. 2010;110:379–85.

3. Konishi M, Lindh C, Nilsson M, Tanimoto K, Rohlin M. Important technical parameters are not presented in reports of intraoral digital radiography in endodontic treatment: recommendations for future studies. Oral Surg Oral Med Oral Pathol Oral Radiol. 2012;114(2):251–8.e1–6. https://doi.org/10.1016/j.oooo.2012.02.015.
4. Heo MS, Choi DH, Benavides E, Huh KH, Yi WJ, Lee SS, Choi SC. Effect of bit depth and kVp of digital radiography for detection of subtle differences. Oral Surg Oral Med Oral Pathol Oral Radiol Endod. 2009;108(2):278–83. https://doi.org/10.1016/j.tripleo.2008.12.053. Epub 2009 Mar 9
5. Farman AG, Farman TT. A comparison of 18 different x-ray detectors currently used in dentistry. Oral Surg Oral Med Oral Pathol Oral Radiol Endod. 2005;99:485–9.
6. de Oliveira ML, Pinto GC, Ambrosano GM, Tosoni GM. Effect of combined digital imaging parameters on endodontic file measurements. J Endod. 2012;38(10):1404–7. https://doi.org/10.1016/j.joen.2012.06.006. Epub 2012 Jul 10
7. Nejaim Y, Gomes AF, Silva EJ, Groppo FC, Haiter NF. The influence of number of line pairs in digital intra-oral radiography on the detection accuracy of horizontal root fractures. Dent Traumatol. 2016;32:180–4. https://doi.org/10.1111/edt.12243.
8. Heo MS, Han DH, An BM, Huh KH, Yi WJ, Lee SS, et al. Effect of ambient light and bit depth of digital radiograph on observer performance in determination of endodontic file positioning. Oral Surg Oral Med Oral Pathol Oral Radiol Endod. 2008;105:239–44.
9. Tsuchida R, Araki K, Endo A, Funahashi I, Okano T. Physical properties and ease of operation of a wireless intraoral x-ray sensor. Oral Surg Oral Med Oral Pathol Oral Radiol Endod. 2005;100(5):603–8.
10. van der Stelt PF. Filmless imaging: the uses of digital radiography in dental practice. J Am Dent Assoc. 2005;136(10):1379–87.
11. Berkhout WE, Beuger DA, Sanderink GC, van der Stelt PF. The dynamic range of digital radiographic systems: dose reduction or risk of overexposure? Dentomaxillofac Radiol. 2004;33:1–5.
12. de Souza TM, de Castro RD, de Vasconcelos LC, Pontual AD, de Moraes Ramos Perez FM, Pontual ML. Microbial contamination in intraoral phosphor storage plates: the dilemma. Clin Oral Investig. 2017;21(1):301–7. https://doi.org/10.1007/s00784-016-1790-7.
13. Durack C, Patel S. Cone beam computed tomography in Endodontics. Braz Dent J. 2012;23(3):179–91.
14. Scarfe WC, Levin MD, Gane D, Farman AG. Use of cone beam computed tomography in Endodontics. Int J Dent. 2009;2009:634567.
15. American Association of Endodontists; American Academy of Oral and Maxillofacial Radiology. Use of cone-beam computed tomography in endodontics joint position statement of the American Association of Endodontists and the American Academy of oral and maxillofacial radiology. Oral Surg Oral Med Oral Pathol Oral Radiol Endod. 2011 Feb;111(2):234–7.
16. SEDENTEXCT guidelines. Safety and efficacy of a new and emerging dental x-ray modality: radiation protection no. 172-cone beam CT for dental and maxillofacial radiology (evidence-based guidelines). http://www.sedentexct.eu/files/radiation_protection_172.pdf
17. Venskutonis T, Plotino G, Juodzbalys G, Mickeviciene L. The importance of cone-beam computed tomography in the management of endodontic problems: a review of the literature. J Endod. 2014;40(12):1895–901.
18. Ee J, Fayad MI, Johnson BR. Comparison of endodontic diagnosis and treatment planning decisions using cone-beam volumetric tomography versus periapical radiography. J Endod. 2014;40(7):910–6.
19. Sakhadari S, Talaeipour AR, Talaeipour M, Pazhutan M, Tehrani SH, Kharazifard MJ. Diagnostic accuracy of CBCT with different voxel sizes and intraoral digital radiography for detection of periapical bone lesions: an ex-vico study. J Dent (Tehran). 2016;13(2):77–84.
20. Balasundaram A, Shah P, Hoen MM, Wheater MA, Bringas JS, Gartner A, Geist JR. Comparison of cone-beam computed tomography and periapical radiography in predicting treatment decision for periapical lesions: a clinical study. Int J Dent. 2012;2012:920815.

21. Nikneshan S, Valizadeh S, Javanmard A, Alibakhshi L. Effect of voxel size on detection of external root resorption defects using cone beam computed tomography. Iran J Radiol. 2016;13(3):e34985.
22. Yi J, Sun Y, Li Y, Li C, Li X, Zhao Z. Cone-beam computed tomography versus periapical radiograph for diagnosis external root resorption: a systematic review and meta-analysis. Angle Orthod. 2017;87(2):328–37.
23. Pinto M, Rabelo KA, Sousa Melo SL, Campos P, Oliveira L, Bento PM, Melo DP. Influence of exposure parameters on the detection of simulated root fractures in the presence of various intracanal materials. Int Endod J. 2017;50(6):586–94.
24. Melo SL, Bortoluzzi EA, Abreu M Jr, Corrêa LR, Corrêa M. Diagnostic ability of a cone-beam computed tomography scan to assess longitudinal root fractures in prosthetically treated teeth. J Endod. 2010;36:1879–82.
25. Neves FS, Freitas DQ, Campos PSF, Ekestubbe A, Lofthag-Hansen S. Evaluation of cone -beam computed tomography in the diagnosis of vertical root fractures: the influence of imaging modes and root canal materials. J Endod. 2014;10:1530–6.
26. Vasconcelos KF, Nicolielo LF, Nascimento MC, Haiter-Neto F, Bóscolo FN, Van Dessel J, EzEldeen M, Lambrichts I, Jacobs R. Artefact expression associated with several cone-beam computed tomographic machines when imaging root filled teeth. Int Endod J. 2015;48(10):994–1000.
27. Schulze R, Heil U, Gross D, Bruellmann DD, Dranischnikow E, Schwanecke U, et al. Artefacts in CBCT: a review. Dentomaxillofac Radiol. 2011;40:265–73.
28. Schulze RK, Berndt D, d'Hoedt B. On cone-beam computed tomography artifacts induced by titanium implants. Clin Oral Implants Res. 2010;21:100–7.
29. Esmaeili F, Johari M, Haddadi P, Vatankhah M. Beam hardening artifacts: comparison between two cone beam computed tomography scanners. J Dent Res Dent Clin Dent Prospects. 2012;6(2):49–53.
30. Bechara B, Alex McMahan C, Moore W, Noujeim M, Teixeira F, Geha H. Cone beam CT scans with and without artefact reduction in root fracture detection of endodontically treated teeth. Dentomaxillofac Radiol. 2013;42(5):20120245.

Complications of Local Anaesthesia in Endodontics

3

Unni Krishnan, Alex Moule, and Tara Renton

3.1 Introduction

Problems resulting from local anaesthesia during endodontic treatment can result from many causes. They can be restricted to a local area or result in systemic signs and symptoms. Problems can arise from a direct (primary) cause involving the injection process or as a reaction to this (secondary cause). Symptoms can be transient or permanent and can be mild to severe in intensity. There are many textbooks that deal with technical aspects of local anaesthesia used in dentistry and complications resulting from its use. There is also excellent visual material available on various internet sites giving detailed explanations of dental anaesthetic techniques. This chapter will deal with complications arising during/after the administration of local anaesthesia with particular reference to its use in endodontics.

Pain management of the patient during endodontic treatment is critical. The clinician and their team must use different resources to holistically manage the patients (and their family or escort) to ensure that they feel well cared for, are in control of the situation, understand fully what is happening to them and realise the risks and benefits of the intended treatment. Research has shown that fear of pain associated with the delivery of local anaesthesia is a common cause of anxiety, and this alone can prevent many from obtaining dental treatment. Dental phobia is the most common phobia reported, and over 80% of patients are anxious about dental treatment, which of course lowers their pain threshold. Most patients with endodontic

U. Krishnan (✉) • A. Moule
School of Dentistry, University of Queensland,
288 Herston Road, Herston, QLD 4006, Australia
e-mail: unni.krishnan@uq.edu.au; a.moule@uq.edu.au

T. Renton
Kings College London Institute,
Denmark Hill Campus, Bessmer Road, London SE59RS, UK
e-mail: tara.renton@kcl.ac.uk

P. Jain (ed.), *Common Complications in Endodontics*,
https://doi.org/10.1007/978-3-319-60997-3_3

emergencies no longer have a choice regarding attendance or the need for anaesthesia. They require profound anaesthesia. Needle fear and also the patient's fear of numbness are issues to consider. Many patients arrive at the operatory anxious, tired and in pain, requiring immediate diagnosis and treatment. Anxiety can be compounded by fear of dental injections. It also influences perception of pain. Thus it is important in endodontic treatment to reduce the anxiety and pain associated with delivery of effective anaesthesia. This delivery should be an almost pain-free process if care is taken with the use of an empathetic gentle patient management and slow delivery of the local anaesthetic. By avoiding block anaesthesia where possible, by adopting an infiltration technique and routinely using aspiration effectively during block anaesthesia, the majority of complications can be avoided.

3.2 Failure to Deliver Pain-Free Local Anaesthesia

Explanation for the need of the injection and reassurance of the patient are important in patient care. Distraction using visual aids, music or any patient preferred media is advised. Pain and burning during anaesthesia can also be minimised by careful anaesthetic technique. Tissues at the injection site should be dried, and a small amount of topical anaesthetic should be applied exactly to the site of the injection. Sixty seconds is a long time when treating an emergency in a busy dental practice. Nevertheless, to be effective, topical anaesthetic should be left in place for at least this long, preferably longer. It is not effective if used for a shorter period of time. To obviate any pH changes in old local anaesthetic solution, ensure solutions are in date before use. The anaesthetic should be kept at and administered at room temperature. Expression of a few drops of anaesthetic from the cartridge before the injection will ensure that the bung is moving freely. If possible tissues at the injection site should be stretched taut at the time of needle insertion. Slow advancement of the needle tip through tissues and slow deposition of solution once the target area is reached are helpful to prevent pain during injection procedures. Positive communication with the patient and keeping the syringe out of sight are important habits along with the technical process itself. Distraction techniques, e.g. involving tugging the tissues over the needle tip or asking a patient 'to see if they can try opening even wider than they are', 'wiggling their toes' are essential parts of the local anaesthetic process. Prewarning the patient of a possible electric-like feeling when administering an inferior alveolar nerve block (IANB) injection can be helpful in patient management.

Disposable anaesthetic needles are invariably sharp on first use. Nevertheless if direct contact is made though with bone, the tip can become damaged. Any tiny barb produced at the tip on the needle can cause needle insertion to become painful if a second delivery is made, or result in bleeding and possibly contribute to nerve injury when the barbed needle is withdrawn from tissues. If contact is made with bone, the needle should be inspected before a second injection is made and replaced if necessary. Block injections should be preferred where local tissues are inflamed or swollen. Palatal infiltrations should be given in areas where the tissues are not tightly attached to the palate.

3.3 Failure to Obtain Adequate Pulpal Anaesthesia in Mandibular Teeth

Failure to obtain adequate pulpal anaesthesia is the most frequent untoward outcome of local anaesthesia in endodontics and is often associated with delivery of an IANB injections. Though it goes without saying that lack of lip numbness is a clear sign of lack of pulpal anaesthesia, lack of pulpal anaesthesia can occur despite the presence of lip numbness, especially in mandibular posterior teeth with symptomatic irreversible pulpitis. Lack of pulpal anaesthesia is often objectively tested as an inability to obtain two consecutive reading of 80 with electric pulp tester (EPT) or after prolonged application of a cold stimulus. However, every endodontist is aware that pulps can be sensitive even when this test appears to confirm complete anaesthesia. Many studies have highlighted the inadequacy of IANB providing sufficient pulpal anaesthesia to allow for restorative treatments with less than 50% of healthy anterior teeth that are likely to be anaesthetised by an IANB. The pulpal anaesthesia rate will further decline with pulpitis and other local factors.

Lack of lip numbness is a sign of a misdirected block and is reported to occur from 5% up to 23% of the time [1, 2]. While lip numbness usually occurs in 4–6 minutes after an IANB, pulpal anaesthesia in a mandibular first molar regularly takes longer (up to 9 min). Lower central incisors may take longer still (up to 19 min) [3]. In addition, 12–20% of patients can have slow onset of pulpal anaesthesia, defined as an 80 EPT reading occurring after 15 min [3]. Thus sufficient time should be allowed for pulpal anaesthesia to develop before endodontic therapy is initiated. The slower onset in anterior teeth should be considered when treating these teeth, though the latter could be mitigated with a buccal infiltration.

Incorrect techniques, failure to identify landmarks, insufficient dosage and anatomical variations such as bifid IAN canals are often cited as the many reasons for lack of lip numbness. An inability to identify the three critical landmarks, namely, the coronoid notch, the pterygomandibular raphe and the occlusal plane of mandibular teeth, are the most common causes for failure of IANB injections. Many anxious patients half open their mouth and posture the jaw forwards. Anecdotally one of the major reasons for missing an IANB injection is identifying injection landmarks while the mouth is not completely open. Injections given in this jaw position often result in the solution being deposited ineffectively distal and below the IAN. Perhaps the single most important adjunct to the delivery of an IANB is to ensure that the patients open their mouth, ‘as wide as they can’, before the injection is placed. Asking the patient if they can open ‘even wider’ just before injection ensures that landmarks can be seen and also provides useful distraction at the time of delivery.

The loss of multiple mandibular posterior teeth can result in confusion regarding the orientation of the cranio-caudal plane of injection site. An unusually larger buccal pad of fat and a larger than usual tongue can also obscure vision, preventing accurate location of the site of insertion. It is worthwhile, especially in these cases, to let the assistant retract the tongue with a mouth mirror to the non-operating side and to identify the cranial end of the pterygomandibular raphe rather than the caudal end. The latter is more difficult to identify when mandibular molars are absent. Simultaneously, the face of the mouth mirror can be used to compress the buccal pad of fat against the medial surface of the ramus of mandible, and this will surprisingly often reveal an otherwise obscured pterygomandibular raphe. While repeating of IANB will often fix problems with anaesthesia, it increases the risk of nerve injury as the usual protective reflexes will no longer be operating effectively.

Popular theories and their drawbacks on causes of failure of an IANB in symptomatic irreversible pulpitis in mandibular teeth are discussed.

Obtaining profound pulpal anaesthesia in mandibular molars with symptomatic irreversible pulpitis is one of the most common problems facing clinicians. Success rates have been reported to be as low as 14–33%. [2]. Before embarking on strategies to manage failed IANB injections in symptomatic irreversible pulpitis, it is important to dispel some of the popular misconceptions:

1. *Misdirected injection*: While a misdirected block injection can lead to lack of anaesthesia, lack of pulpal anaesthesia following an IANB in the presence of lip numbness is not necessarily due to an inaccurate injection site [1]. IANBs performed using an ultrasound or peripheral nerve stimulator to accurately locate the neurovascular bundle have not always increased the success rate of mandibular first molar pulp anaesthesia when compared to conventional techniques [4, 5].
2. *Accessory innervation*: The two sources of accessory innervation to the mandible that are considered to be associated with failed pulpal anaesthesia are the mylohyoid nerve and the cutaneous branches of the cervical plexus. Contrary to popular belief, accessory innervation from mylohyoid nerve is unlikely to be the cause of failure of an IANB in symptomatic irreversible pulpitis or even in healthy subjects. Blocking of the mylohyoid nerve has not been associated with increased success of an IANB in healthy subjects [6, 7] or in patients with irreversible pulpitis [8]. A recent systematic review concluded that additional lingual infiltrations of mandibular teeth did not improve the anaesthetic success of pulpal anaesthesia in mandibular molars, premolars and canines irrespective of whether 2% lignocaine or 4% articaine was used [9]. However, it did increase success rates for mandibular incisors [9]. Accessory innervation from the cervical plexus has been shown to play a role in pulpal anaesthesia, but in a recent study, only 60% of subjects with symptomatic irreversible pulpitis were shown to have gained pulpal anaesthesia with an IANB coupled with intraoral cervical plexus anaesthesia [10]. Anaesthesia of the cervical plexus is made by depositing the solution by infiltration distal and below the apex of the mandibular first molar.
3. *Ion trapping hypothesis*: Diffusibility and binding are two critical factors in the clinical effectiveness of local anaesthesia [11].The lipid soluble, uncharged

base form (RN) of the local anaesthetics is responsible for the diffusion of the solution into a nerve sheath. The amount of base form in the solution is determined by the pKa (dissociation constant) of the solution and the pH of extra-cellular environment. The ion trapping hypothesis states that the lower pH associated with infection reduces the amount of active RN of the local anaesthetic. This does not in itself explain why IANB can fail in infected teeth, as the site of infection is away from the injection site and often only limited to the tooth apex [1].

The use of buffered lignocaine, which should theoretically result in significantly higher amount of available RN, has not been shown to increase the success rate of IANBs in symptomatic irreversible pulpitis using either 2 or 4% lignocaine formulations [12, 13]. The lack of sufficient RN of local anaesthesia due to low pH within or around the tooth is unlikely to be the reason for a failed IANB. This may nevertheless be of significant in infiltrations where the site of injection and location of abscess may be in close proximity.

4. *Central core theory*: This is based on the anatomy of IAN, where central fibres have been shown to supply the molars and peripheral fibres, supplying the anterior teeth. Additionally, the lip is supplied by the external and myelinated A β fibres of the IAN, which are relatively easily anaesthetised as compared to the core fibres and the unmyelinated C fibres, and the unregulated nociceptive elements in symptomatic irreversible pulpitis. While the inability of a solution to diffuse through the entire nerve bundle, particularly if the block is misdirected or if there is insufficient solution deposited at the site, may seem a plausible explanation why IANB anaesthesia may fail, it does not explain failure to anaesthetise inflamed pulps in molar teeth [14].
5. *Difference in susceptibility of different category of nerve fibres to anaesthesia*: A negative response to an EPT does not correspond with pain-free treatment. In one study over 40% of pulps in patients with irreversible pulpitis were not completely anaesthetised, even though teeth did not react to an EPT [15]. This may be because local anaesthetic solutions are four times more effective in blocking the myelinated Aδ fibres, which are stimulated by EPT, than the unmyelinated C fibres, which are often involved in the dull, boring, radiating pain associated with symptomatic irreversible pulpitis [16, 17]. This difference in susceptibility to local anaesthetic of a nerve fibre group might be a contributing factor in lack of pulpal anaesthesia in symptomatic irreversible pulpitis.

Most likely explanation for failure of IANB in symptomatic irreversible pulpitis:

1. *Flow of anaesthetic to path of least resistance*: Considering the failure to obtain profound pulpal anaesthesia in up to 23% of healthy mandibular molars anaesthesia, it is important to recognise that a single factor is unlikely to cause anaesthetic failure in irreversible pulpitis [3]. Hence some of the factors which may play a role in failure to achieve anaesthesia in healthy molars, such as the flow of anaesthetic along the path of least resistance away

from the pterygomandibular space, may contribute to failure in symptomatic molar teeth [3].

2. *Neurogenic inflammation and susceptibility to local anaesthetic*: There is evidence to suggest that nerves arising from the inflamed tissue have altered resting potentials and lower thresholds for excitability and that they release neuropeptides capable of maintaining neurogenic inflammation [18]. A plausible explanation of anaesthetic failure in inflamed pulps is that local anaesthetic administration may thus not prevent evocation of central cortical action potentials in such situations [19–21]. There is also enhanced expression of Nav 1.8 tetrodotoxin-resistant Na + (TTX-R) voltage-gated sodium channels (VGSCs) in inflamed pulps [22, 23]. TTX-R Na + channels have been shown to be four times less sensitive to lignocaine [24]. Hyperalgesic agents such as prostaglandin E2 are also able to increase the activation-inactivation rate, decrease the threshold and increase maximal conductance of TTX-R Na + channels [25]. Injury to peripheral nerves which occurs in pulpitis may in addition result in a dramatic shift in transcription of neuropeptides, thus resulting in neuroplasticity (axon sprouting) to a variable length along the inflamed nerve [18].
3. *Demyelination and susceptibility to local anaesthesia*: Recently, pulp tissue extracted from human subjects with severe spontaneous pulpal pain has been shown to exhibit increased accumulations of multiple isoforms of sodium channels at atypical nodal sites with evidence of demyelination [26, 27]. These sites of demyelination could theoretically change the axon excitability characteristics with spontaneous nerve activity and pain paroxysms, which may not be blocked by local anaesthetic agents [17, 27].
4. *Central sensitisation*: Increased excitability of central neurons caused by a barrage of impulses sent to the trigeminal nucleus and brain from a tooth with severe pulpitis could result in exaggerated CNS responses to minimal peripheral stimuli and widening of the sensory receptive field [17]. Local anaesthetics are unable to block these signals transmitted from the brain and are considered by some to contribute to anaesthetic failure [17, 19]. Central changes such as increased c-fos expression in brain have been used as precise indicator of acute and persistent central neuronal reaction to peripheral nerve injury, inflammation and neuropathy [28]. It has been shown that c-fos expression is upregulated with pulpal inflammation. The role of central sensitisation in teeth with symptomatic irreversible pulpitis is well documented [18, 29]. Local anaesthesia can produce only partial and slow reversal of expansion in receptive fields and hyperexcitability associated with post-injury central sensitisation [30, 31].

From a practical perspective, it is unlikely that any of these processes act independently, in isolation to one another. It is more likely that multiple factors contribute to failure to achieve pulpal anaesthesia. Hence the strategies to manage should also be multipronged.

Strategies to manage failure of pulpal anaesthesia with an IANB in symptomatic irreversible pulpitis:

1. Premedication: Antibiotics have no role in the treatment of symptomatic irreversible pulpitis [32]. However, oral non-steroidal anti-inflammatory agents, particularly 600 mg ibuprofen administered 1 hour before an injection, have consistently been shown to be effective in improving the efficacy of an IANB in painful teeth [33, 34]. This technique should be employed whenever practically possible.

   Supplementary injections:
2. Several supplemental injections can be considered when block injections fail to provide sufficient anaesthesia. Options include:
   (a) *Block reinjection*: Where there is a suspicion that a block has been unsuccessful after a reasonable length of time, reinjection is warranted. However, if a patient has profound lip numbness, but still experiences pain with the endodontic treatment, reinjection is usually an unsuccessful procedure. Alternative block techniques, including a Gow-Gates block, can be sometimes helpful.
   (b) *Buccal infiltration*: Supplementing an IANB with a buccal infiltration of articaine has been shown to be more successful than using an IANB alone in difficult cases [35]. Two recent systematic reviews have confirmed that the odds of getting successful pulpal anaesthesia with supplemental buccal infiltration with 4% articaine are higher compared to buccal infiltration with 2% lignocaine [33, 36]. However, with inflamed pulps there are still around 20% of patients who still experience operative pain even after premedication and using a buccal infiltration with articaine.
   (c) *Intraligimentary injection*: This involves firm administration of an anaesthetic solution into the periodontal ligament adjacent to the symptomatic tooth, either with a standard syringe, with a proprietary intraligimentary injection devices or with computer controlled devices, e.g. The Wand® or CompuDent® (CompuDent®, Milestone Scientific Inc., Deerfield, IL). Intraligimentary injections can provide immediate but short-term anaesthesia of a painful pulp.

       An intraligimentary injection is the most common supplementary injection used by endodontists when block anaesthesia does not provide sufficient anaesthesia.
   (d) *Intraosseous injection*: Correctly given, an intraosseous injection delivers a solution directly into the cancellous bone immediately adjacent to a painful tooth. An intraosseous injection given in the region of the first molar, after an IANB, will usually provide effective anaesthesia sufficient for pulp extirpation [37]. While this technique is not without problems, is cumbersome, requires special armamentarium and can increase the heart rate when administered with adrenaline-containing anaesthetic, it is nevertheless a very effective supplemental injection technique for anaesthetising a symptomatic tooth when IANB injections have proved to be unsuccessful. Anatomical considerations prevent its use in all parts of the mouth. A number of proprietary devices are available, e.g. Stabident and X-tip intraosseous systems.

(e) *Intra-pulpal injection*: This technique, which involves the administration of local anaesthesia directly into a pulp, with sufficient back pressure, results in 100% success, but the duration of action is only short lived (10–20 min) [38]. While used as last resort, when properly administered, it is an extremely useful anaesthetic technique, particularly where the pulp is large and the exposure point is small. The patient must be prewarned that 'they will experience sharp pain' for just an instant. The jaw should be the firmly stabilised with firm finger rests. When the pulp is not exposed and all reasonable attempts have been made to anesthetise the pulp, access to the pulp can be obtained relatively atraumatically with a small thin bur. Once this drops into the chamber, it can be withdrawn and the local anaesthetic administered through this, using as much force as the syringe allows. Anaesthesia is obtained by the pressure applied to the pulp and not by the solution used. The success rate depends on whether adequate back pressure is maintained [1]. If the operator does not notice any back pressure, then it is unlikely that the procedure will be effective. Anecdotally the use of this technique is far less stressful to the patient than multiple attempts at anaesthesia, testing each time whether the tooth is 'completely numb now'.

(f) *Intracanal injection*: On occasions, removal of the coronal pulp can be completed, but the patient continues to experience sensitivity in one or other root canal. Anaesthesia can be obtained usually without pain in the same way making sure sufficient back pressure is developed.

(g) *Combination techniques*: Intraligimentary and intraosseous injections can provide pulpal anaesthesia but sometimes for only a short duration of time. Where it has been possible to gain sufficient anaesthesia to access the pulp through one of these techniques, it is still advantageous to immediately proceed to an intra-pulpal injection to ensure complete anaesthesia for pulp removal.

(h) *Sedation*: Managing a very nervous or uncooperative patient with a very painful molar can be stressful for both the operator and the patient, particularly when local anaesthesia has initially proved unsuccessful. Where oral and intravenous sedation or similar facilities are available, the use of these at least during the initial stages of treatment is a good adjunct to treatment ease and patient management.

3.3.1 Achieving Anaesthesia in Maxillary Teeth

Failure to gain satisfactory anaesthesia with maxillary teeth with acute pulpitis is not as common as with mandibular teeth. This is primarily due to the ease of access to the neural system via infiltrations. Nevertheless, problems still occur and supplemental anaesthesia may be required. There is no evidence to support the use of both buccal and palatal injections, although there is also no reason not to do so in difficult cases, provided the palatal injections are given slowly and not into tissues that are firmly attached to the tissues. Sloughing can occur

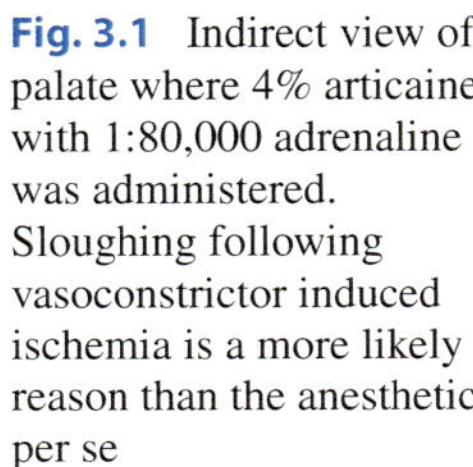

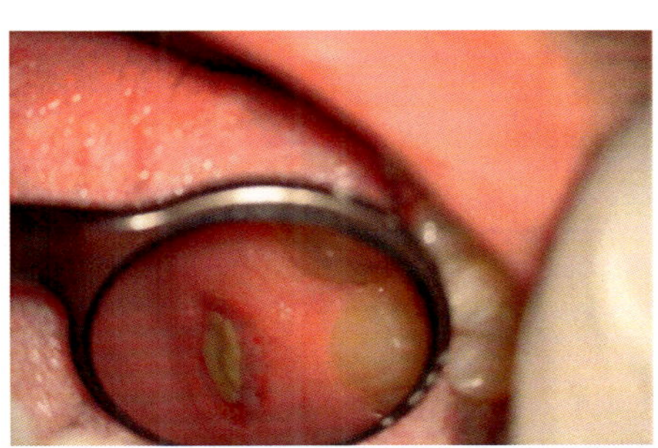

Fig. 3.1 Indirect view of palate where 4% articaine with 1:80,000 adrenaline was administered. Sloughing following vasoconstrictor induced ischemia is a more likely reason than the anesthetic per se

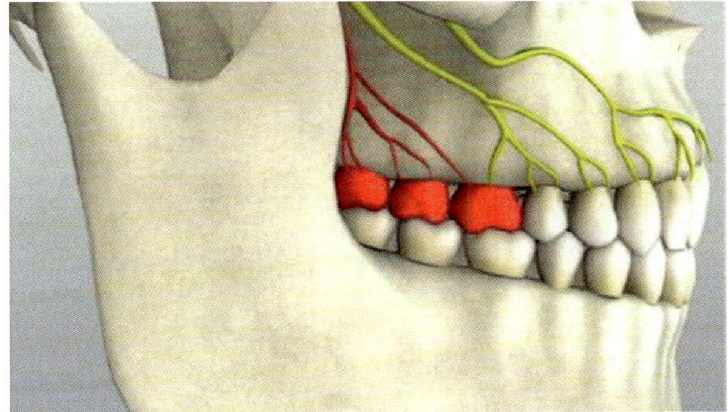

Fig. 3.2 Diagrammatic representation of nerve supply to apices of apices of maxillary teeth http://www.merckmanuals.com/professional/dental-disorders/symptoms-of-dental-and-oral-disorders/toothache-and-infection

(Fig. 3.1) due to prolonged ischemia, especially with use of higher concentration of adrenaline (1:50,000). The management is symptomatic and it resolves in a few days.

When anaesthetising symptomatic maxillary teeth, it is important to appreciate that the nerves to the teeth pass postero-anteriorly and that infiltrations for a first molar must be given both mesially and distally to anaesthetise all buccal roots (Fig. 3.2). Where pulpal anaesthesia is difficult for a molar, the injection should be given more distally and apically to the tooth.

Of note also that with long maxillary teeth, e.g., some canines, failure to achieve anaesthesia may be due the fact that the anaesthetic has not been delivered sufficiently close enough to the apex of the tooth.

With many maxillary teeth, infection and inflammation are in the area where an injection would normally be made. Effectiveness of a local anaesthetic solution is pH dependant. For a local anaesthetic solution to work effectively, the pH should be closer to physiological levels. Infected tissues usually have a lower pH. Thus, if local anaesthesia is delivered to a site that is inflamed or infected, its effectiveness may be severely diminished. The use of block injections, particularly an infraorbital block, is often necessary in these events.

Ophthalmic complications of maxillary injections and inferior alveolar nerve block can occur. Most of the reported cases are from single injections and due to inadvertent intravascular injections. If these do occur, it is important to reassure the patient about the transient nature of the problem and cover the eye until the corneal reflex returns. The patient should be escorted home and not drive until vision returns completely to normal. Ophthalmic advice should be sought if symptoms persist for more than 6 hours.

3.4 Complications of Local Anaesthesia and Endodontic Treatment

3.4.1 Possible Mechanism of LA Nerve Injury

Nerve injury due to LA is complex. The nerve injury may be physical (needle, compression due to epineural or perineural haemorrhage) or chemical (haemorrhage or LA contents). Thus the resultant nerve injury may be a combination of peri-, epi- and intraneural trauma causing subsequent haemorrhage, inflammation and scarring resulting in demyelination (loss of nerve lining (Fig. 3.3) [39]. Local anaesthesia practice can cause injury to nerves in many ways. The location of nerve injury may also be important as well as mechanism. Factors that need to be considered are that only 1.3–8.6% of patients get an 'electric shock' type sensation on application of an IAN block and 57% of patients who suffer from prolonged neuropathy have not experienced the discomfort on injection, thus this is not a specific sign [78].

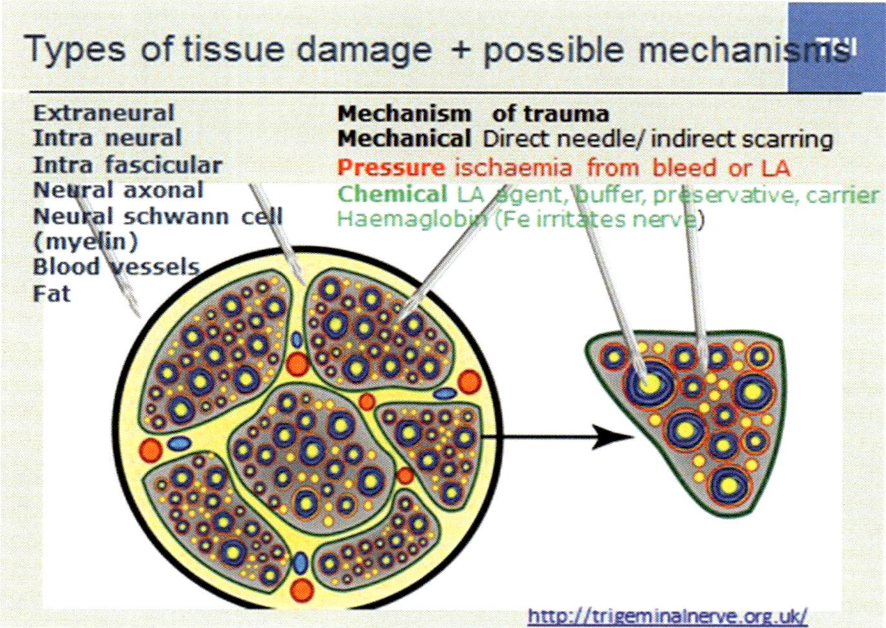

Fig. 3.3 Diagrammatic representation of mechanisms of nerve injury from IANB

3.4.2 Damage to the IANB

3.4.2.1 Neuropathy

Any damage to sensory nerve tissue may cause a mixture of anaesthesia (numbness), paraesthesia (altered sensation which is not painful), dysaesthesia (altered sensation which is uncomfortable/painful) and neuropathic pain. Neuropathy in the orofacial region must be taken seriously and the cause established, as there are some serious conditions that need to be eliminated if a cause is not obvious [42]. Often there is a history that helps determine the origin. Sensory deficits should be mapped on the face so that an estimate can be made of resolution or expansion of the deficit. Any patient with an expanding area of paraesthesia for which a cause has not been established should be referred for specialist evaluation. Amongst other things, paraesthesia can result from trauma, nerve injury, surgery, infections and prolonged reactions to local anaesthesia, viruses, malignancy or serious pathoses. If a dental cause is suspected, patients require reassurance, careful documentation and follow-up.

Unilateral paraesthesia and facial paralysis can occur in a misdirected block where local anaesthetic solution is deposited in the parotid gland. It usually occurs when the depth of needle penetration is nearly to the hub of a long needle. It is more likely to happen when the ramus of the mandible is flared laterally making it difficult for the operator to 'hit the bone'. The unilateral paralysis of facial muscles is reversible. This resolves over hours. The patient needs to be reassured, and the eye has to be protected until the blink reflex returns, as corneal reflex is often lost.

3.4.2.2 Neurological Injuries Resulting from Untreated Periapical Infections

It is not uncommon in endodontic practice to encounter patients with apical periodontitis of endodontic origin leading to sensory impairment of the inferior alveolar or mental nerve. This invariably resolves with the reduction in inflammation and local swelling. A number of authors have reviewed and documented clinical cases of neurological disorder with paraesthesia and hypaesthesia of the mental nerve resulting as a sequel of apical periodontitis of a mandibular second premolar and second molar teeth [40–42].

3.4.2.3 Motor Nerve Palsy Due to Endodontic Treatment

There are reports of facial motor nerve deficit as a result of endodontic treatment due to extrusion of endodontic irrigants, hydrogen peroxide and ethanol rinses [43, 44].

3.4.2.4 Paraesthesia and Pain Associated with Endodontically Related Nerve Injuries

Endodontic treatment of premolar and mandibular teeth has the potential to damage the inferior alveolar nerve via direct trauma, pressure or neurotoxicity. Trigeminal nerve injury is the most problematic consequence of dental surgical procedures with major medicolegal implications [44]. While incidence of lingual nerve injury has remained static over many years, the incidence of inferior alveolar nerve injury has increased; the latter likely being due to implant surgery and endodontic therapy [45].

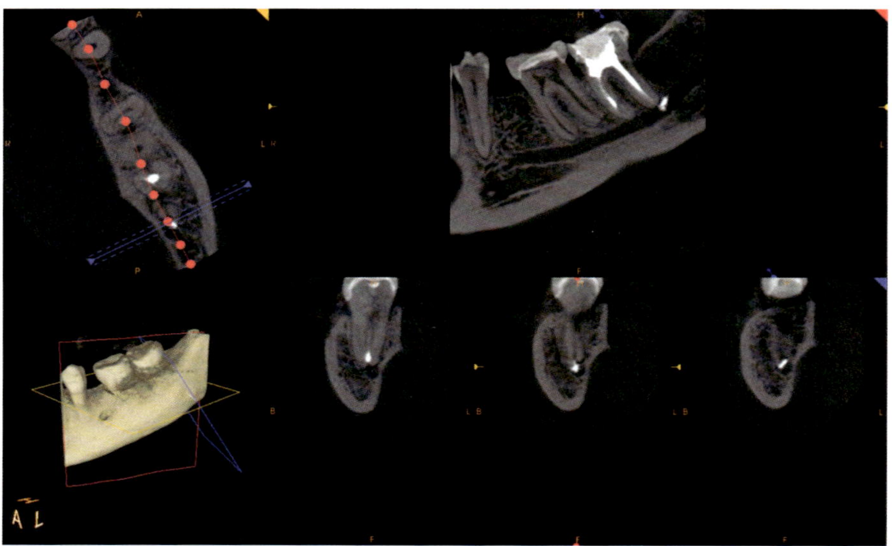

Fig. 3.4 CBCT imaging of a tooth that shows extrusion of endodontic sealant into the inferior alveolar canal causing pain and paraesthesia

Iatrogenic injuries to the third division of the trigeminal nerve remain a common and complex clinical problem (Fig. 3.4). Altered sensation and pain in region may interfere with speaking, eating, kissing, shaving, applying make-up, tooth brushing and drinking, in fact just about every social interaction we take for granted [46, 78]. Thus these injuries have a significant negative effect on the patient's quality of life, and the iatrogenesis of these injuries lead to significant psychological effects [47].

Persistence of any peripheral sensory nerve injury depends on the mechanisms, the severity of the injury, the increased age of the patient, the time elapsed since the injury and the proximity of the injury to the cell body (the more proximal lesions are having a worse prognosis). Most sensory nerve injuries related to dentistry are permanent. LA-induced nerve injuries have nearly 80% likelihood of recovery. Many authors recommend referral of injuries before 4 months [50], but this may be too late for many endodontically related peripheral sensory nerve injuries. Inferior alveolar nerve injuries related to endodontic treatment, particularly where there is extrusion of filling material, require immediate attention with permanency likely after 24–30 h [50]. After 3 months, permanent central and peripheral changes occur within the nervous system subsequent to such injury, and they are unlikely to respond to surgical intervention [48].

The IAN is at risk from a variety of endodontic procedures. The IAN is contained within a bony canal, predisposing it to ischemia, trauma and subsequent injury in relation to dental procedures. This may explain the higher incidence of permanent damage for inferior alveolar nerve injuries compared with lingual nerve injuries [45]. Inferior alveolar nerve injury during endodontic treatment can result from local anaesthetic accidents, from irrigant extrusion and from over instrumentation or overfilling, in all cases resulting in one or a combination of mechanical injury, haemorrhagic, ischaemic or chemical injury to the nerve.

There are relatively few detailed reports on nerve injuries resulting from endodontic treatment [42]. The largest series of endodontic-related trigeminal nerve injuries included 61 patients reviewed over an 8-year period [9], with most of these patients presenting with persistent pain. There are relatively few reports of persistent pain subsequent to endodontic procedures [49]. In a recent study of 216 patients with trigeminal nerve injuries related to dentistry, 70% are reported to have chronic neuropathic post-traumatic pain [50].

Neuropathic pain (NP) syndromes are chronic pain disorders that develop after a lesion involving the peripheral or central nervous structures that are normally involved in signalling pain. The characteristics of NP differ substantially from those of other chronic pain states, i.e. chronic nociceptive pain, which develops while the nervous system that is involved in pain processing is intact. Apart from the existence of negative somatosensory signs (deficit in function), there are other features that are characteristic of neuropathic conditions (allodynia, hyperalgesia and hyperpathia) [51]. Paraesthesia is typically described by patients as bothersome but not painful. Furthermore, NP states require different therapeutic approaches such as anticonvulsants, which are not effective in nociceptive pain [52].

Thus symptoms experienced by patients with post-traumatic neuropathy of the trigeminal nerve can range from next to no symptoms, such as minimal anaesthesia in a small area to devastating effects on the patient's quality of life [53].

3.4.2.5 Local Anaesthesia-Related Neuropathy During Endo Procedures

As stated earlier, local anaesthesia is often complex in endodontics as the patients often experience difficulty in achieving analgesia. Patients undergoing endodontic treatment often have multiple injections and may be more at risk of local anaesthetic-related nerve injuries [54]. More recently the incidence of nerve injury in relation to IANBs has been calculated as 1:609,000 but with a reported increase in injury rate when 4% anaesthetic agents are used [55]. These LA injuries are associated with a 34–70% incidence of neuropathic pain, which is lower when compared with endodontic-related nerve injuries. Recovery is reported to take place at 8 weeks for 85–94% of cases [56].

LA injuries may have a better prognosis than nerve injuries resulting from endodontic treatment. In both cases, the nerve injury may be physical (compression due to epineural or perineural haemorrhage or extruded material) or chemical (haemorrhage or local anaesthetic or endodontic compound contents). There may be elements of direct mechanical trauma, which generally would be worse in endodontically caused nerve injuries.

Intraoperatively all clinicians should document unusual patient reactions occurring during application of local analgesic blocks (such as sharp pain or an electrical shock-like sensation), and multiple blocks should be avoided if possible as they may also increase the risk of local anaesthetic-related nerve injuries.

3.4.3 Assessment of Trigeminal Nerve Injuries

The emphasis in trigeminal neuro-functional studies has been on using conventional mechanical tests, which are subjective. Due to the variability in methodology and reporting, they are of limited value for inter-study comparisons and little clinical significance in relation to a patient's pain and functionality. Recently several investigators have recommended the use of the patient's report alone [53], in combination with subjective and objective neurosensory tests [50] or utilising quality of life questionnaires (OHIP 14–31) for a more holistic approach for the assessment of patients with trigeminal nerve injury [57]. In this way hopefully to make studies easier to compare.

3.4.4 Management of Neuropathy Related to Endodontics

Differentiation between the possible causes of nerve injury, whether it is of local anaesthetic, periapical inflammation [50] or endodontically origin, is difficult. An accurate diagnosis is dependent on a thorough history and specific identification of the neuropathic area distribution. On occasions the use of adjunctive antibiotics or NSAIDS and paracetamol may enable the clinician to exclude inflammatory or infection-related pain as against post-traumatic NP.

3.4.4.1 Management

There is limited evidence base for managing dental LA-related nerve injuries. Unfortunately, a quarter of the cases are permanent and never recover. There is no 'magic bullet' to fix them; we have to wait and reassure the patient. In order to maximise resolution of any sensory neuropathy, it has been recommended to institute early medical intervention. The general medical practitioner should be involved and should prescribe the medication:

- *Steroids*: Step-down 5-day course of prednisolone, oral 50 mg, 40 mg, 30 mg, 20 mg and10 mg for 5 days
- *NSAIDs:* Ibuprofen oral 400–600 mg 6 hourly
- *Vitamin B* complex

Patients who report severe electric-like pain (though it is not a definite sign) following the administration of an IANB should be followed up [63]. What is important, however, is to inform all patients of the risks of problems that may result from IANB, however slight the risk, beforehand and do everything in your power to minimise the risks. Such as minimising repeat blocks and using supplementary techniques.

Some factors to consider in planning procedures which may influence the safety of the procedures include:

- *Block anaesthesia*: **Consider first whether block anaesthesia is really required**. By avoiding IANBs there is less risk of injury to the lingual and inferior alveolar nerves, which though rare, is debilitating to the patients and has no cure. Infiltrations provide more localised and shorter lasting anaesthesia which is of benefit to the patients. This technique requires less skill and less discomfort for the patient during the injection and avoids unnecessary lingual anaesthesia after dental treatment. Recent studies [9, 59–62] have suggested that infiltration of 4% articaine in the mandibular molar region can result in anaesthesia of the lower first molar that is in most cases as effective as an inferior dental block.
- *Concentration of LA*: Any increased concentration of any agent leads to increased neural neurotoxicity [64].
- *Volume of LA*: There is no evidence to support the suggestion that increased volumes of solution result in more nerve damage, but as all chemicals are neurotoxic, it is dependent upon the proximity to the nerve, concentration, neural damage and additional volumes that add to potential neurotoxicity.
- *Multiple injections*: Second or subsequent injections that impede directly on or in neural tissue may not be associated with the usual 'funny bone' neuralgic pain. Thus the patient does not self-protect as effectively possibly rendering the nerves more at risk of direct damage. Alternatives to block injections may be indicated.
- *Type of LA agent*: Bupivacaine is the most neurotoxic of all LA agents.
- *Type of vasoconstrictor*: The role of vasoconstrictor in nerve damage is unknown.
- *Sedated or anaesthetised patients*: There is no evidence to support unresponsive patients are prone to nerve injury as they are less likely to protect themselves when the IDB needle encroaches too close to the nerve.
- *Lack of LA aspiration*: There is no evidence to support that aspiration during an IANB results in lower persistent neuropathies though it is always advisable.
- *Patient factors*: Patient factors include age (>50 years of age), migraines, patients with existing neuropathic pain conditions (fibromyalgia) and those predisposed to developing peripheral neuropathy.

Acute Management

Should endodontically induced nerve injuries be suspected, acute management involves urgent referral. Some patients may require surgery. The largest series reported to date is by Pogrel [65], who described the management of 61 patients with endodontically induced nerve injuries over an 8-year period. Eight patients were asymptomatic and received no treatment. Forty-two patients exhibited only mild symptoms or were seen more than 3 months after undergoing root canal therapy. They received no surgical treatment. Only 10% of these patients experienced any resolution of symptoms. Eleven patients underwent surgical exploration. Five of these patients underwent exploration and received treatment within 48 h, and all recovered completely. The remaining six patients underwent surgical exploration and received treatment between 10 days and 3 months after receiving endodontic therapy. Of these six patients, four experienced

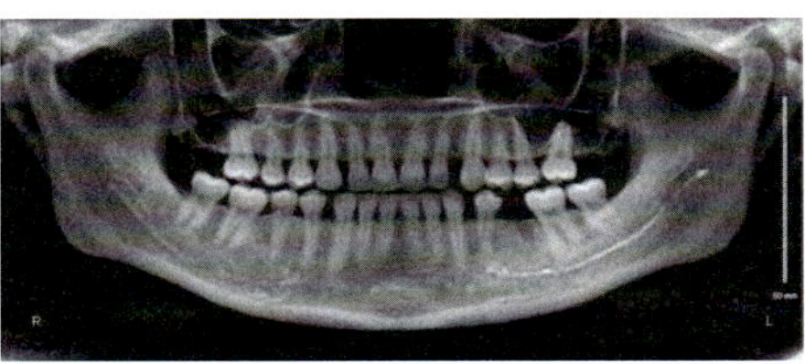

Fig. 3.5 Panoramic radiograph showing extruded sealer material in the left inferior alveolar canal resulting from endodontic treatment

partial recovery and two experienced no recovery at all. Thus Pogrel [65] concludes that early surgical exploration and débridement may reverse the side effects (pain and paraesthesia) of endodontic treatment on the inferior alveolar nerve. If the patient has continued symptoms of paraesthesia or pain once the local anaesthetic has worn off and the radiograph obtained after endodontic therapy shows sealant in the inferior alveolar canal (Fig. 3.5), then immediate referral to an oral and maxillofacial surgeon is indicated. Immediate surgical exploration and débridement may provide satisfactory results.

Escoda-Francoli et al. [66] described a case of endodontic treatment of a permanent right mandibular first molar in which the sealer cement overextended in large amounts and damaged the right inferior alveolar nerve. The condition reverted a few months after the surgical removal of the material. There are several reports of nerve injury in relation to over instrumentation and overfilling [67, 68]. Endodontic retreatment for inferior alveolar nerve injury was also reported by Yatsuhashi et al. [67]. Gatot and Tovi [68] recommended steroid therapy for early postoperative neuritis. More recently Grotz et al. [69] described the management of 11 patients with endodontic-associated neuropathy. They similarly reported that the neurological findings were dominated by hypaesthesia and dysaesthesia with 50% of patients reporting pain. Initial X-rays showed root filling material in the area of the mandibular canal. Nine cases were treated with apicectomy and decompression of the nerve; in two cases, extraction of the tooth was necessary. Only one patient reported persistent pain after surgery. Both Scolozzi et al. [70] and Brkic et al. [71] describe a limited series of patients successfully treated with surgical decompression (removal of material within the canal or apicecting the tooth) resulting in resolution of the endodontically related nerve injury. As stated earlier, patients must be assessed on a case-by-case basis, but immediate surgical exploration and débridement may provide satisfactory results.

Delayed Management

If the neuropathy is longer standing and the patient has chronic pain, then post-traumatic neuropathy must be diagnosed and appropriate treatment prescribed. Most patients accept a full explanation and reassurance for their symptoms. Many patients can find the explanation for their neuropathic pain symptoms very helpful. Antibiotics may be prescribed to exclude apical infection. NSAIDs and paracetamol will also exclude inflammatory pain, but neuropathic pain due to post-traumatic nerve injury will not respond to these medications.

Oshima et al. [72] reported that 16 patients of 271 patients presenting with chronic orofacial pain were diagnosed with chronic neuropathic tooth pain subsequent to endodontic retreatment. Most of these patients were treated for maxillary teeth, and 70% of the patients responded to tricyclic antidepressant therapy which highlights the importance of establishing whether the patient has neuropathic pain to start with. A recent Cochrane review highlights the lack of robust evidence in managing trigeminal nerve injuries [73]. Recommendations for treatment of trigeminal neuropathic pain are also well described by Truelove [52].

3.4.5 Recommendations Based on the Current Evidence

Before undertaking endodontic care, practitioners should:

1. Preoperatively, identify teeth proximal to the IAN and take special care in preventing over instrumentation or extrusion of irritants.
2. Intraoperatively, recognise and record certain events that may be indicative of nerve injury, e.g. extreme patient discomfort during treatment including:
   - Intraoperative pain during irrigation
   - Intraoperative pain during preparation and filling
   - Inferior alveolar vessel bleed during preparation and delay filling
3. Postoperatively, continue to support and reassure your patient and advise them to visit websites designed to assist by post-traumatic neuropathy related to dentistry. *Always* undertake a *Homecheck* and arrange to contact your patients postsurgically the following morning. Neuropathy related to endodontics can be delayed, and the patient must be encouraged to report any change in sensation up to 3–4 days post-treatment (Renton et al. unpublished). If nerve injury is suspected, due to over instrumentation or deposition of endodontic material into the canal, the apex and/or tooth must be removed within 48 hours of placement in order to maximise recovery from nerve injury [65].
4. If the patient is insistent on keeping the tooth, urgent referral of the patient may be indicated for mandibular decompression and saline irrigation of the nerve and canal (Fig. 3.6) [65].

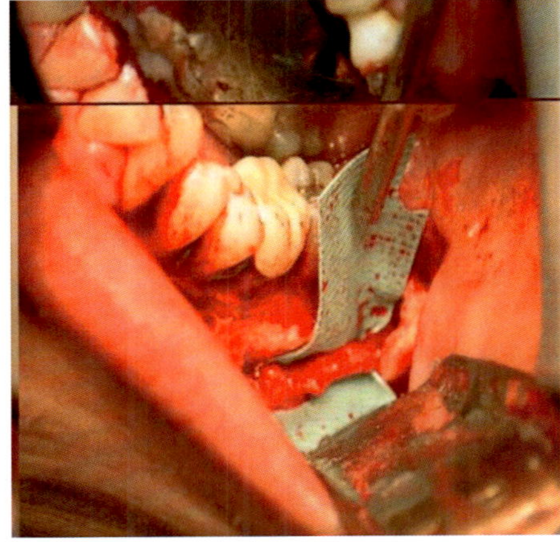

Fig. 3.6 Clinical picture of traditional approach for decorticating buccal aspect of mandible to gain access to inferior dental canal and IAN. This technique was recommended for IAN injuries presenting late, but some authors prefers access via the socket for recent injuries

Pain following root filling a tooth is a common occurrence, and this usually responds well to occlusal adjustment and the prescription of anti-inflammatory medication. If there is no evidence of overfill present, then pain may be due to:

- Apical inflammation (neuritis) confirmed by prescription of anti-inflammatories
- Chemical nerve injury from irrigants or filling material
- Thermal damage

However in the any event once neuropathy is identified, the clinician must reassure the patient, prescribe steroids (prednisolone step down such as 15 mg 5 days, 10 mg 5 days, 5 mg 5 days and high-dose NSAIDs and 600 mg ibuprofen) and make a timely referral to an appropriately trained micro-neurosurgeon if necessary; the clinical evidence is poor but despite this remains recommended practice; however, in vitro studies have demonstrated the possible benefit of these regimes [74].

3.4.6 Incidence of LA Nerve Injuries

Nerve injuries related to local anaesthetic injections are thankfully rare. Incident reports vary considerably. The incidence of IANB nerve injuries was first comprehensively reported by a retrospective examination of voluntary reported nonsurgical paraesthesia cases in Ontario, Canada, during the period from 1973 to 1993 [55]. Based on the number of cartridges used, these authors reported an incidence to be between 1.2 and 2.27 per 1 million injections depending on the type of anaesthetic used. The frequency of paraesthesia with articaine being twice that observed with other agents. Sambrook and Goss [64] estimated the incidence to be 1 in 27,415 cases of prolonged neuropathy related to IAN blocks per year in Australia. On the other hand, Haas and Lennon [55] found the incidence to be 1 in 785,000 injections, while Garisto et al. reported a rate of IANB paraesthesias to be 1 in 13,800,970. Renton et al. [75] reported a much higher incidence based upon surveys of dentists and specialists.

Two studies examining reports of paraesthesia from 1994 to 1998 and 1999 to 2008 have reported similar findings, implicating the local anaesthetics 4% articaine and 4% prilocaine with paraesthesia [76]. Other studies have corroborated these findings [56, 58, 76, 77]. All of the above studies found that the lingual nerve was most often affected during mandibular anaesthesia as compared to the inferior alveolar nerve.

3.4.6.1 Significance of IANB Nerve Injuries

The long-term significant problems seen in patients are severe. There is no ‘fix’ for these injuries, only prevention. Thus we can only wait for resolution, while managing the patient therapeutically, using medical and psychological interventions. Eighty-one percent of the IAN block nerve injuries resolve in 2 weeks [78]. Those with permanent injury often result in high levels of dysaesthesia and pain, mainly affecting the tongue with attendant social and psychological impacts [78].

While with consent, a patient may be aware of these rare but possible injuries, as no one else has ever heard of them or understands their nature; the resultant isolation for the patient is severe. There is significant stress to both dentist and patients.

3.5 Needle Breakage and Equipment Failures

With modern delivery systems, needle breakage is now a very rare complication. If breakage occurs, it invariably does so where the needle meets the hub. The needle may break if there is forceful contact made with bone or if the patient moves suddenly. Almost all needle breakages reported in the literature involve using 30 gauge needles used in block injections or in posterior superior nerve blocks. Long needles should therefore be used for block injections. Needles should not be inserted to the hub or bent at the hub prior to the injection in order to gain a better anaesthetic result. Both these procedures invite needle breakage if the patient moves suddenly. *Treating stressful patients with painful pulps is stressful, and care should not to rush any procedure, including anaesthetic procedures, as this may lead to problems including needle breakage and nerve injury.*

Should needle breakage occur during a block injection, it is imperative to keep the patient's mouth opening wide (mouth prop). If a long needle has been used and if the needle is visible, it can be grasped with a needle holder and removed. If the needle is not visible, then immediate referral is mandatory.

Conclusion

In this chapter, complications with dental anaesthesia in endodontics have been discussed. By far the greatest complication is failure to obtain good anaesthesia, particularly in mandibular molars with symptomatic irreversible. The causes and management of anaesthetic failure have been discussed. Complications relating to paraesthesia including that due to nerve injury from the delivery of local anaesthesia and endodontic treatment have been discussed in detail. These are often serious injuries. Guidelines are given for the prevention and management of these.

References

1. Nusstein JM, Reader A, Drum M. Local anesthesia strategies for the patient with a "hot" tooth. Dent Clin N Am. 2010;54(2):237–47.
2. Monteiro MR, Groppo FC, Haiter-Neto F, Volpato MC, Almeida JF. 4% articaine buccal infiltration versus 2% lidocaine inferior alveolar nerve block for emergency root canal treatment in mandibular molars with irreversible pulpits: a randomized clinical study. Int Endod J. 2015;48(2):145–52.
3. Reader A, Nusstein J, Drum M. Successful local anaesthesia for restorative dentistry and endodontics. Chicago: Quintessence Books; 2011.
4. Simon F, Reader A, Drum M, Nusstein J, Beck M. A prospective, randomized single-blind study of the anesthetic efficacy of the inferior alveolar nerve block administered with a peripheral nerve stimulator. J Endod. 2010;36(3):429–33.
5. Hannan L, Reader A, Nist R, Beck M, Meyers WJ. The use of ultrasound for guiding needle placement for inferior alveolar nerve blocks. Oral Surg Oral Med Oral Pathol Oral Radiol Endod. 1999;87(6):658–65.
6. Clark S, Reader A, Beck M, Meyers WJ. Anesthetic efficacy of the mylohyoid nerve block and combination inferior alveolar nerve block/mylohyoid nerve block. Oral Surg Oral Med Oral Pathol Oral Radiol Endod. 1999;87(5):557–63.

7. Foster W, Drum M, Reader A, Beck M. Anesthetic efficacy of buccal and lingual infiltrations of lidocaine following an inferior alveolar nerve block in mandibular posterior teeth. Anesth Prog. 2007;54(4):163–9.
8. Dou L, Luo J, Yang D. Anaesthetic efficacy of supplemental lingual infiltration of mandibular molars after inferior alveolar nerve block plus buccal infiltration in patients with irreversible pulpitis. Int Endod J. 2013;46(7):660–5.
9. Dou L, Luo J, Yang D, Wang Y. The effectiveness of an additional lingual infiltration in the pulpal anesthesia of mandibular teeth: a systematic review. Quintessence Int. 2013;44(5):457–64.
10. Bitner DP, Uzbelger Feldman D, Axx K, Albandar JM. Description and evaluation of an intraoral cervical plexus anesthetic technique. Clin Anatomy (New York, NY). 2015;28(5):608–13.
11. Malamed SF. Handbook of local anesthesia. 6th ed. Amsterdam: Elsevier; 2011.
12. Saatchi M, Khademi A, Baghaei B, Noormohammadi H. Effect of sodium bicarbonate-buffered lidocaine on the success of inferior alveolar nerve block for teeth with symptomatic irreversible pulpitis: a prospective, randomized double-blind study. J Endod. 2015;41(1):33–5.
13. Schellenberg J, Drum M, Reader A, Nusstein J, Fowler S, Beck M. Effect of buffered 4% lidocaine on the success of the inferior alveolar nerve block in patients with symptomatic irreversible pulpitis: a prospective, randomized double-blind study. J Endod. 2015;41(6):791–6.
14. Virdee SS, Seymour D, Bhakta S. Effective anaesthesia of the acutely inflamed pulp: part 1. The acutely inflamed pulp. Br Dent J. 2015;219(8):385–90.
15. Nusstein J, Reader A, Nist R, Beck M, Meyers WJ. Anesthetic efficacy of the supplemental intraosseous injection of 2% lidocaine with 1:100,000 epinephrine in irreversible pulpitis. J Endod. 1998;24(7):487–91.
16. Huang JH, Thalhammer JG, Raymond SA, Strichartz GR. Susceptibility to lidocaine of impulses in different somatosensory afferent fibers of rat sciatic nerve. J Pharmacol Exp Ther. 1997;282(2):802–11.
17. Hargreaves KM, Keiser K. Local anesthetic failure in endodontics. Endod Top. 2002;1(1):26–39.
18. Byers MR, Suzuki H, Maeda T. Dental neuroplasticity, neuro-pulpal interactions, and nerve regeneration. Microsc Res Tech. 2003;60(5):503–15.
19. Wallace JA, Michanowicz AE, Mundell RD, Wilson EG. A pilot study of the clinical problem of regionally anesthetizing the pulp of an acutely inflamed mandibular molar. Oral Surg Oral Med Oral Pathol. 1985;59(5):517–21.
20. Modaresi J, Dianat O, Soluti A. Effect of pulp inflammation on nerve impulse quality with or without anesthesia. J Endod. 2008;34(4):438–41.
21. Byers MR, Taylor PE, Khayat BG, Kimberly CL. Effects of injury and inflammation on pulpal and periapical nerves. J Endod. 1990;16(2):78–84.
22. Renton T, Yiangou Y, Plumpton C, Tate S, Bountra C, Anand P, et al. BMC Oral Health. 2005;5(1):5.
23. Esmaeili A, Akhavan A, Bouzari M, Mousavi SB, Torabinia N, Adibi S. Temporal expression pattern of sodium channel Nav 1.8 messenger RNA in pulpitis. Int Endod J. 2011;44(6):499–504.
24. Roy ML, Narahashi T. Differential properties of tetrodotoxin-sensitive and tetrodotoxin-resistant sodium channels in rat dorsal root ganglion neurons. J Neurosci. 1992;12(6):2104–11.
25. Gold MS, Reichling DB, Shuster MJ, Levine JD. Hyperalgesic agents increase a tetrodotoxin-resistant Na+ current in nociceptors. Proc Natl Acad Sci U S A. 1996;93(3):1108–12.
26. Henry MA, Luo S, Foley BD, Rzasa RS, Johnson LR, Levinson SR. Sodium channel expression and localization at demyelinated sites in painful human dental pulp. J Pain. 2009;10(7):750–8.
27. Luo S, Perry GM, Levinson SR, Henry MA. Pulpitis increases the proportion of atypical nodes of Ranvier in human dental pulp axons without a change in Nav1.6 sodium channel expression. Neuroscience. 2010;169(4):1881–7.
28. Byers MR, Chudler EH, Iadarola MJ. Chronic tooth pulp inflammation causes transient and persistent expression of Fos in dynorphin-rich regions of rat brainstem. Brain Res. 2000;861(2):191–207.

29. Huang J, Lv Y, Fu Y, Ren L, Wang P, Liu B, et al. Dynamic regulation of delta-opioid receptor in rat trigeminal ganglion neurons by lipopolysaccharide-induced acute pulpitis. J Endod. 2015;41(12):2014–20.
30. Dahl JB, Brennum J, Arendt-Nielsen L, Jensen TS, Kehlet H. The effect of pre- versus postinjury infiltration with lidocaine on thermal and mechanical hyperalgesia after heat injury to the skin. Pain. 1993;53(1):43–51.
31. Woolf CJ. Evidence for a central component of post-injury pain hypersensitivity. Nature. 1983;306(5944):686–8.
32. Agnihotry A, Fedorowicz Z, van Zuuren EJ, Farman AG, Al-Langawi JH. Antibiotic use for irreversible pulpitis. Cochrane Database Syst Rev. 2016;2:Cd004969.
33. Corbella S, Taschieri S, Mannocci F, Rosen E, Tsesis I, Del Fabbro M. Inferior alveolar nerve block for the treatment of teeth presenting with irreversible pulpitis: a systematic review of the literature and meta-analysis. Quintessence Int. 2017;48(1):69–82.
34. Li C, Yang X, Ma X, Li L, Shi Z. Preoperative oral nonsteroidal anti-inflammatory drugs for the success of the inferior alveolar nerve block in irreversible pulpitis treatment: a systematic review and meta-analysis based on randomized controlled trials. Quintessence Int. 2012;43(3):209–19.
35. Kanaa MD, Whitworth JM, Meechan JG. A prospective randomized trial of different supplementary local anesthetic techniques after failure of inferior alveolar nerve block in patients with irreversible pulpitis in mandibular teeth. J Endod. 2012;38(4):421–5.
36. Kung J, McDonagh M, Sedgley CM. Does articaine provide an advantage over lidocaine in patients with symptomatic irreversible pulpitis? A systematic review and meta-analysis. J Endod. 2015;41(11):1784–94.
37. Guglielmo A, Reader A, Nist R, Beck M, Weaver J. Anesthetic efficacy and heart rate effects of the supplemental intraosseous injection of 2% mepivacaine with 1:20,000 levonordefrin. Oral Surg Oral Med Oral Pathol Oral Radiol Endod. 1999;87(3):284–93.
38. VanGheluwe J, Walton R. Intrapulpal injection: factors related to effectiveness. Oral Surg Oral Med Oral Pathol Oral Radiol Endod. 1997;83(1):38–40.
39. Pogrel MA, Bryan J, Regezi J. Nerve damage associated with inferior alveolar nerve blocks. J Am Dental Assoc. 1995;126(8):1150–5.
40. von Ohle C, ElAyouti A. Neurosensory impairment of the mental nerve as a sequel of periapical periodontitis: case report and review. Oral Surg Oral Med Oral Pathol Oral Radiol Endod. 2010;110(4):e84–9.
41. Shadmehr E, Shekarchizade N. Endodontic periapical lesion-induced mental nerve paresthesia. Dent Res J (Isfahan). 2015;12(2):192–6.
42. Krishnan U, Moule A. Mental nerve paraesthesia: A review of causes and two endodontically related cases. Saudi Endodontic J. 2015;5(2):138–45.
43. Kruse A, Hellmich N, Luebbers HT, Gratz KW. Neurological deficit of the facial nerve after root canal treatment. Oral Surg Oral Med Oral Pathol Oral Radiol Endod. 2009;108(2):e46–8.
44. Guivarc'h M, Ordionic U, Ahmed HMA, Cohen S, Catherine J-H, Bukiet F. Sodium hypochlorite accident: a systmatic review. J Endod. 2017;43(1):16–24.
45. Caissie R, Goulet J, Fortin M, Morielli D. Iatrogenic paresthesia in the third division of the trigeminal nerve: 12 years of clinical experience. J Can Dent Assoc. 2005;71(3):185–90.
46. Hillerup S. Iatrogenic injury to oral branches of the trigeminal nerve: records of 449 cases. Clin Oral Investig. 2007;11(2):133–42.
47. Pogrel MA, Thamby S. The etiology of altered sensation in the inferior alveolar, lingual, and mental nerves as a result of dental treatment. J Calif Dent Assoc. 1999;27(7):531. 4–8
48. Kiyak HA, Beach BH, Worthington P, Taylor T, Bolender C, Evans J. Psychological impact of osseointegrated dental implants. Int J Oral Maxillofac Implants. 1990;5(1):61–9.
49. Ziccardi VB, Zuniga JR. Nerve injuries after third molar removal. Oral Maxillofac Surg Clin North Am. 2007;19(1):105–15. vii

50. Polycarpou N, Ng YL, Canavan D, Moles DR, Gulabivala K. Prevalence of persistent pain after endodontic treatment and factors affecting its occurrence in cases with complete radiographic healing. Int Endod J. 2005;38(3):169–78.
51. Renton T, Yilmaz Z. Managing iatrogenic trigeminal nerve injury: a case series and review of the literature. Int J Oral Maxillofac Surg. 2012;41(5):629–37.
52. Costigan M, Scholz J, Woolf CJ. Neuropathic pain: a maladaptive response of the nervous system to damage. Annu Rev Neurosci. 2009;32:1–32.
53. Truelove E. Management issues of neuropathic trigeminal pain from a dental perspective. J Orofac Pain. 2004;18(4):374–80.
54. Renton T, Yilmaz Z. Profiling of patients presenting with posttraumatic neuropathy of the trigeminal nerve. J Orofac Pain. 2011;25(4):333–44.
55. Mohammadi Z. Endodontics-related paresthesia of the mental and inferior alveolar nerves: an updated review. J Canad Dental Assoc. 2010;76:a117.
56. Haas DA, Lennon D. A 21 year retrospective study of reports of paresthesia following local anesthetic administration. J Canad Dental Assoc. 1995;61(4):319–20. 23–6, 29–30
57. Pogrel MA, Thamby S. Permanent nerve involvement resulting from inferior alveolar nerve blocks. J Amer Dental Assoc. 2000;131(7):901–7.
58. Renton T, Thexton A, Crean SJ, Hankins M. Simplifying the assessment of the recovery from surgical injury to the lingual nerve. Br Dent J. 2006;200(10):569–73. discussion 5
59. Hillerup S, Jensen RH, Ersboll BK. Trigeminal nerve injury associated with injection of local anesthetics: needle lesion or neurotoxicity? J Amer Dental Assoc. 2011;142(5):531–9.
60. Meechan JG. The use of the mandibular infiltration anesthetic technique in adults. J Amer Dental Assoc. 2011;142(Suppl 3):19s–24s.
61. Kanaa MD, Whitworth JM, Corbett IP, Meechan JG. Articaine and lidocaine mandibular buccal infiltration anesthesia: a prospective randomized double-blind cross-over study. J Endod. 2006;32(4):296–8.
62. Corbett IP, Kanaa MD, Whitworth JM, Meechan JG. Articaine infiltration for anesthesia of mandibular first molars. J Endod. 2008;34(5):514–8.
63. Jung IY, Kim JH, Kim ES, Lee CY, Lee SJ. An evaluation of buccal infiltrations and inferior alveolar nerve blocks in pulpal anesthesia for mandibular first molars. J Endod. 2008;34(1):11–3.
64. Smith MH, Lung KE. Nerve injuries after dental injection: a review of the literature. J Can Dent Assoc. 2006;72(6):559–64.
65. Kingon A, Sambrook P, Goss A. Higher concentration local anaesthetics causing prolonged anaesthesia. Do they? A literature review and case reports. Aust Dent J. 2011;56(4):348–51.
66. Pogrel MA. Damage to the inferior alveolar nerve as the result of root canal therapy. J Am Dent Assoc. 2007;138(1):65–9.
67. Escoda-Francoli J, Canalda-Sahli C, Soler A, Figueiredo R, Gay-Escoda C. Inferior alveolar nerve damage because of overextended endodontic material: a problem of sealer cement biocompatibility? J Endod. 2007;33(12):1484–9.
68. Yatsuhashi T, Nakagawa K, Matsumoto M, Kasahara M, Igarashi T, Ichinohe T, et al. Inferior alveolar nerve paresthesia relieved by microscopic endodontic treatment. Bull Tokyo Dent Coll. 2003;44(4):209–12.
69. Gatot A, Tovi F. Prednisone treatment for injury and compression of inferior alveolar nerve: report of a case of anesthesia following endodontic overfilling. Oral Surg Oral Med Oral Pathol. 1986;62(6):704–6.
70. Grotz KA, Al-Nawas B, de Aguiar EG, Schulz A, Wagner W. Treatment of injuries to the inferior alveolar nerve after endodontic procedures. Clin Oral Investig. 1998;2(2):73–6.
71. Scolozzi P, Lombardi T, Jaques B. Successful inferior alveolar nerve decompression for dysesthesia following endodontic treatment: report of 4 cases treated by mandibular sagittal osteotomy. Oral Surg Oral Med Oral Pathol Oral Radiol Endod. 2004;97(5):625–31.
72. Brkic A, Gurkan-Koseoglu B, Olgac V. Surgical approach to iatrogenic complications of endodontic therapy: a report of 2 cases. Oral Surg Oral Med Oral Pathol Oral Radiol Endod. 2009;107(5):e50–3.

73. Oshima K, Ishii T, Ogura Y, Aoyama Y, Katsuumi I. Clinical investigation of patients who develop neuropathic tooth pain after endodontic procedures. J Endod. 2009;35(7):958–61.
74. Coulthard P, Kushnerev E, Yates JM, Walsh T, Patel N, Bailey E, et al. Interventions for iatrogenic inferior alveolar and lingual nerve injury. Cochrane Database Syst Rev. 2014;4:Cd005293.
75. Sun H, Yang T, Li Q, Zhu Z, Wang L, Bai G, Li D, Li Q, Wang W. Dexamethasone and vitamin B (12) synergistically promote peripheral nerve regeneration in rats by upregulating the expression of brain-derived neurotrophic factor. Arch Med Sci. 2012;8(5):924–30. https://doi.org/10.5114/aoms.2012.31623. Epub 2012 Nov 7
76. Renton T, Janjua H, Gallagher JE, Dalgleish M, Yilmaz Z. UK dentists' experience of iatrogenic trigeminal nerve injuries in relation to routine dental procedures: why, when and how often? Br Dent J. 2013;214(12):633–42.
77. Gaffen AS, Haas DA. Retrospective review of voluntary reports of nonsurgical paresthesia in dentistry. J Can Dent Assoc. 2009;75(8):579.
78. Garisto GA, Gaffen AS, Lawrence HP, Tenenbaum HC, Haas DA. Occurrence of paresthesia after dental local anesthetic administration in the United States. J Am Dent Assoc. 2010;141(7):836–44.
79. Renton T, Adey-Viscuso D, Meechan JG, Yilmaz Z. Trigeminal nerve injuries in relation to the local anaesthesia in mandibular injections. Br Dent J. 2010;209(9):E15.

Part II

Endodontic Complications During Procedure

4 Access-Related Complications

Bradford R. Johnson

4.1 Introduction

Endodontic access is the first mechanical step of root canal therapy, and its importance is often underestimated, that is, until something goes wrong. With proper case selection and risk assessment, it should be possible to minimize the risk of access-related complications. Recognition of the variables associated with complications, both tooth related and patient related, during the history and diagnosis phase is a critical element of prevention and successful treatment. The purpose of this chapter is to present some useful tools for risk assessment and describe strategies for successful endodontic access.

4.2 Case Selection and Risk Assessment for Endodontic Access

Prevention of complications during endodontic access starts with proper diagnosis and case selection. The AAE Endodontic Case Difficulty Assessment Form and Guidelines [1] is a useful reference for preoperative case evaluation and determining potential risk for complications during endodontic access. Each of the following findings increases the degree of difficulty for endodontic access: limitation in mouth opening, position of the tooth in the arch (e.g., second and third molars), full coverage or large pin-retained restoration (Fig. 4.1), bridge abutment, rotation or tipping of the tooth (Fig. 4.2), receded pulp chamber (Fig. 4.3), calcified canal space(s) or canals not visible on radiograph (Figs. 4.4 and 4.5), pulp stones or calcifications, internal or external resorption, and atypical coronal anatomy (e.g., dens evaginatus, taurodont, or "C"-shaped canal anatomy) (Fig. 4.6). Figure 4.7 demonstrates a three-rooted

B.R. Johnson, D.D.S., M.H.P.E.
Professor and Head, Department of Endodontics, University of Illinois at Chicago, Chicago, IL, USA
e-mail: bjohnson@uic.edu

P. Jain (ed.), *Common Complications in Endodontics*,
https://doi.org/10.1007/978-3-319-60997-3_4

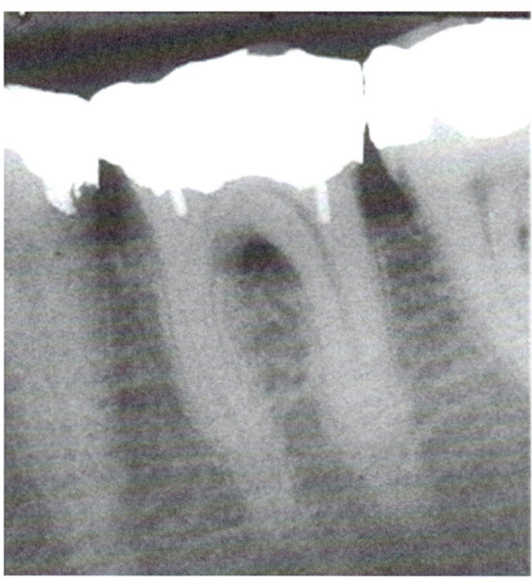

Fig. 4.1 Large MODB pin-retained amalgam restoration. The loss of original occlusal anatomy landmarks and pulp canal space calcification will make this a more challenging tooth to access for root canal therapy

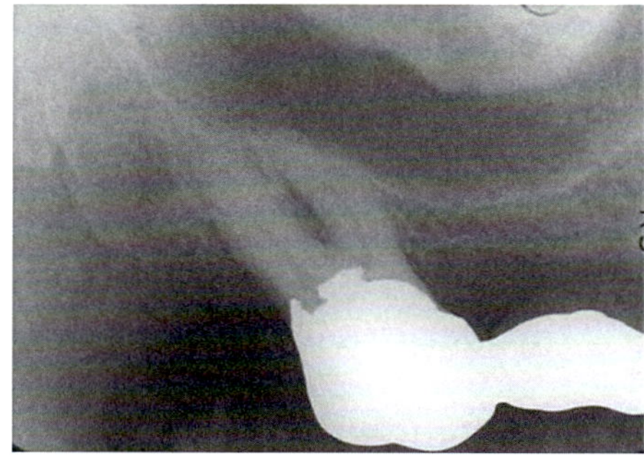

Fig. 4.2 Maxillary second molar fixed partial prosthesis abutment that is mesially inclined. Endodontic access for this tooth will require careful attention to the inclination of the tooth. It may be helpful to draw a line on the facial surface of the tooth for reference during access since a typical access preparation made perpendicular to the occlusal plane would almost certainly result in a perforation through the mesial surface of the tooth

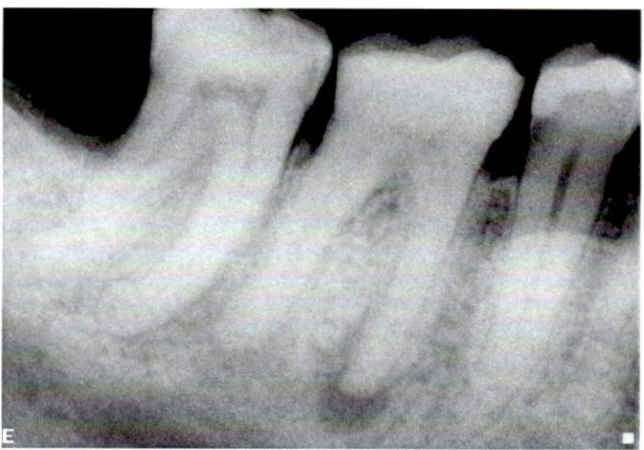

Fig. 4.3 Mandibular right first molar with necrotic pulp and asymptomatic apical periodontitis. Canals are faintly visible, but the vertical height of the pulp chamber has receded. In this situation, the normal tactile sense of a bur "dropping" into the pulp chamber is not expected

maxillary second premolar. Although it is not possible to visualize all three canals on a standard periapical radiograph, close inspection of the image suggests the possibility of atypical anatomy, which could then be confirmed by limited field of view cone beam computed tomography (CBCT) imaging prior to access.

In addition, a tooth that has been previously accessed, with or without complete treatment, presents the risk of preexisting perforation, canal blockage, or loss of

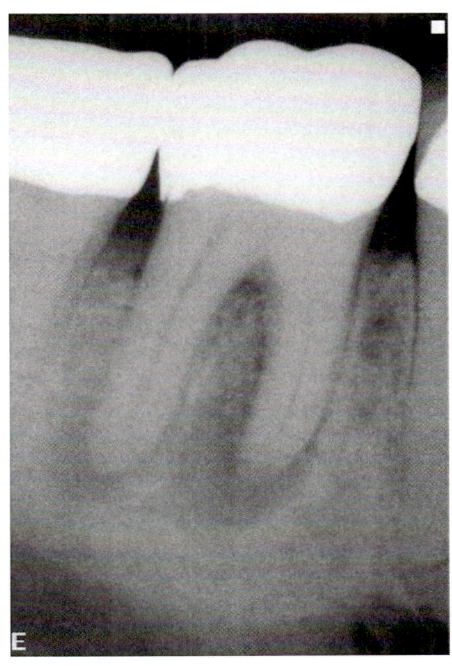

Fig. 4.4 Mandibular right first molar with full occlusal coverage restoration and diagnosis of pulpal necrosis and acute apical abscess. The pulp chamber and coronal portion of the canal space in the mesial root are not visible on the radiograph

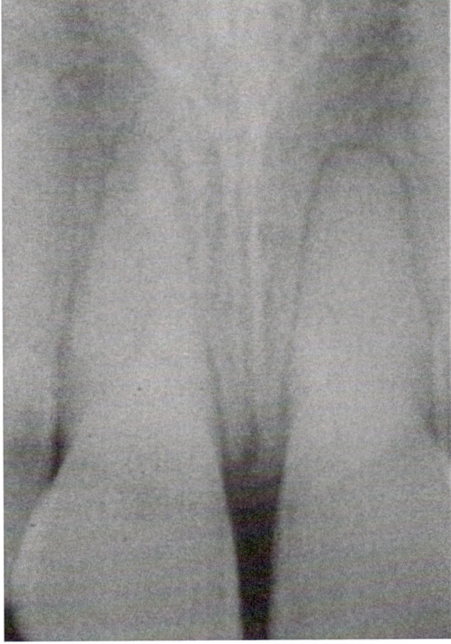

Fig. 4.5 Both maxillary central incisors have undergone calcific metamorphosis (pulp canal obliteration) secondary to trauma many years ago. The left maxillary central incisor has evidence of a widened PDL space and has recently become symptomatic. Root canal therapy should be possible, but use of a dental operating microscope is essential

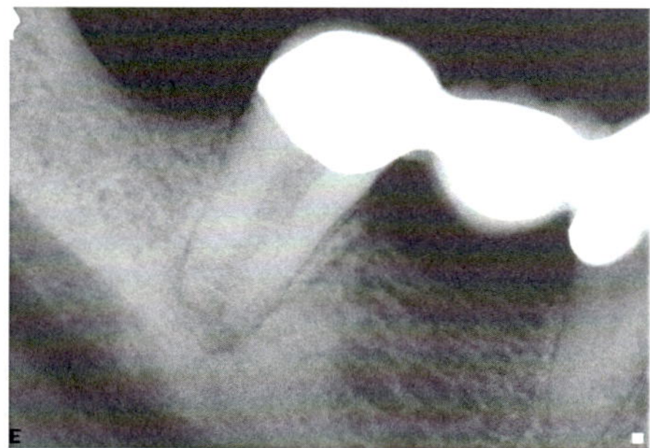

Fig. 4.6 Mandibular second molar that is an abutment for a fixed partial prosthesis. The diagnosis is necrotic pulp and asymptomatic apical periodontitis. Unusual canal space anatomy is obvious from the initial periapical radiograph, and CBCT imaging is recommended prior to initiating endodontic access

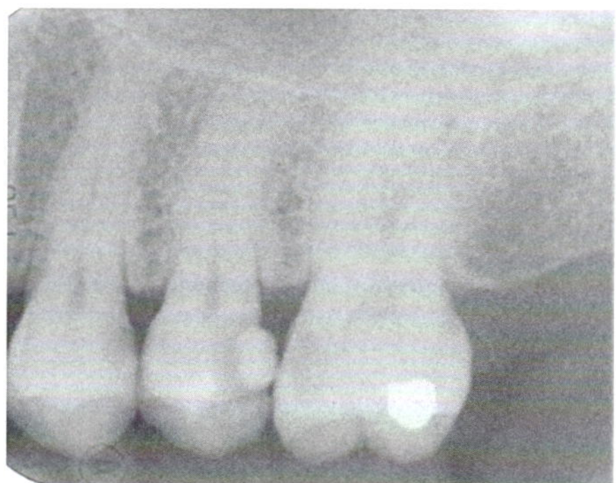

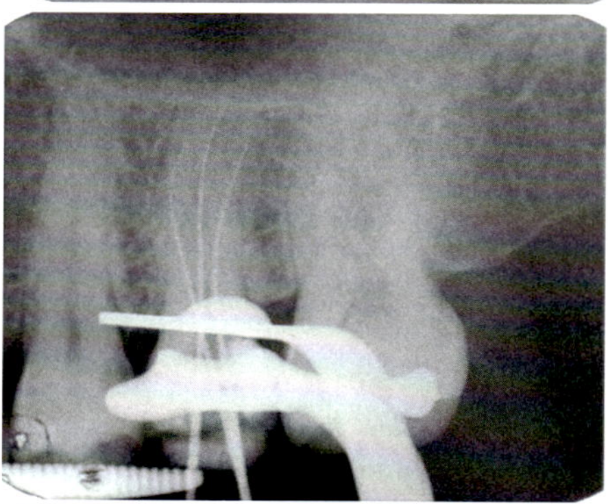

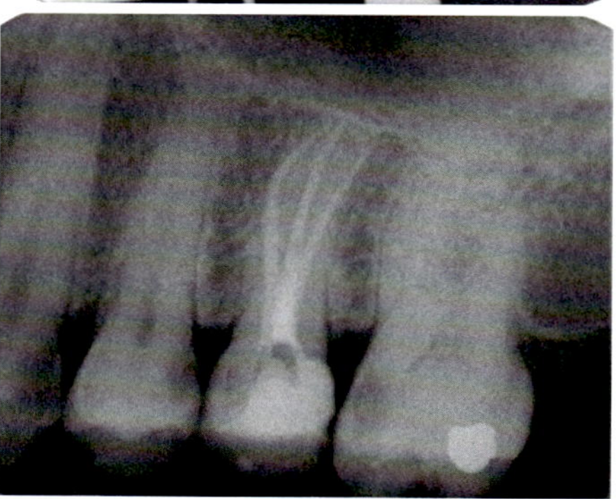

Fig. 4.7 Maxillary second premolar with three canals (two facial and one palatal). Even though the anatomy is not obvious on the periapical image (top), close inspection should alert the clinician to the probability of unusual canal anatomy. The presence and location of the canals can be determined with a preoperative CBCT scan

normal pulpal floor anatomical landmarks. Gouging of the floor and walls of the pulp chamber during access can obliterate normal internal anatomy that could otherwise be used to help locate canal orifices.

4.3 Goals of Endodontic Access

4.3.1 Traditional Access Preparation Compared to Minimally Invasive Access

In the traditional approach to endodontic access, there are three primary goals: conservation of tooth structure, complete unroofing of the pulp chamber, and straight-line access to the apical third of the canal [2]. While all three of these goals are reasonable and supported by decades of clinical practice, new technology in endodontics, such as super flexible nickel-titanium (NiTi) instruments and dental microscopes, has resulted in a shift in the primary focus of access to preservation of coronal tooth structure to avoid possible predisposition to future root fracture. It is still important to completely remove any remnants of pulp tissue from the pulp horns and to have an access opening large enough to locate all canals. Failure to remove all pulp tissue can cause discoloration of the coronal tooth structure and, in addition, provide a potential source of nutrition for any remaining microorganisms. Examples of a traditional molar access are shown in Figs. 4.8 and 4.9.

The concept of minimally invasive access and focus on preservation of coronal tooth structure, also referred to as *directed dentin conservation* [3] and *conservative endodontic cavity* [4], is a relatively new idea, and there are no long-term clinical studies to either support or reject this approach. However, anecdotally, there is a growing concern among many endodontists that root fracture of endodontically treated teeth, often occurring years after initial root canal treatment, is a significant cause of treatment failure and should be addressed to improve the probability of long-term survival of endodontically treated teeth. Some preliminary in vitro research suggests that a conservative endodontic

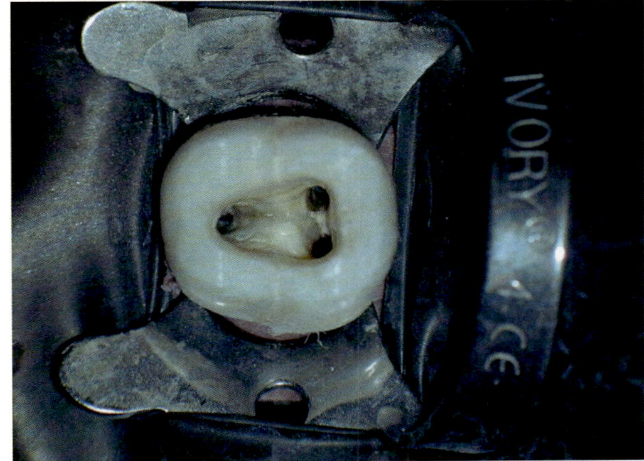

Fig. 4.8 Example of a traditional endodontic access preparation in a mandibular molar. All canal orifices are visible and straight-line access is provided. The distal canal (left on image) is centered between the two mesial canals and on an imaginary mesiodistal midline drawn through the occlusal surface of the tooth. If the distal canal was not centered, the presence of a second distal canal should be considered likely

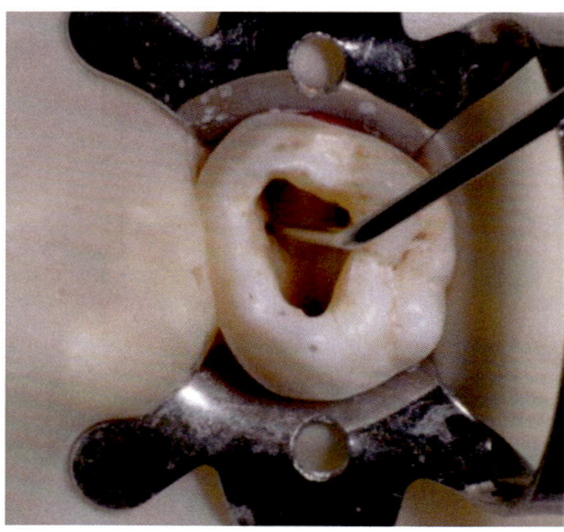

Fig. 4.9 Example of a traditional endodontic access preparation in a maxillary first molar. Note the rhomboid shape with an explorer in the often elusive MB2 canal orifice. The occlusal outline of the access is skewed to the mesial of the tooth to parallel the cross section of the tooth at the CEJ (also refer to Fig. 4.13)

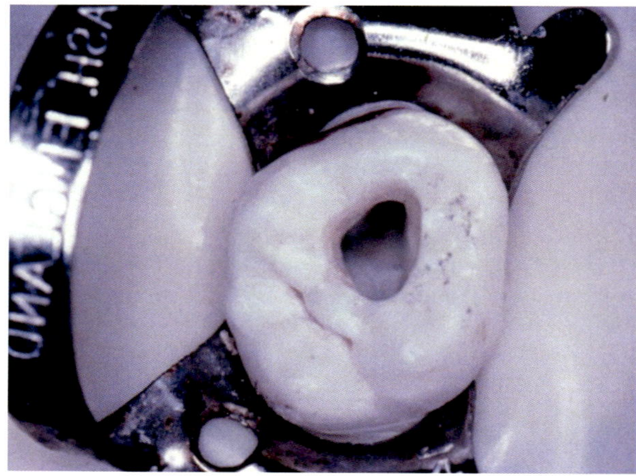

Fig. 4.10 A minimally invasive access on a maxillary first molar. Although the canal orifices cannot be directly visualized, the magnification and illumination provided by a dental operating microscope, along with the use of super flexible nickel-titanium instruments, would allow for safe completion of root canal therapy on this tooth

cavity approach is probably worthy of additional study and consideration [4, 5]. Without the enhanced magnification and illumination offered by a dental operating microscope, a conservative endodontic access presents greater risk of perforation and missed anatomy than a traditional access preparation. Figures 4.10, 4.11, and 4.12a–c demonstrate variations of a minimally invasive endodontic access preparation.

4.3.2 General Rules for Establishing the Outline and Depth of an Endodontic Access Cavity

Krasner and Rankow [6] proposed three rules derived from the sectioning and observation of the pulp chambers of 500 extracted teeth:

- Law of centrality
- Law of concentricity
- Law of the CEJ

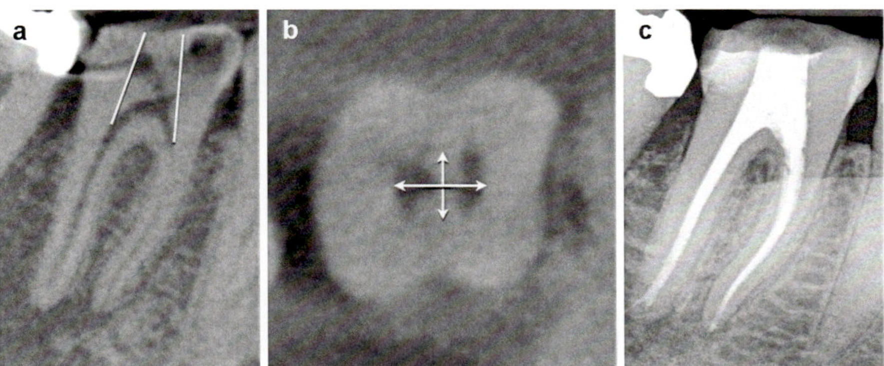

Fig. 4.11 Use of CBCT to plan a minimally invasive access. (**a**) Sagittal view showing vertical approach. (**b**) Axial view to determine the mesial-distal and facial-lingual dimensions. (**c**) Periapical radiograph of completed root canal with composite resin restoration (Case courtesy of Dr. William Nudera)

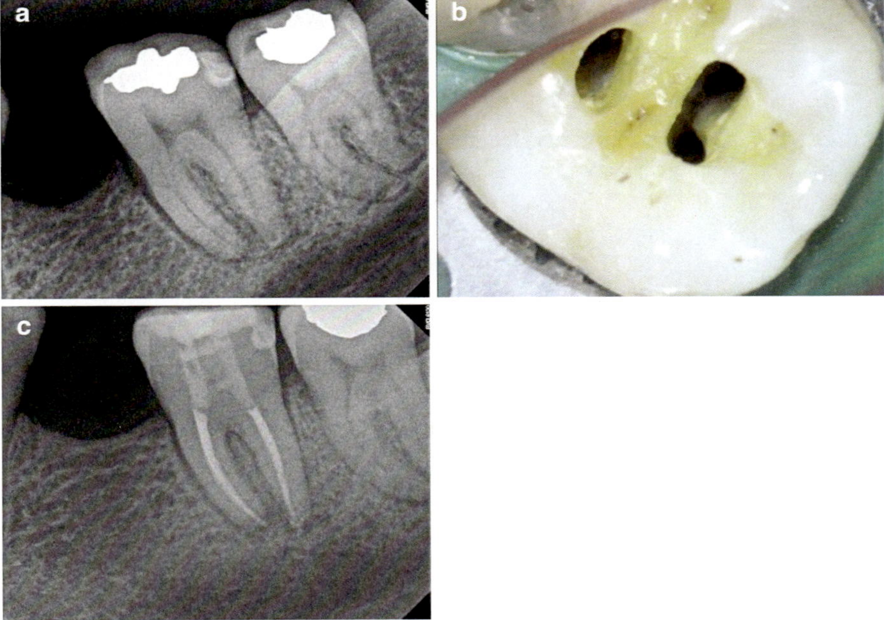

Fig. 4.12 (**a**) Preoperative periapical radiograph of mandibular left first molar. A minimally invasive access was planned (Case courtesy of Dr. Jon Ee). (**b**) A variation of a minimally invasive access that preserves a section of solid dentin connecting the facial and lingual aspects of the tooth (sometimes referred to as a "truss" access), with two smaller occlusal access preparations, one to access each of the two roots. (**c**) Final completion periapical radiograph demonstrating gutta-percha fill and bonded composite resin filling the pulp chamber. Note how a dentin "beam" was preserved in the middle of the tooth and the pulp chamber was not completely unroofed by the occlusal access (although all pulp tissue was removed from the pulp chamber using special ultrasonic instruments)

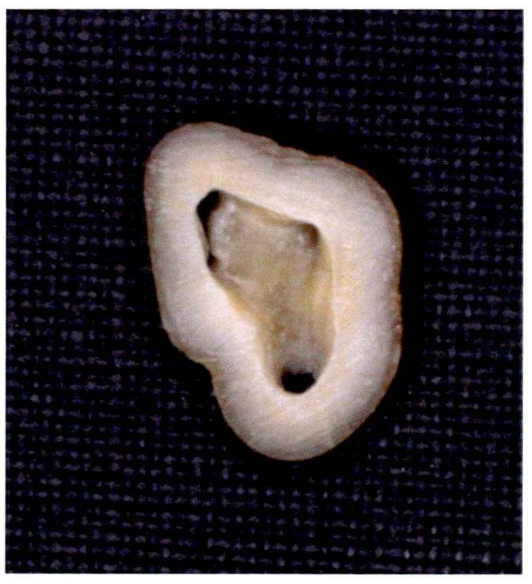

Fig. 4.13 Cross section at the CEJ of a maxillary first molar demonstrating Krasner and Rankow's law of concentricity

The law of centrality states that the floor of the pulp chamber is located in the center of the tooth at the CEJ. This often varies from the center of the occlusal surface of the tooth, so it is important to be able to visualize the cross section of the tooth at the CEJ. The law of concentricity states that the walls of the pulp chamber are concentric with the external surface of the tooth at the CEJ (Fig. 4.13). That is, the occlusal outline of the access cavity should mimic the general shape, on a smaller scale, of a cross-sectional slice through the tooth at the CEJ. For example, a tooth that is wider in the facial-lingual/palatal dimension than mesial-distal at the CEJ (such as a mandibular incisor or maxillary premolar) should have a similar occlusal outline to assist in locating all canals. Krasner and Rankow [5] noted that canals were typically located at the angle formed by the junction of two canal walls in a multi-rooted tooth. Finally, the law of the CEJ states that the CEJ is the most predictable landmark for determining the depth of the pulp chamber (Fig. 4.14). Even in teeth with calcified and/or receded pulp chambers, the roof of the pulp chamber can be found at the level of the CEJ [7]. This finding applies primarily to molars since the roof of the pulp chamber for anterior teeth and premolars often extends coronal to the CEJ in younger patients and can recede apical to the CEJ with increasing age and restorative treatment. The CEJ landmark can serve as an excellent guide to help prevent perforation through the pulpal floor or lateral surface of the tooth. If the pulp chamber has not been located after bur penetration to the estimated depth of the CEJ, it is appropriate to stop and expose a radiograph (a bitewing image is often the most useful) to determine the actual location of the pulp space in relation to the initial access cavity (Fig. 4.15). Another general rule to help prevent a pulpal floor perforation is to recognize that the dentin on the floor of the pulp chamber is usually darker in color than the more coronal dentin. It may be difficult to precisely determine the location of the CEJ in teeth with full occlusal coverage restorations. These teeth often present a greater risk for pulpal floor perforation (Fig. 4.16) and should be approached with caution. The enhanced magnification and illumination provided by a dental operating microscope is particularly important when performing endodontic access on teeth with full occlusal coverage restorations.

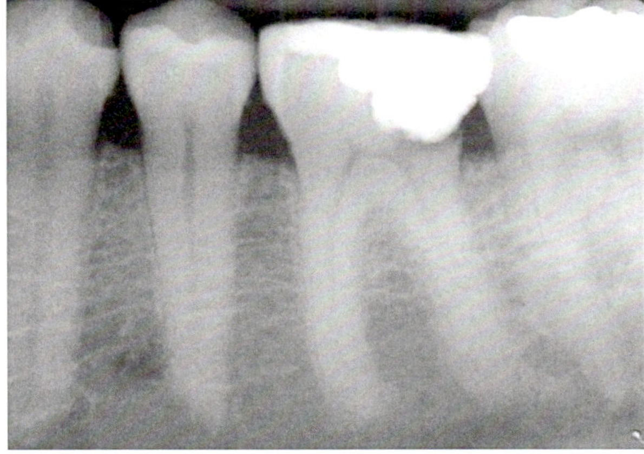

Fig. 4.14 Periapical radiograph of mandibular left first molar demonstrating the finding that the CEJ is a predictable landmark for determination of the roof of the pulp chamber in molars, even after the pulp chamber becomes constricted in a vertical dimension (the level of the CEJ can be seen on the mesial of this tooth and would also be apparent—and measurable—on clinical exam)

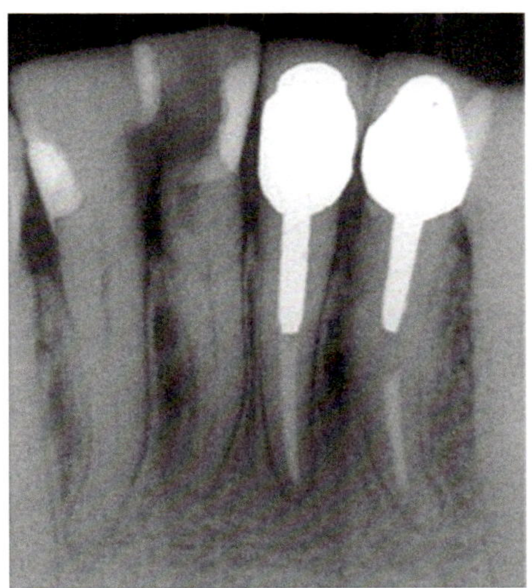

Fig. 4.15 During endodontic access of the mandibular right central incisor, the clinician stopped, removed the rubber dam, and exposed a radiograph to help confirm location of the canal in relation to the access cavity. In this case, a perforation was avoided, and the canal was easily located after reviewing the radiograph

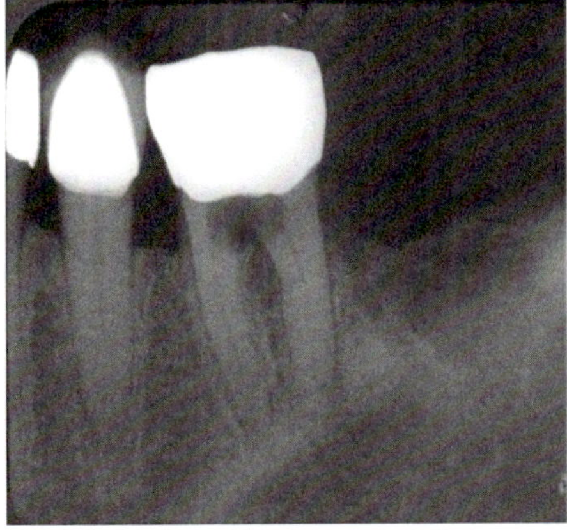

Fig. 4.16 The patient presented on an emergency basis for evaluation and treatment of left mandibular pain. A diagnosis of symptomatic irreversible pulpitis, mandibular first molar, was established. The clinician was unable to achieve adequate anesthesia and attempted to rapidly enter the pulp chamber to allow for an intrapulpal injection. Unfortunately, visibility was impaired by bleeding from a hyperemic pulp, and appropriate depth of bur penetration was not determined prior to initiating access. A furcal floor perforation occurred. Although an attempt can be made to repair this perforation, the prognosis is questionable due to size and location

Limited field of view cone beam computed tomography (CBCT) can also be useful to assist in the location of calcified or receded canals, both for preoperative evaluation and intra-treatment use [8]. Figures 4.11 and 4.17a, b demonstrate the use of preoperative CBCT to assist in treatment planning and access design and location of extra canals.

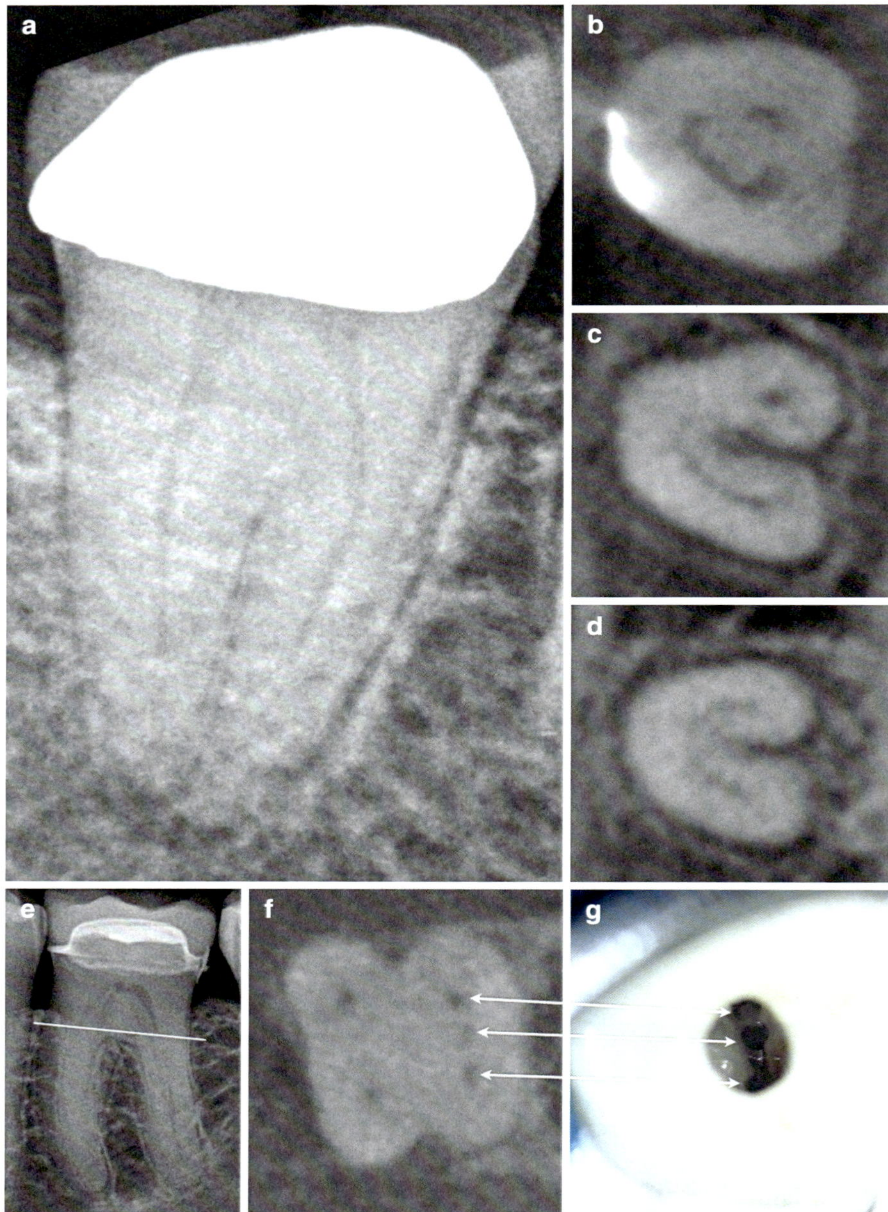

Fig. 4.17 (**a**), (**b**) A CBCT was taken for both of these teeth prior to initiated access to assess suspected complex anatomy. (**a**) A complex "C-shaped" canal configuration was confirmed. (**b**) The presence of five canals (three in the mesial root) was detected

4.3.3 When *Not* to Use a Rubber Dam

Although use of a rubber dam during root canal therapy is considered the standard of care [9], there are special situations that justify initial access of a tooth prior to placement of the rubber dam. However, placement of the rubber dam should always occur prior to use of endodontic files or any other instruments or materials that could potentially be swallowed or aspirated. The rubber dam is also essential to assure treatment in an aseptic environment, but this is secondary to patient safety.

It may be beneficial to start access on teeth that are heavily restored, rotated, or tipped without the initial use of a rubber dam. When the pulp chamber is located, place the rubber dam and confirm that the pulp chamber and/or canal has been located by tactile sense and with a small stainless steel file connected to an electronic apex locator (EAL). The EAL is an excellent tool to determine if the presumed canal space has been located or, alternatively, if a perforation was created. Small perforations are easier to repair and have a better prognosis than large perforations. A tooth that could be easily confused with a similar adjacent tooth should either be marked prior to access or accessed without a rubber dam to prevent treatment of the wrong tooth—one of the most obvious and preventable access complications. It is often safer to access a mandibular incisor prior to placement of the rubber dam due to the narrow mesial-distal dimension and facial inclination of these teeth.

4.4 Selection of Burs and Instruments for Initial Access

No single bur is the best choice for all circumstances; rather, specific conditions and tooth type can help determine the most appropriate bur for endodontic access cavity preparation. Figures 4.18 and 4.19 show some of the many burs available, most of which were designed specifically for access preparation. Selection will depend in part on the presence and type of dental restoration present. Access through porcelain or ceramic-type materials can be particularly challenging, and diamond-coated burs are typically most appropriate. Copious water spray during access will help prevent fracture of the ceramic material, although this is also a risk when accessing through porcelain fused to metal or all ceramic restorations. The patient should always be warned that a replacement crown may be necessary. Zirconia has recently become a more popular all-ceramic material for single crowns and relatively short-span fixed prostheses. The material is very strong and esthetic and also a very hard material to penetrate with most burs if endodontic access is needed [10]. Special burs have been specifically designed for use on zirconia.

After initial penetration through the roof of the pulp chamber, switching to a non-end-cutting bur is often the best choice for refining the access while minimizing risk of pulpal floor perforation. The Endo-Z bur (Fig. 4.18) and LA Axxess bur (Kerr) are two examples of non-end-cutting burs that are useful for refining an endodontic access. Long shank burs with relatively narrow shafts and a small, cone-shaped cutting tip provide greater visibility and precision when accessing small teeth such as mandibular incisors (Fig. 4.20). These burs are also useful when searching for calcified or receded canals.

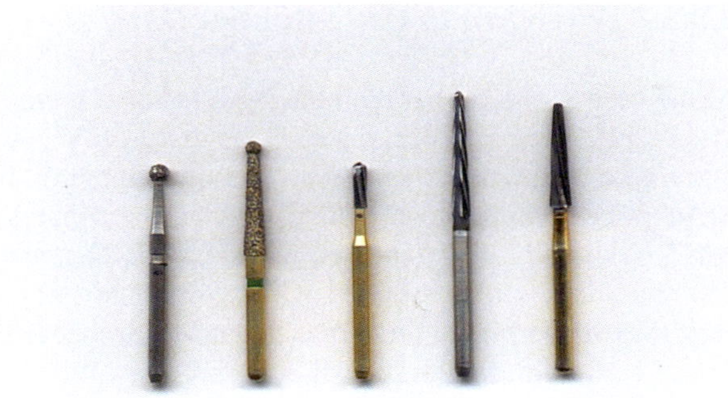

Fig. 4.18 Examples of high-speed burs that may be used for endodontic access. From L to R: round diamond, tapered diamond with round head, Transmetal bur, Multi-Purpose bur, Endo-Z bur (Dentsply Maillefer, Johnson City, TN)

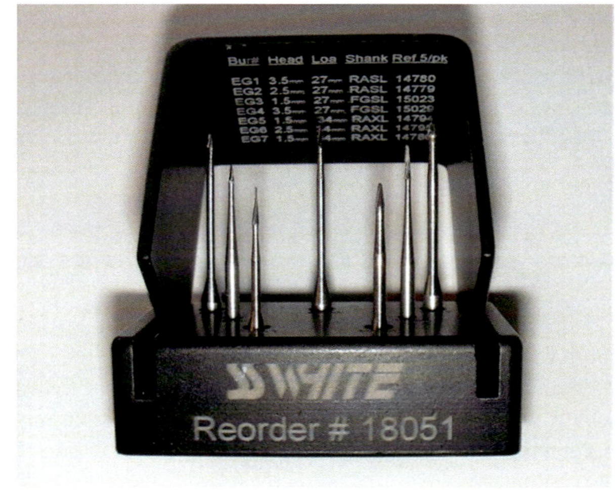

Fig. 4.19 Special long shank burs with cone-shaped cutting tips can be very useful for accessing small teeth and troughing for hidden canals (SS White). Burs are available in a variety of lengths and for both high-speed and low-speed handpieces

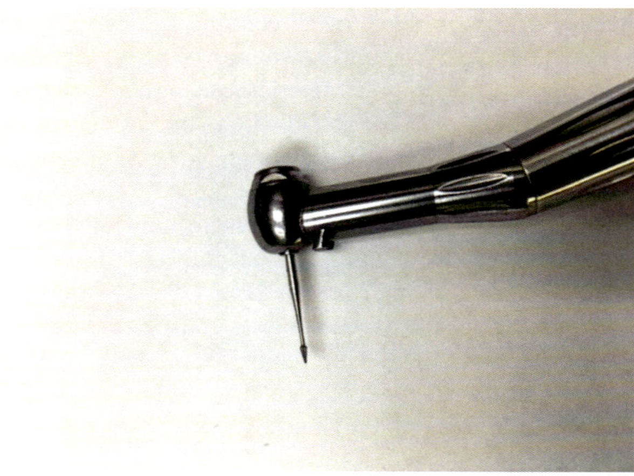

Fig. 4.20 The extra length of this high-speed bur (EG1; SS White) allows for much greater visibility when preparing an access opening in a small or narrow tooth or searching for calcified canals. The EG1 bur has a 3.0 mm cutting tip and the shaft extends 17.0 mm beyond the head of the high-speed handpiece

4.5 Locating Calcified Canals

4.5.1 Value of Magnification and Illumination

4.5.1.1 Loupes and Microscopes

It is difficult to overestimate the value of enhanced magnification and illumination for the safe preparation of an endodontic access and location of small canals [11, 12]. Although the use of magnifying loupes with a dedicated light source is a definite improvement over unaided vision and standard dental operatory light, the dental operating microscope provides even greater utility for the prevention of iatrogenic mishaps, creation of an ideal access form, location of all canals, and visualization of aberrant anatomy and cracks.

4.5.1.2 Fiber Optics

Transillumination with a fiber-optic light source directed through the facial or lingual/palatal aspect of a tooth at the level of the CEJ can be used to highlight differences in dentin color and therefore assist in canal location. This is similar in principle to transillumination with a fiber-optic light source to help in the visualization of incomplete coronal fractures (Fig. 4.21).

4.5.2 Intra-treatment Supplemental Radiographs and Cone Beam Computed Tomography

Even with enhanced magnification and illumination, some canals will remain elusive. Additional intra-treatment radiographs are often useful to assist in the location of all canals (Figs. 4.22a–d and 4.23). Since the rubber dam clamp may obscure the area in question, it may be necessary to remove the clamp prior to exposing a radiograph (Fig. 4.15). The potential value of CBCT is illustrated in Figs 4.11, 4.17, and 4.24a, b.

4.5.3 Ultrasonics and Special Burs

As mentioned in the previous section, narrow long shank burs, both low speed and high speed, can be very useful for assisting in the location of calcified canals (Fig. 4.19).

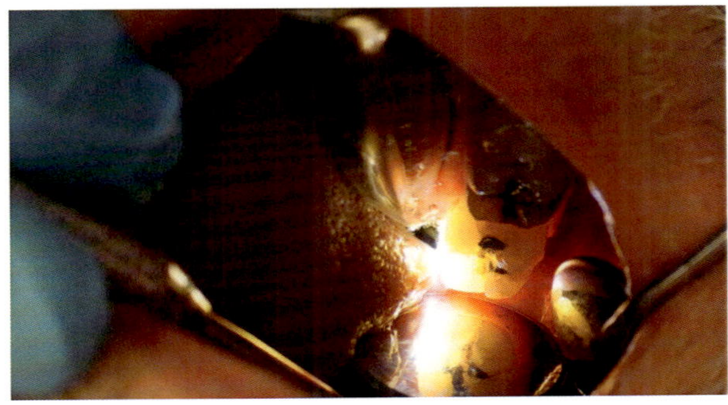

Fig. 4.21 Fiber-optic transillumination of a mandibular second molar to determine the extent of a fracture. A similar approach can be readily adapted to highlight differences in dentin density when looking for a receded or calcified pulp canal space

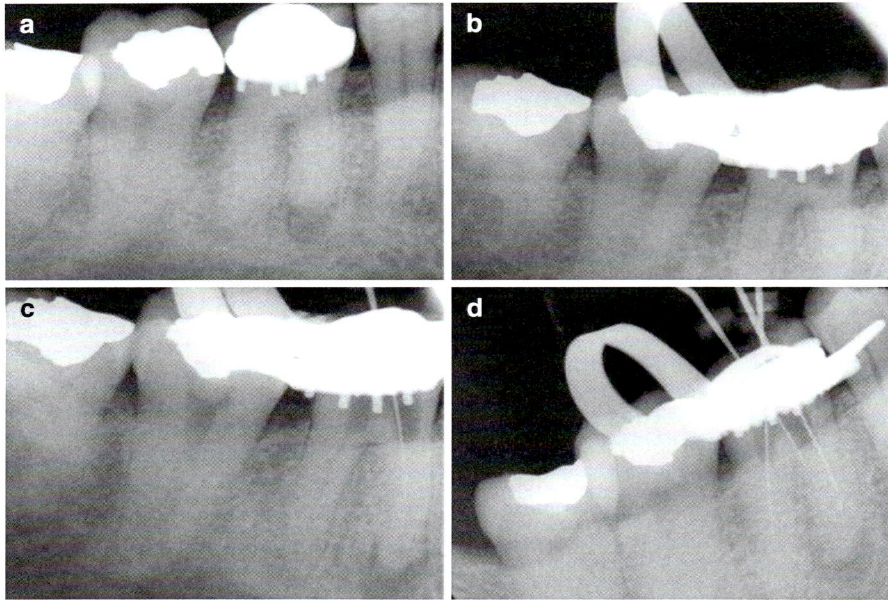

Fig. 4.22 (**a**) Preoperative radiograph of a mandibular right first molar. The tooth has a pin-retained foundation core buildup and full occlusal coverage restoration. Canals are not visible. (**b**) An intraoperative radiograph was exposed to evaluate depth and direction of access to help assist in location of the canals. (**c**) An additional intraoperative radiograph was exposed when the first canal was located. (**d**) Radiograph showing that three canals have been located. An electronic apex locator was also used when each suspected canal was found to confirm that a true canal had been found and not a perforation

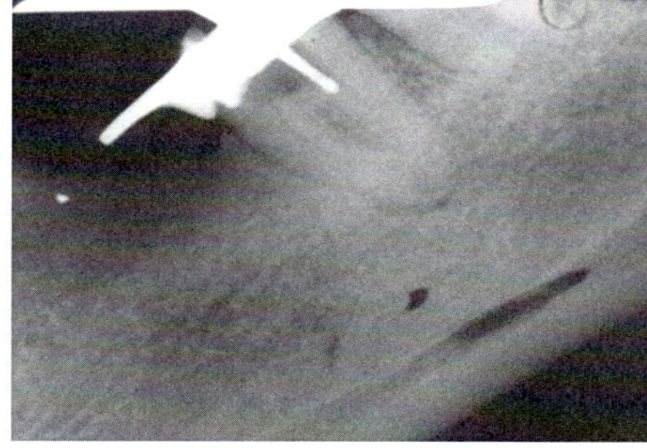

Fig. 4.23 Intraoperative radiograph with small round bur in place to assist in orientation while searching for calcified canals

Ultrasonic tips are specifically designed to assist with endodontic access by dislodging calcific deposits and pulp stones, as well as troughing for calcified canals.

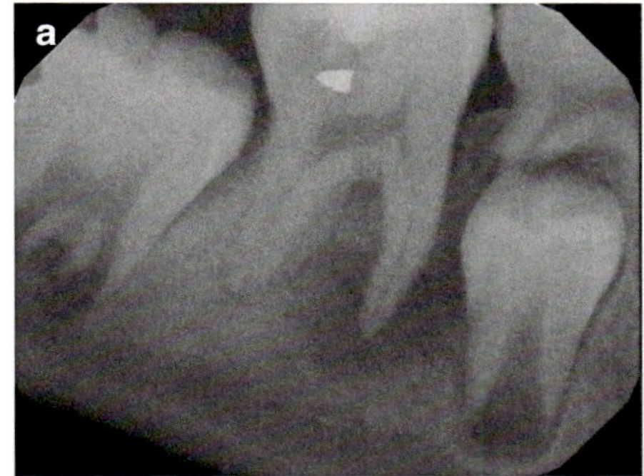

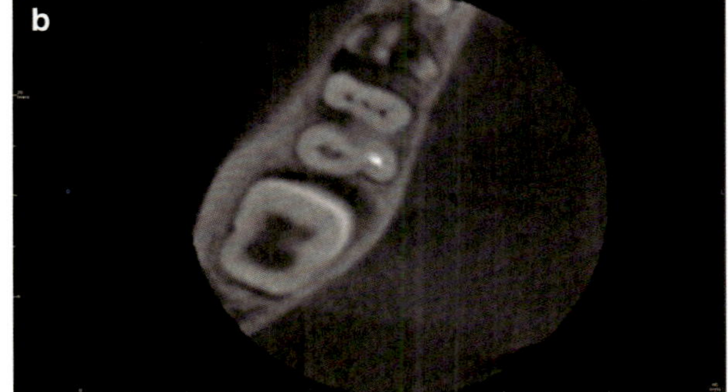

Fig. 4.24 (**a**) Preoperative radiograph of a mandibular right first molar on a 10-year-old Hispanic male. The diagnosis was pulp necrosis and chronic apical abscess. A CBCT scan was obtained mid-treatment due to suspected unusual anatomy. In an axial section, three canals are visible in the mesial root, and a fused distolingual root (white material in this canal is calcium hydroxide) is present and two possible canals in the main distal root

4.6 Managing Teeth that Are Rotated, Crowded, Tilted, or Heavily Restored

Teeth that are not heavily restored and in normal position in the dental arch can also present challenges if attention is not paid to usual tooth inclination and anatomy. The most common perforation sites by tooth type are listed in Table 4.1.

If a crown is present, removal prior to endodontic treatment is sometimes indicated and can greatly facilitate caries excavation, evaluation of restorability, proper isolation of the tooth, and location of calcified canals. Figure 4.2 shows a maxillary second molar with moderate mesial inclination and full occlusal coverage restoration. If the fixed partial prosthesis is treatment planned for replacement, safe and efficient endodontic therapy is best assured by removal and temporization prior to root canal treatment. If replacement is not planned, then access through the bridge abutment should proceed carefully, with constant attention to proper angulation of the bur and depth of penetration. As in many cases, intraoperative radiographs can be useful although it will not be possible to determine the precise location of the bur until the tip of the bur is apical to the crown margin.

Table 4.1 Common perforation sites

Tooth type	Common perforation site	Reason
Maxillary incisors	Facial	Inclination of the tooth
Mandibular incisors	Mesial or distal most common, facial also possible	Narrow mesial-distal width, inclination of the tooth
Maxillary premolars	Mesial or distal	Narrow mesial-distal width and natural mesial concavity on first premolars
Mandibular premolars	Facial	Lingual inclination of crown with relatively vertical alignment of the root in the alveolus; therefore, an access perpendicular to the lingually inclined occlusal surface can perforate on the facial surface before reaching the canal space
Mandibular molars	Lingual	Lingual inclination of the entire tooth in relation to the occlusal plane
Maxillary and mandibular molars with receded pulp chambers and calcified canals	Furcation	Failure to identify floor of the pulp chamber during access

4.7 Management of Complications During Access

Bur separation during access is a fairly uncommon complication unless excessive pressure is applied during access and/or the bur is dull from multiple previous uses. If this happens prior to reaching the pulp chamber, the rubber dam and high-speed suction should prevent possible aspiration or ingestion of the separated fragment. Obviously, the potential for aspiration or ingestion is greater if the initial access is being performed prior to placement of the rubber dam. In this situation, the main consideration is location of the separated piece or confidence that it was removed from the oral cavity by the high-speed suction. Once the pulp chamber is unroofed, a separated bur can drop into the pulp canal space and may be challenging to remove. Figure 4.25 shows a nickel-titanium orifice opener that separated during refinement of the molar access and coronal shaping and was subsequently pushed deeper into the mesiobuccal canal during an attempt to remove it (note another separated nickel-titanium rotary file is present in the mesiolingual canal).

Excessive bleeding from the pulp during access can be disconcerting and greatly diminishes the ability to visualize all internal aspects of the preparation. It is important to be able to recognize whether the bleeding is due to a highly inflamed pulp or a pulpal floor perforation. This is one of the many reasons why a pulpal diagnosis must be established prior to access. In teeth with highly inflamed pulps, the bleeding often observed during initial access is normal. The solution is to remove all coronal pulp tissue with a non-end-cutting high-speed bur, a low-speed large round bur, or a sharp spoon excavator. If bleeding still persists, it may be necessary to remove the bulk of the coronal pulp tissue from the canal(s). This can be safely accomplished with rotary nickel-titanium orifice opener instruments, carefully advanced

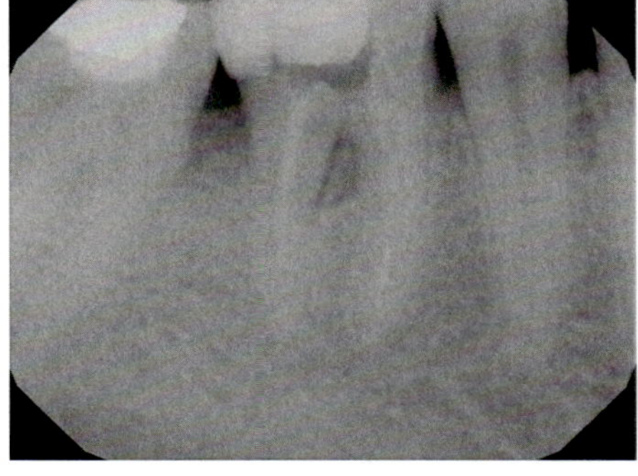

Fig. 4.25 Mandibular right first molar with separated nickel-titanium access opener file in the mesiobuccal canal and a smaller separated instrument in the mesiolingual canal

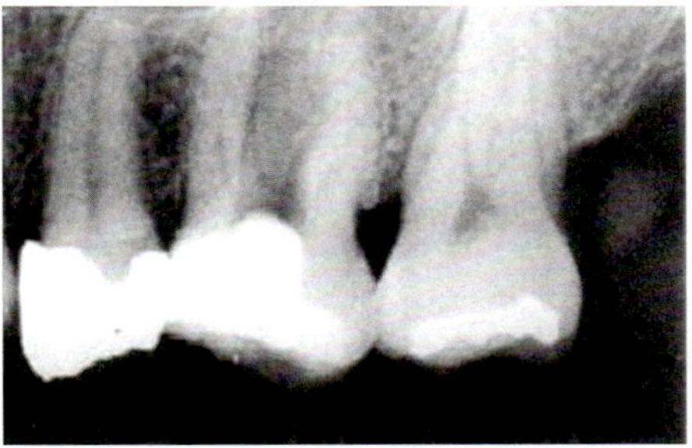

Fig. 4.26 Maxillary left first molar with a large perforation in the furcal floor of the pulp chamber. Although repair could, and probably should, be attempted, the prognosis is unfavorable due to size and location

approximately one-third to one-half the estimated canal length. If done properly, the bulk of the pulp tissue will be removed, bleeding will be controlled to allow for refinement of the access, and the risk of creating a ledge in the canal is minimal. A greater concern is bleeding due to a perforation. This should always be suspected if sudden bleeding is observed in a tooth with a diagnosis of pulp necrosis. The amount of bleeding from a perforation is usually less than that seen from highly inflamed pulp and can be controlled by applying direct pressure with a small cotton pellet soaked in local anesthetic solution containing 1:100,000 epinephrine. If a perforation is confirmed, referral to a specialist for evaluation and management is recommended.

Perhaps the most serious complication during endodontic access is creating an unintended communication (perforation) through the pulpal floor (Fig. 4.26) or an external surface of a tooth at or below the level of the periodontal attachment. The three primary variables for predicting outcome of a repaired perforation are location, size, and timeliness of repair (decreasing the risk of microbial contamination). That is, a better outcome can be expected if the perforation is small, located apically and distant from potential communication with the oral cavity, and repaired as soon as possible after occurrence. A perforation coronal to the periodontal attachment can often be adequately sealed by the final coronal restoration. As the perforation site moves apically, into or just apical to the periodontal attachment, options include surgical flap reflection and external repair with a resin-modified glass ionomer restorative material, orthodontic extrusion to expose the perforation area prior to repair (assuming

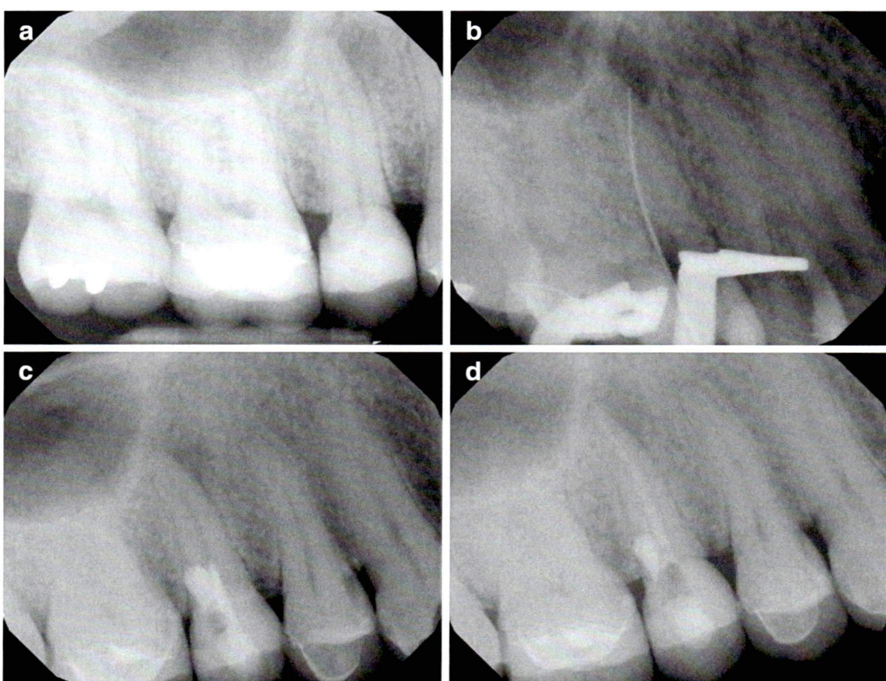

Fig. 4.27 (**a**) Preoperative radiograph of maxillary right second premolar with full occlusal coverage ceramic restoration. The diagnosis was necrotic pulp and asymptomatic apical periodontitis. (**b**) A perforation on the distal aspect of the tooth occurred during access. This radiograph shows a file in place confirming the perforation. Strategies to prevent this iatrogenic mishap include initial access without the rubber dam and careful attention to the long axis of the tooth. (**c**) The perforation was immediately repaired via an orthograde approach using a dental operating microscope for visualization of the perforation and placement of EndoSequence® BC RRM™ (root repair material) (Brasseler, USA). Note that a small piece of gutta-percha was temporarily placed in the main canal to prevent inadvertent blockage of the canal. The gutta-percha was removed after perforation repair and instrumentation of the canal space continued. (**d**) Immediate postoperative image of repaired perforation and calcium hydroxide placed in main canal

adequate crown/root ratio), or a surgical crown-lengthening procedure to allow for access to the perforation site. If the perforation is in the furcation or apical to the periodontal attachment, an internal repair through an orthograde approach should be the first choice (Figs. 4.27a–d). Fortunately, several highly biocompatible materials are currently available for perforation repair (e.g., mineral trioxide aggregate [MTA], BC putty, and Biodentine). All of these are calcium silicate-based bioceramic materials and actually encourage bony healing. Internal perforation repair is best performed under a dental operating microscope for optimum visualization of the area and material placement. If the perforation extends beyond the root surface into the bone, packing a resorbable collagen material (e.g., CollaCote) beyond the external root surface to form a matrix is often recommended. This matrix allows for adequate condensation of the repair material without excessive extrusion into the PDL and bone.

References

1. AAE Endodontic Case Difficulty Assessment Form and Guidelines. American Association of Endodontists, 211 E. Chicago Ave., Suite 1100, Chicago, IL 60611–2691.
2. Johnson BR. Endodontic access. Gen Dent. 2009;57:570–7.
3. Clark D, Khademi J. Modern molar endodontic access and directed dentin conservation. Dent Clin N Am. 2010;54:249–73.
4. Krishan R, Paque F, Ossareh A, Kishen A, Dao T, Friedman S. Impacts of conservative endodontic cavity on root canal instrumentation efficacy and resistance to fracture assessed in incisors, premolars, and molars. J Endod. 2014;40:1160–6.
5. Moore B, Verdelis K, Kishen A, Dao T, Friedman S. Impacts of contracted endodontic cavities on instrument efficacy and biomechanical responses in maxillary molars. J Endod. 2016;42:1779–83.
6. Krasner P, Rankow HJ. Anatomy of the pulp-chamber floor. J Endod. 2004;30:5–16.
7. Deutsch AS, Musikant BL. Morphological measurements of anatomic landmarks in human maxillary and mandibular pulp chambers. J Endod. 2004;30:388–90.
8. Fayad M, Johnson BR, editors. 3D imaging in endodontics: a new era in diagnosis and treatment. New York: Springer; 2016.
9. Ingle JI, Bakland LK, Baumgartner CJ, editors. Ingle's endodontics. 6th ed. Hamilton: BC Decker, Inc.; 2008.
10. Christensen RP, Ploeger BJ. A clinical comparison of zirconia, metal and alumina fixed-prosthesis frameworks veneered with layered or pressed ceramic: a three-year report. J Am Dent Assoc. 2010;141:1317–29.
11. Buhrley LJ, Barrows MJ, BeGole EA, Wenckus CS. Effect of magnification on locating the MB2 canal in maxillary molars. J Endod. 2002;28:324–7.
12. Monea M, Hantoiu T, Stoica A, Situ D, Sitaru A. The impact of operating microscope on the outcome of endodontic treatment performed by postgraduate students. Eur Sci J. 2015;11:305–11.

5 Instrumentation-Related Complications

Obadah H. Attar, Sami M. Chogle, and Tun-Yi Hsu

5.1 Introduction

Similar to other disciplines of advanced dentistry, a clinician may encounter complications or unforeseen circumstances during endodontic therapy. Every clinician performing endodontic procedures would have experienced a range of outcomes ranging from a case well done to an unfavorable prognosis related to a procedural accident. Examples of complications during the root canal procedure include ledge formation, separated instruments, and over-instrumentation. However, fear of procedural accidents should not deter a practitioner from performing root canal treatment. An experienced clinician uses knowledge, clinical skill and acumen, experience, and awareness of his or her own limitations to minimize these accidents.

It is important to adhere to the biological and mechanical objectives for shaping canals and cleaning root canal systems [1, 2] to minimize needless complications such as blocks, ledges, over-instrumentation, and periapical tissue damage. Regrettably, these events are clinically encountered and can drastically reduce the prognosis of the treatment. Although prevention is the key (due to their irreversible nature), in the presence of such complications, the role of perseverance and patience cannot be overemphasized. With the aid of magnification, illumination, advanced techniques, and appropriate instruments, the experienced clinician can negotiate most blocks and ledges within the root canal system. However, over-instrumentation and the ensuing damage to apical tissues require additional corrective measures and an assessment of the prognosis before continuing the treatment.

During root canal preparation, another risk included is that of instrument breakage or fracture. Although most clinicians associate a "broken instrument" with a

O.H. Attar, B.D.S., D.Sc.D. (✉) • S.M. Chogle, M.S.D. • T.-Y. Hsu, D.D.S., D.Sc.D., D.M.D.
Henry M. Goldman School of Dental Medicine, Boston University, Boston, MA, USA
e-mail: attar@bu.edu; schogle@bu.edu; thsu@bu.edu

P. Jain (ed.), *Common Complications in Endodontics*,
https://doi.org/10.1007/978-3-319-60997-3_5

separated file, this may even include a silver point segment, a broken Lentulo instrument, a Gates-Glidden drill (GG drill), or a portion of a carrier-based obturator [3, 4]. In terms of frequency, the addition of rotary NiTi files to almost every cleaning and shaping technique has contributed to a higher number of fractured NiTi instruments [5, 6]. Over the years a variety of approaches for managing broken instruments have been presented. Specifically, the increasing utilization of the dental operating microscope and ultrasonic devices into clinical practice has allowed for visualization and manipulation of the fractured instrument, favorably affecting the probability of instrument segment removal and the prognosis of such teeth [7, 8].

Treating similar teeth in patients with comparable medical and dental histories does not ensure similar outcomes. Some patients may experience postoperative discomfort after initiation or recent completion of an endodontic procedure while others may not. The contrasting clinical outcomes may lead to false conclusions about the cause-effect relationship of endodontic procedures to the "flare-up." The development of inter-appointment pain, with or without swelling, is an infrequent but challenging problem. Multiple complex factors may be involved including mechanical, microbial, chemical, immunological, gender, and psychological components [9, 10]. Prospective studies show an overall incidence of 1.8–3.2% [11, 12]. Even though the overall occurrence is low, flare-ups represent such a significantly stressful situation to the patient that it demands concern and attention to its resolution and possible prevention. It is especially distressing for a previously asymptomatic or minimally symptomatic patient to experience moderate to severe pain and swelling after treatment.

This chapter outlines the causes, prevention, treatment, and prognosis of various types of procedural accidents that may occur in root canal instrumentation. The role of factors including proper case selection, treatment planning, and attainment of advanced skills in the prevention of complications will be addressed. When an incident does occur during root canal instrumentation, the importance of communication with the patient regarding the incident, the procedures necessary for correction, the alternative treatment modalities, and the effect of this accident on prognosis, all of these, will also be discussed.

5.2 Reversible Errors

Iatrogenic errors discussed in this section are referred to as "reversible" because most often complete or partial recovery from the problem can be successfully established. The ability to recover from iatrogenic misadventures and render them "reversible" depends largely on the timing of identification of the problem during root canal therapy. If errors undergo unrecognized, this may lead not only to inability to correct the error but also to creating other errors that may or may not be correctable in a "domino effect." Clinical expertise plays an important role in recognizing and recovering from errors as they happen. Expert clinicians are not only able to correct errors but most importantly identify potential challenges and try to avoid them, which happens during the diagnostic phase of the root canal therapy. Such errors are discussed below.

5.2.1 Blockage

Blockage of the root canal system occurs when the original working length is lost, leading to an "immature" stop within the root canal system short of the anatomical canal length. This can be recognized clinically by using the electronic apex locator, which will show loss of canal potency and ability to establish the working length to the minor constriction zone, or radiographically by showing the initial file short of the working length. Clinically, iatrogenic blockage happens after a glide path has been established to the working length. Blockage can happen because of:

1. Pushing dentinal shavings and other root canal debris such as pulp stones apically and creating a blockage at any level of the root canal system
2. Introducing foreign materials within the root canal system such as separated files, ultrasonic tips, restorative materials from the access cavity, etc.

Blockage of the root canal system can be avoided by taking proactive measures starting at access cavity preparation and removing any weak or undermined restorative material that can be dislodged and introduced deep within the root canal system. Amalgam or other restorative materials such as composite or glass ionomer can break down during instrumentation phase of root canal therapy and can be dislodged within the canals, with greater risk after coronal preferring of the canals and when the orifices are at a larger size. Complete removal of any suspicious restorative material or pulp stones that may get dislodged from the access walls is essential to avoid disintegration of the restorative materials and establishment of a straight line access that is free from contact with access cavity walls. All access cavity refinement is advised to be completed before coronal preflaring of the root canal system to minimize the possibility of foreign materials to fall into the canal space. Preflaring with rotary instruments such as Gates-Glidden burs for orifice shapers should be done to a length short of the length established with hand files. Rotary instruments should not be taken further than what hand instruments have already achieved. Early introduction of rotary instruments without establishing a glide path or exploring the canal anatomy with hand files may lead to blockage or loss of canal anatomy continuity, which renders finding and negotiating narrow canals difficult.

Maintaining enough canal lubrication and copious irrigation during hand and rotary instrumentation is essential to avoid iatrogenic errors such as file separation and blockage. Several instrumentation techniques have been introduced to minimize packing debris apically as the root canal systems are being instrumented, especially when canal size closely approximates the file size. For example, crown-down technique with coronal preflaring facilitates irrigation of the coronal portion of the canal early during instrumentation and removes pulp tissue debris from the coronal portion of the canal, which often packs the most significant amount of the pulp tissue and debris. It facilitates working length establishment by removal of canal irregularities and allows proper gauging of the apical foramen by elimination of coronal constriction that may provide a false gauging of the apical area [13].

Blockage can also be avoided during instrumentation by frequent recapitulation of the canal to the working length using potency files. Goldberg et al. define a potency file as a small K-type file which can be passively introduced through the apical constriction without actively widening it [14]. This will prevent accumulation of dentinal shavings at the apical area and help clean any potential blockage as it happens. If dentinal blockage is identified, it should be carefully negotiated with smaller hand files that can gently "bind" at the blockage level and instrumented until bypassed.

Other types of canal blockage can happen when rotary instruments and ultrasonic tips separate within the root canal system. Prevention, management, and outcomes will be discussed in the following section.

5.2.2 Separated Instruments

Modern rotary instruments and instrumentation technique minimized instrument separation significantly that nowadays it's considered a safe and predictable way to clean and shape the root canal system predictably. Instrument separation can be prevented by following manufacturer's recommendation for operational speed, torque, and sequence of usage. Two types of fatigue result in rotary file separation, cyclic and torsional. Cyclic fatigue happens when the rotary file is kept around the curve for too long. Torsional fatigue happens when the file tip at any length is partially or completely locked within the canal while the shaft continues to move at the set torque and speed. This can happen if excessive pressure is applied to the file, leading to increased friction to canal walls, or if the operator skips files resulting in increased stresses to files. Canal instrumentation without proper irrigation increases the amount of stress on the file by blocking the flutes.

How to prevent:

1. If using *rotary* instruments:
   (a) Follow manufacturer's recommendation (speed, torque, use, etc.).
   (b) Never keep rotating files in canals for too long (especially in curved canals).
   (c) Don't push the file into the canal or exert pressure. Let the file guide you.
   (d) Never skip file sizes.
   (e) Use copious irrigation in between instrumenting.
   (f) Dispose used files.
   (g) Adequate access preparation to achieve straight line access is very important.
   (h) Manually instrument root canal systems first to create a glide path for rotary instruments.
   (i) Keep in mind that larger files are more susceptible to fatigue failure.
   (j) 0.06 has less resistance to fracture than 0.04 tapered instruments.
2. If using *hand* instruments:
   (a) Use copious irrigation/lubrication.
   (b) Do not force or wedge instruments into a canal. Instead, they should be teased gently into place.

(c) Sequential instrumentation—using the quarter-turn technique and increasing file size only after the current working file fits loosely into the canal without binding.
(d) Gradual increase in file sizes.
(e) Flutes should be cleaned regularly.
(f) Use alternative instrumentation techniques such as balanced force technique.
(g) An instrument that cannot be inserted to the desired depth should be removed and the tip modified to slightly bend before resuming the pathfinding process.
(h) Inspect rotary and hand instruments before use. Unwinding or overwinding of hand instruments should be identified, and files should not be inserted into the canal. Remember that rotary files may not show early signs of fatigue like stainless steel hand files.
(i) The degree of rotation of hand files within the root canal system is the major factor in file separation. Overturning a hand file is what usually breaks the file, not the pull strokes.

3. If using *ultrasonics*:
   (a) Use manufacturer's recommendation (power setting, use, etc.).
   (b) Inspect ultrasonic tips: if the diamond coating is gone, dispose the instrument to avoid applying more pressure on the instrument to make it cut.

Management of separated instruments depends on the size, type, stage of cleaning and shaping during which the instrument was separated, and the clinical ability to retrieve or bypass the separated instrument (Table 5.1). Instruments separated before the completion of the biomechanics preparation of the canal can impact the success of the treatment [15]. Cases with pulp necrosis, periapical lesions, and instruments separated short of the working length are expected to have lower success rate than vital cases with no periapical lesions at the working length [16].

Several techniques have been introduced to retrieve separated instruments. Files can be loosened using ultrasonic instruments especially those that break at the coronal or middle third of the canal and can be visualized under the surgical operating

Table 5.1 Protocol for fractured instruments

Fractured instrument (can it be bypassed?)			
Yes	No (consider the location)		
Continue biomechanical preparation. Do not attempt to remove the fractured part of the instrument	Apical third	Middle/coronal third	
	Removal is not advisable	Is straight line access possible?	
		Yes	*No*
		Consider attempt at removal keeping in mind the risks vs. benefits	Do not attempt removal

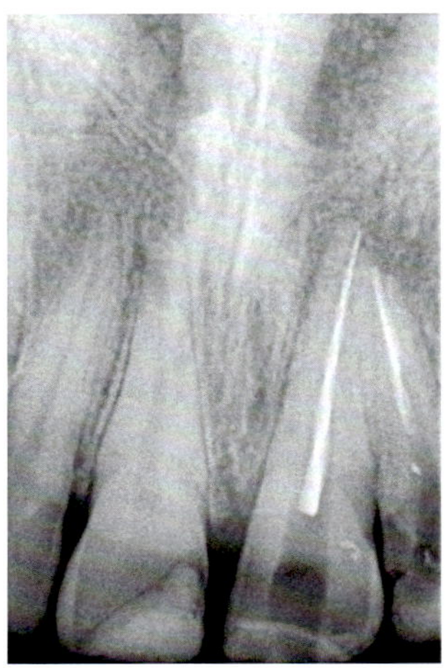

Fig. 5.1 *Separated rotary endodontic file*. Separated rotary file in tooth #9 that was retrieved using ultrasonics to loosen the file coronally

microscope (Fig. 5.1). Other systems are designed specifically for that purpose, such as Instrument Removal System or "IRS," Masseran system, Terauchi File Retrieval Kit, etc. Cone beam volumetric tomography analysis can help to determine the exact location of the separated instrument and certain anatomical challenges that can be encountered during instrument retrieval such as root curvature and concavities. Proper understanding of the limitations and indications for each technique is essential for the success of the procedure and to avoid introducing additional problems to the endodontic treatment rendered.

5.3 Irreversible Errors

Irreversible errors often are the product of reversible errors that were ignored or unidentified, compromising the endodontic treatment outcomes. Some of these errors can have greater impact than others depending on the magnitude, location, and stage at which they were introduced into the procedure. Errors discussed in this section include ledging, zipping, transportation, gouging, over-instrumentation, damage to the periapical tissues, and flare-ups.

5.3.1 Transportation

Transportation of the canal can be defined as "the initial deviation of the original root canal pathway by the removal of dentinal wall on the outer curve and may result in creation of a new canal pathway" (Fig. 5.2). Rotary files vary in the cutting efficiency at their tip. The more aggressive the tip is, the more likely it is to start creating its own path or "transport" the canal. Excessive pressure during rotary instrumentation of introducing larger files in smaller canals can result in aggressive cutting at the tip and loss of the flexibility of the file to be able to follow the original path of the canal. Files

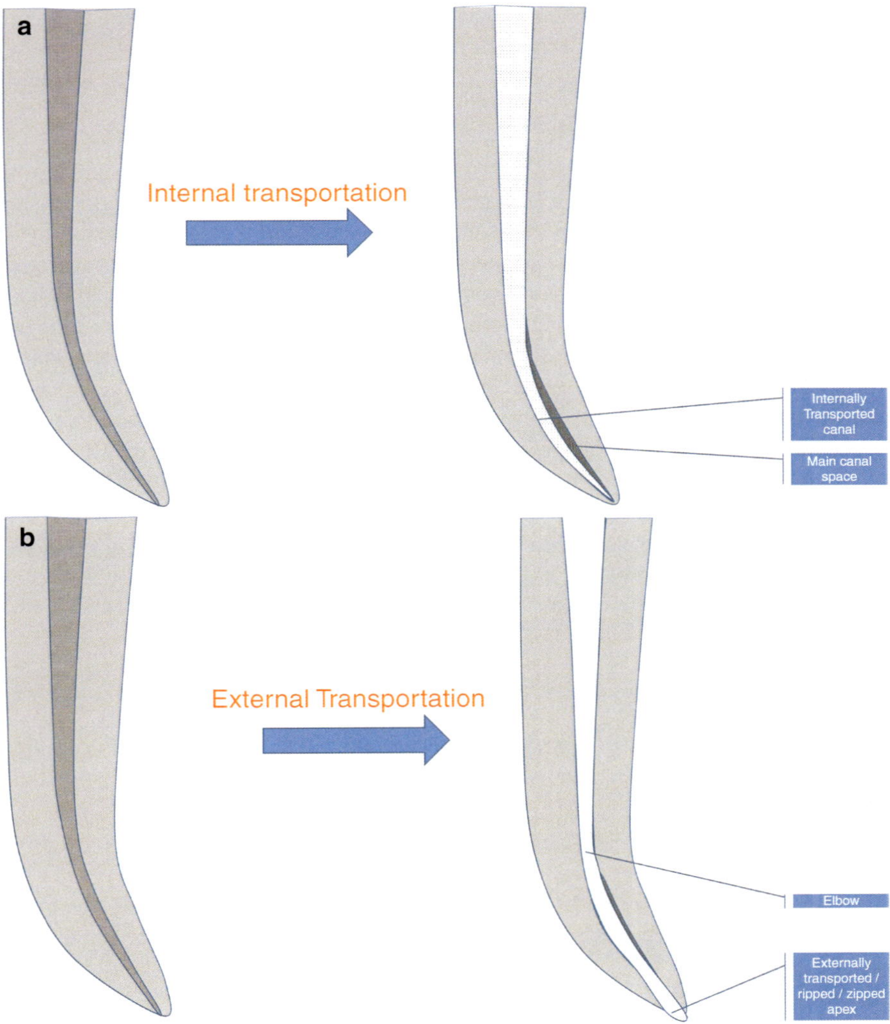

Fig. 5.2 *Transportation/ledge formation*: tooth #19 with ledge formation at the distal canal that was bypassed. Note the external transportation of the mesial root canal system. (**a**) *Internal transportation*: internally transported canal deviating from the natural canal curvature. (**b**) *External transportation*: external transportation beyond the working length compromising the minor/major constriction zone. Note elbow area above the transported area

with a radial land behind the cutting edge are referred to as "landed files" and that geometric feature can help in keeping the file centered within the root canal system and preventing the file from deviating from the canal curvature to some degree. Holding rotary files at rotation short of the working length results in excessive grinding on the outer walls as the file tries to resolve to its original linear shape, especially files with less flexibility. If undetected, transportation may lead to hedging, zipping, gouging, or even perforation of the root canal wall.

5.3.2 Ledge

Canal ledge can be defined as "an iatrogenic error created during instrumentation of the root canal system resulting in an irregularity in the surface of the root canal system—often times the outer wall of the curvature - that result in the creation of an artificial step within the root canal wall that prevents file placement beyond the irregularity" (Fig. 5.3). Continuous instrumentation short of the working length can force the file tip to start deviating from the original canal anatomy and start creating its own path, which starts with a ledge. This will create a "step" within the root canal system which makes it difficult to bypass into the remainder of the canal especially with rotary files that cannot be precurved to bypass the ledge (Fig. 5.4). A ledge can be removed by successive enlargement of the canal to eliminate irregularities, but it depends largely on the size of the ledge. Ledges usually occur on the outer curvature of the canal walls where the file tip tends to straighten the canal and may result in the file abruptly stopping short of the working length since it's hitting the step created every time the file glides through the canal. If unidentified, ledges can proceed into a larger gouging or elbow and eventually into apical perforation into the outer canal wall.

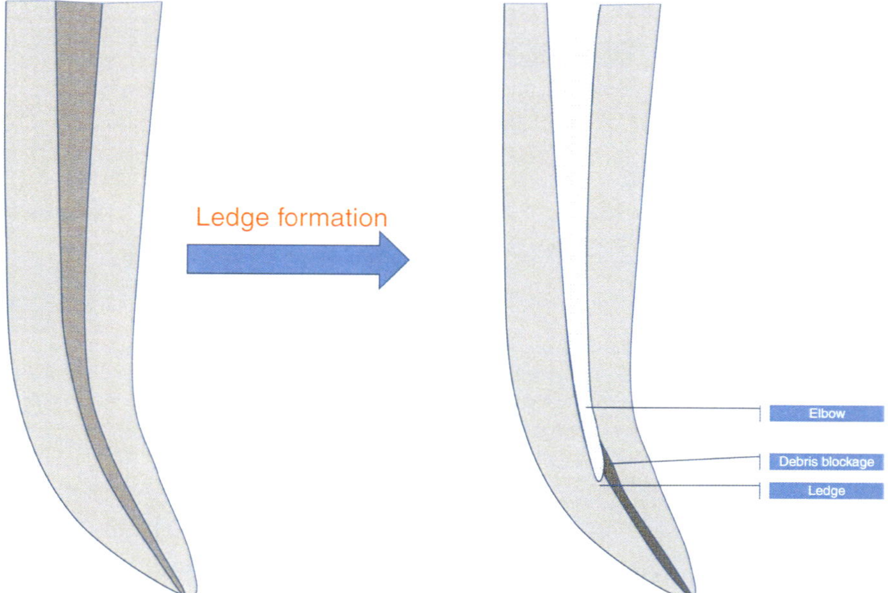

Fig. 5.3 *Ledge formation*: canal blockage results in ledge formation

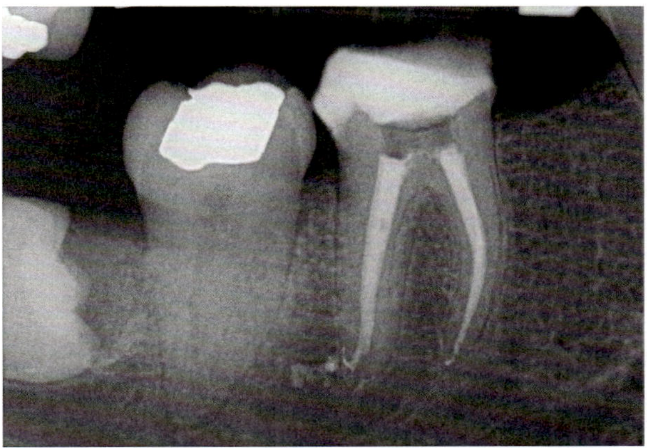

Fig. 5.4 *Ledge*: tooth #30 with ledged distal canal that was bypassed

5.3.3 Zipping

A zip can be defined as an "iatrogenic error created during instrumentation of the root canal system resulting in a tear-drop irregularity in the outer wall of the apical third of a curved root canal system, it's basically a transportation of the outer wall that results in a reverse-taper at the apical third." The term "apical zip" was first introduced by Weine and Kelly in 1975 [17]. Zipping can result from introducing large size files to the working length and keeping the rotary file rotating around the curve close to or at the apex resulting in excessive grinding into the outer canal walls. Over-instrumentation of a curved canal beyond the apical foramen can also result in zipping since the file tip has no guidance within the inner walls of the canals, creating its own path by straightening the canal. Zipping the canal poses a challenge in establishing an apical stop at the working length and preventing extrusion of the materials beyond the apex. Precautions should be taken to prevent pushing obturation materials beyond the apex, and sometimes apexification with the creation of an artificial stop at the apical third of the canal should be considered to avoid overextension of obturation materials, especially if thermo-plasticized obturation techniques are to be used.

5.3.4 Gouging/Elbow

Gouging the root canal walls can happen at any level beyond the orifice and can be the result of forcing rotary instruments such as Gates-Glidden burs beyond the resistance level. Canal elbows are "the area of the root canal system immediately coronal to the transported or zipped irregular area." The curved canal morphology shows an hourglass appearance.

5.3.5 Damage to the Periapical Tissues/Flare-ups

Defined by *American Association of Endodontists* [18], flare-up is the acute exacerbation of an asymptomatic pulpal and/or periradicular pathosis after the initiation or continuation of root canal treatment. The term has been generously used for situations not only limited to the abovementioned but also any significant additional development of symptoms or signs after procedure, whether it was initially symptomatic or asymptomatic and whether the treatment was still in progress or completed.

Flare-up complicates the treatment course. It is an undesired situation that makes the patient suffer both physically and psychologically. Although mostly minor to moderate [11], flare-up may turn into more severe and systemic complication, such as acute alveolar abscess and cellulitis. With the positive expectation after treatment, patient usually is frustrated and anxious when they experience flare-up. Patient may question the validity of the treatment and the competency of the practitioner. Practitioner, on the other hand, needs to arrange the unscheduled emergency, to repair the potentially undermined patient-doctor relationship and to manage the adverse clinical situation.

The frequency of flare-up varies from as low as 1.58% [12] to an average 8.4% by meta-analysis between 1966 and 2007 [19]. The older studies tend to have higher incidence, while the more recent ones generally have lower number with modern approach. The unclear definition of flare-up and different inclusion/exclusion criteria explain part of the variation. Risk factors such as sex, age, systemic diseases, preoperative pulp and periapical conditions, treatment modalities, inter-appointment medicament, and one- or multiple-visit treatment were widely investigated [11]. Among those, patient factors, such as necrotic pulp, symptomatic apical periodontitis, and acute apical abscess [20], and treatment factors, such as retreatment, over-instrumentation, and hyper-occlusion, have been associated with higher incidence of flare-up.

The etiologies of flare-up can be categorized into mechanical, chemical, and microbial [10]. A flare-up incident can be contributed to any one or a combination of any other two reasons. If not performed in a controlled manner, the mechanically insulted tissue would have increased but not reduced inflammation after procedure. The direct injury to the periapical tissue by extending instrumentation beyond apical foramen is a common reason for the development of postoperative pain. Once the inflammation is initiated, it takes 24–48 h before it subsides if without sustaining factors. In vital cases, the incidence of postoperative flare-up is similar between pulpotomy and incomplete/complete cleaning and shaping [11]. Hyper-occlusion directly challenges the periapical area and worsens the existing condition. Chemical agents including irrigation solutions, inter-appointment medicament, and obturation material bring significant inflammation to the periapical tissue if overextended. Both the mechanical and chemical insults usually result in immediate development of postoperative pain and/or swelling. The lack of continuing sustaining factors usually renders this situation self-limiting.

Microbial cause, however, requires close attention as it has greater association with flare-ups that develop into abscess and more. The microbial cause includes both the microorganisms and their by-products [21]. The changes of both the quality and quantity of microbial composition in root canal system and the periapical tissue after procedure, the increase of microbial loading by extruded infected debris, and the introduction of secondary infection from procedure or coronal leakage all account for flare-ups of microbial cause. Once active infection is established, it triggers a complex immune/inflammatory cascade locally and/or systemically, which turns into pain, swelling, abscess, or cellulitis depending upon host susceptibility [22].

The preventive measures should focus on minimizing mechanical, chemical, and microbial factors. Preoperative radiographs need to be of diagnostic quality with distinct contrast and correct proportion at different angles for anatomy assessment. Working length verification requires both radiographs and electronic apex locator for better accuracy [23]. Within the confine of root canal system and being passive, effective irrigation needs working concentration above threshold and sufficient volume, frequency, and adjunct effort such as mechanical or ultrasonic agitation to ensure and enhance its efficiency and efficacy [24, 25]. Early introduction and constant irrigation into root canal system, along with coronally directed instrumentation, minimize debris buildup and extrusion [26]. The dispensing of inter-appointment medicament prefers to have maximal contact area reaching full working length but not to be extruded to damage apical tissue [27]. The choice and design of the temporary restoration are based on the clinical situation for the protection of the integrity of the tooth structure and the prevention of secondary coronal infection before the tooth is permanently restored.

Contrary to the common practice [28], antibiotic prophylaxis has been shown to have no value to decrease the incidence of flare-ups [29]. However, pretreatment 30 minutes to 1 h before procedure and posttreatment for 24–48 h of NSAID (nonsteroidal anti-inflammatory drugs) or acetaminophen have been proven to reduce the incidence and intensity of postoperative pain significantly [30–32]. Long-lasting anesthesia such as bupivacaine block anesthesia also showed significant relief from central sensitization and decreased incidence and intensity of postoperative pain [33]. Occlusion reduction only helps if there were preexisting periapical symptoms [34].

As all the treatment risk and options, the best moment to inform and communicate with the patient is before the procedure. The potential incident of flare-up and its management should always be an essential part of postoperative instruction. Patient can therefore make an informed decision with full disclosure and mentally be prepared in the infrequent event of a flare-up. Once occurred, being suffered from the discomfort and distressed from the disruption of the recovery course, it is important to reassure the patient with genuine empathy, availability of timely care, reiteration of etiology and treatment outcome, and adequate effective management.

It is critical that whenever there is persistent, worsening, or additional symptom and/or sign, a differential diagnosis needs to be reestablished to rule out other offending source. A major part of the management has to do with the identification of infection in addition to inflammation. In the case of vital pulps, whether debrided completely or not, it is mostly inflammation by nature at least initially. Strategy to reduce inflammation is the goal. Pharmacological management such as the use of NSAID or intra-canal/systemic steroid has shown significant results [35, 36]. If incompletely debrided at the first place, a thorough pulpectomy should be considered to remove the remaining inflamed tissue. If completely debrided already, reentering the root canal system may not address the periapical inflammation unless there is drainage needed. Other identifiable factors such as history of overextended irrigants, inter-appointment medicament, and obturation materials share similar approach. Hyper-occlusion of the temporary restoration is another common irritating factor.

Cases that are initially vital when treated but without follow-up treatments or challenged by secondary infection because of inappropriate or overdue temporary restorations are susceptible to apical infection as in the necrotic cases. The clinical presentation includes typical signs of infection which include locally with significant exudation, swelling, abscess, and cellulitis or systemically with fever, chill, malaise, etc. This may require incision and drainage, drainage through the tooth, and antibiotic treatment.

Conclusion

Complications related to instrumentation may arise from different iatrogenic errors and may progress in terms of difficulty to recover and implications of the success of the root canal treatment. It is important to note that complications during instrumentation may result in challenges and complications during irrigation and obturation of the root canal systems. Patient should be informed before treatment of the possible problems that may arise during treatment, and proper documentation is necessary to prevent legal and ethical dilemmas. Prevention, early identification, and proper management may improve the overall success rate of the root canal treatment, and proper follow-up intervals relevant to the complexity of the error improve the overall quality of care provided to the patient.

References

1. Schilder H. Cleaning and shaping the root canal. Dent Clin N Am. 1974;18(2):269–96.
2. Ruddle CJ. The Protaper technique. Endod Topics online. 2005;10:187–90.
3. Fors UG, Berg JO. Endodontic treatment of root canals obstructed by foreign objects. Int Endod J. 1986;19(1):2–10.
4. Chenail BL, Teplitsky PE. Orthograde ultrasonic retrieval of root canal obstructions. J Endod. 1987;13(4):186–90.
5. Berutti E, et al. Comparative analysis of torsional and bending stresses in two mathematical models of nickel-titanium rotary instruments: ProTaper versus ProFile. J Endod. 2003;29(1):15–9.
6. Wong R, Cho F. Microscopic management of procedural errors. Dent Clin N Am. 1997;41(3):455–79.

7. Mines P, et al. Use of the microscope in endodontics: a report based on a questionnaire. J Endod. 1999;25(11):755–8.
8. Ward JR, Parashos P, Messer HH. Evaluation of an ultrasonic technique to remove fractured rotary nickel-titanium endodontic instruments from root canals: clinical cases. J Endod. 2003;29(11):764–7.
9. Naidorf IJ. Endodontic flare-ups: bacteriological and immunological mechanisms. J Endod. 1985;11(11):462–4.
10. Seltzer S, Naidorf IJ. Flare-ups in endodontics: I. Etiological factors. J Endod. 1985;11(11):472–8.
11. Walton R, Fouad A. Endodontic interappointment flare-ups: a prospective study of incidence and related factors. J Endod. 1992;18(4):172–7.
12. Imura N, Zuolo ML. Factors associated with endodontic flare-ups: a prospective study. Int Endod J. 1995;28(5):261–5.
13. Morgan LF, Montgomery S. An evaluation of the crown-down pressureless technique. J Endod. 1984;10(10):491–8.
14. Goldberg F, Massone EJ. Patency file and apical transportation: an in vitro study. J Endod. 2002;28(7):510–1.
15. Feldman G, et al. Retrieving broken endodontic instruments. J Am Dent Assoc. 1974;88(3):588–91.
16. Crump MC, Natkin E. Relationship of broken root canal instruments to endodontic case prognosis: a clinical investigation. J Am Dent Assoc. 1970;80(6):1341–7.
17. Weine FS, Kelly RF, Lio PJ. The effect of preparation procedures on original canal shape and on apical foramen shape. J Endod. 1975;1(8):255–62.
18. American Association of Endodontists. Glossary of endodontic terms. 9th ed. St. Louis: Mosby; 2015.
19. Tsesis I, et al. Flare-ups after endodontic treatment: a meta-analysis of literature. J Endod. 2008;34(10):1177–81.
20. Torabinejad M, et al. Factors associated with endodontic interappointment emergencies of teeth with necrotic pulps. J Endod. 1988;14(5):261–6.
21. Dahlen G, Magnusson BC, Moller A. Histological and histochemical study of the influence of lipopolysaccharide extracted from Fusobacterium nucleatum on the periapical tissues in the monkey Macaca fascicularis. Arch Oral Biol. 1981;26(7):591–8.
22. Siqueira JF Jr. Microbial causes of endodontic flare-ups. Int Endod J. 2003;36(7):453–63.
23. Tsesis I, et al. The precision of electronic apex locators in working length determination: a systematic review and meta-analysis of the literature. J Endod. 2015;41(11):1818–23.
24. Siqueira JF Jr, et al. Chemomechanical reduction of the bacterial population in the root canal after instrumentation and irrigation with 1%, 2.5%, and 5.25% sodium hypochlorite. J Endod. 2000;26(6):331–4.
25. Hulsmann M, Hahn W. Complications during root canal irrigation--literature review and case reports. Int Endod J. 2000;33(3):186–93.
26. al-Omari MA, Dummer PM. Canal blockage and debris extrusion with eight preparation techniques. J Endod. 1995;21(3):154–8.
27. Siqueira JF Jr, Lopes HP. Mechanisms of antimicrobial activity of calcium hydroxide: a critical review. Int Endod J. 1999;32(5):361–9.
28. Yingling NM, Byrne BE, Hartwell GR. Antibiotic use by members of the American Association of Endodontists in the year 2000: report of a national survey. J Endod. 2002;28(5):396–404.
29. Pickenpaugh L, et al. Effect of prophylactic amoxicillin on endodontic flare-up in asymptomatic, necrotic teeth. J Endod. 2001;27(1):53–6.
30. Gopikrishna V, Parameswaran A. Effectiveness of prophylactic use of rofecoxib in comparison with ibuprofen on postendodontic pain. J Endod. 2003;29(1):62–4.
31. Menke ER, et al. The effectiveness of prophylactic etodolac on postendodontic pain. J Endod. 2000;26(12):712–5.

32. Moore PA, et al. Analgesic regimens for third molar surgery: pharmacologic and behavioral considerations. J Am Dent Assoc. 1986;113(5):739–44.
33. Gordon SM, et al. Blockade of peripheral neuronal barrage reduces postoperative pain. Pain. 1997;70(2–3):209–15.
34. Rosenberg PA, et al. The effect of occlusal reduction on pain after endodontic instrumentation. J Endod. 1998;24(7):492–6.
35. Krasner P, Jackson E. Management of posttreatment endodontic pain with oral dexamethasone: a double-blind study. Oral Surg Oral Med Oral Pathol. 1986;62(2):187–90.
36. Ehrmann EH, Messer HH, Adams GG. The relationship of intracanal medicaments to postoperative pain in endodontics. Int Endod J. 2003;36(12):868–75.

Complications due to Root Canal Filling Procedures

6

Gianluca Plotino, Mauro Venturi, and Nicola Maria Grande

6.1 Introduction

Microorganisms and their by-products are the major cause of pulpal and periapical disease [1]. The purpose of root canal treatment is either to maintain asepsis of the root canal system or to disinfect it adequately, in order to preserve normal periradicular tissues or when apical periodontitis has occurred to restore them to health [2].

These objectives are pursued by removing remaining pulp tissue and by eliminating debris and microorganisms through instrumentation and irrigation [2]. However, it is often impossible to achieve the complete elimination of bacteria from infected root canal systems [3]. For this reason, the proper placement of an adequate tight root canal filling has been recognized as an important aspect for a successful outcome in endodontic treatments [4–7] aiming to prevent recolonization of the root canal system by oral microbiota [8, 9] and to block the portal of exit to the periapex for organisms that, even after instrumentation and disinfection, have survived in the pulp cavity, thus preventing the coronal and apical penetration of tissue fluids into the canal space that may serve as a source of substrate for persistent bacteria [10, 11] (Figs. 6.1 and 6.2).

Unfortunately, root canal filling does not invariably provide a complete seal of root canals [12], although it may entomb many microorganisms remained within them.

G. Plotino (✉)
Private Practice, GPT Clinic, Rome, Italy
e-mail: endo@gianlucaplotino.com

M. Venturi
Private Practice, Bologna, Italy
e-mail: info@endodonziamauroventuri.it

N.M. Grande
Professor of Endodontics, Catholic University of Sacred Heart - Rome, Italy and Magna Grecia University, Catanzaro, Italy
e-mail: nmgrande@gmail.com

P. Jain (ed.), *Common Complications in Endodontics*,
https://doi.org/10.1007/978-3-319-60997-3_6

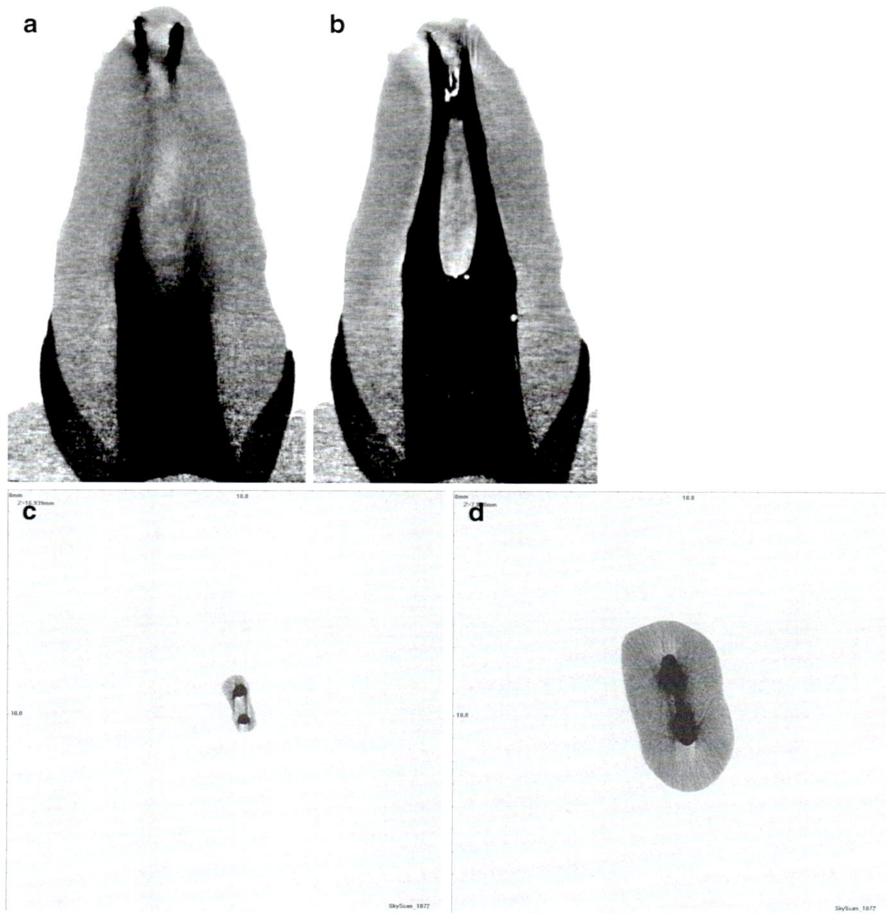

Fig. 6.1 (**a**) Micro-computed tomography axial section of a tooth with the root canals filled. The material appears in *black* color and shows a good filling of the root canals. (**b**) Micro-computed tomography axial section of the same tooth showing a lack of flow of the filling material in the apical isthmus between the root canals and the presence of some voids (in *white*). (**c**) Microcomputed tomography cross section of the same tooth within the two root canals in the apical third, showing a good filling of the prepared root canals. (**d**) Micro-computed tomography cross section of the same tooth within the two root canals and the isthmus in the coronal third showing a good filling of the endodontic space

Nevertheless, the combined effects of both host immune responses and operating procedures allow to obtain high percentages of success of endodontic treatment [13–15]. However, in relation to the endodontic treatment, complications may occur, some of which may also be caused by the filling techniques and the materials used.

Some complications of endodontic treatment depend on the difficulties with tools and materials that dental practitioners have to use within complex spaces [16–19]. A correct diagnosis, a treatment plan, and the knowledge of anatomical variations of the root canal system are necessary to obtain a favorable outcome of the endodontic treatment [20, 21].

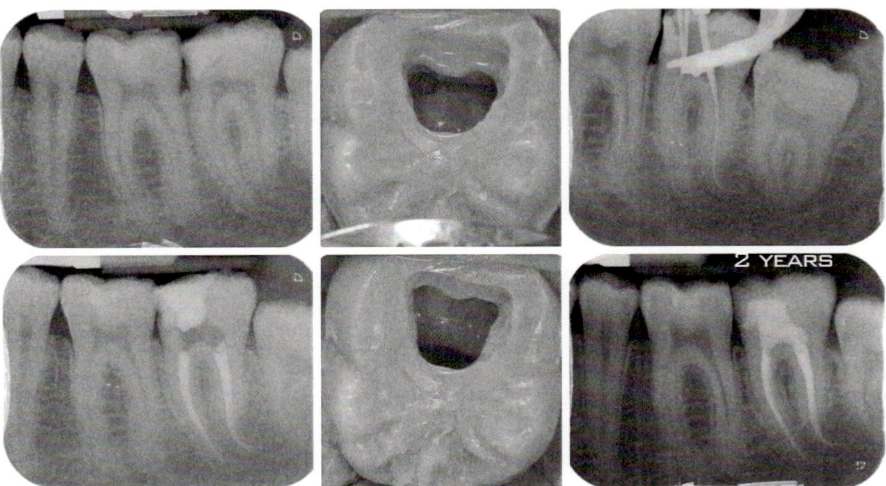

Fig. 6.2 A second left lower molar has been treated showing a root canal filling flush to the apex and obtaining a good seal without any filling material extrusion

Many studies have demonstrated that mechanical instrumentation and intracanal irrigation during root canal therapy result in a reduction of bacterial counts [22–24]. Indeed, most of the studies fail to adequately report clinically important and potentially patient-relevant outcomes [25], and there is currently insufficient reliable evidence showing the superiority of any one individual irrigant [25]. Moreover, there are no studies showing that the use of irrigants currently available, as well of any instrumentation technique, allows for a root canal space free of bacteria [25–28]. During mechanical instrumentation, an amorphous layer of tissue remnants is deposited on the surface of the root canal. This "smear layer," consisting of organic and inorganic materials as well of bacteria and their by-products, may prevent adhesion of sealers to the canal wall and seems to serve as a substrate for bacterial growth. The current opinion is that removing the smear layer is useful and that the removal should be carried out before root canal filling [25–27, 29–32]. White et al. [33] observed that plastic filling materials and sealers penetrated dentinal tubules after removal of smear layer. Okşan et al. [34] also found that smear layer prevented the penetration of sealers into dentinal tubules. Tubular penetration increases the interface between the filling and the dentinal structures, which may improve the ability of a filling material to prevent leakage [35].

6.2 Root Canal Filling Materials

6.2.1 Characteristics of Ideal Root Canal Filling Materials

The quality guidelines for endodontic treatment of the *European Society of Endodontology* state that materials used to fill the root canal system should be biocompatible, dimensionally stable, able to seal, unaffected by tissue fluids, insoluble, nonsupportive of bacterial growth, radiopaque, and easily removed from the canal if retreatment is needed [2, 36].

Grossman [37] listed the characteristics of an ideal root canal filling material as follows:

1. It should be easily introduced into the root canal.
2. It should seal the canal laterally as well as apically.
3. It should not shrink after being inserted.
4. It should be impervious to moisture.
5. It should be bacteriostatic or at least not encourage bacterial growth.
6. It should be radiopaque.
7. It should not stain tooth structure.
8. It should not irritate periradicular tissues.
9. It should be sterile, or easily and quickly sterilized, immediately before insertion.
10. It should be removed easily from the root canal, if necessary.

Historical Background

The Beginning of the Use of the Gutta-Percha

Information about the use of the gutta-percha as root canal filling material before the beginning of the twentieth century are scarce and vague.

In the 1800s and before, materials such as medicated cotton pellets, tin foil, oxychloride of zinc, lead foil, plaster of Paris, gold foil, wood, spunk, oxyphosphate of zinc, zinc oxide, paraffin, copper points, and various others were used to fill root canals.

In 1847, Hill developed the first root canal filling material containing gutta-percha, called "Hill's stopping". The compound, which mainly contained bleached gutta-percha, calcium carbonate, and quartz, was patented in 1848 and then made available for dental use [38, 39].

In 1867, Bowman was credited with using gutta-percha points to fill root canals by the St. Louis Dental Society [38, 39].

In 1883, Perry declared that he had used a point of gold wire coated with softened gutta-percha, a sort of anticipation of modern techniques for the use of the gutta-percha delivered by a carrier. He also softened strips of gutta-percha with a lamp and rolled them, thus preparing gutta-percha points. Then the points were heated and compacted into the canals in which it introduced alcohol, realizing something similar to a chemical softening technique [40].

In 1887, the S.S. White Company began to produce gutta-percha points [41]. In 1893, Rollins introduced gutta-percha to which was added vermilion, which contains mercury. However, the use of this material was not considered acceptable [42].

Callahan in 1914 introduced the use of resin to soften and dissolve gutta-percha so that it could be used as a cementing agent [43].

The Silver Points

In 1933, Jasper introduced the silver points [44] that were widely used to fill the root canals in the 1930s to the 1960s, particularly in smaller canals. They had the same size as instruments used in the preparation of the canal. Silver points could be inserted easily and allow for easy working length control. The main disadvantage of silver points is that they do not seal laterally or apically due to their lack of plasticity. They left too much space to be filled by sealer, thus leading to leakage, that caused corrosion of the silver points and formation of cytotoxic silver salts [45–47].

Silver points used in smaller canals could be successful, but their use in larger canals was inappropriate and gave rise to failures. The silver point use declined because of their inherent disadvantages, and currently there are no indications for their use.

The Medicated Materials

The use of X-rays progressively is made possible to better evaluate the root canal fillings, and it was evident that other materials suitable to fill the observed gaps should be used. At first zinc oxide- and eugenol-based cements, which were able to harden in the root canals, were used, but the results obtained with these materials were unsatisfactory. So it was thought appropriate to propose the use of fillings with antiseptics and medicated cements, and pastes were proposed, containing phenol, formaldehyde, antibiotics, and endomethasone.

In 1965, Sargenti introduced a paste originally marketed as N-2, containing 6.5% paraformaldehyde, lead, and mercury [48–50]. Lead has subsequently been reported in distant organ systems when N-2 is placed within the radicular space [51]. In another study, the investigators reported the same results regarding systemic distribution of the paraformaldehyde component of N-2 [51, 52]. Removal of the heavy metals from N-2 resulted in a new formulation: RC2B. Other paraformaldehyde sealers include endomethasone, SPAD, and Reibler's paste.

In general, the toxic and adverse in vivo effects of these materials on the pulp and periapical tissues have been demonstrated over time [53, 54]. In addition to the toxic nature of these materials, clinicians placed them with a lentulo spiral. Overextension often resulted in osteomyelitis and paresthesia. One clinician reported irreversible neurotoxicity, manifested as dysesthesia, in cases where paraformaldehyde pastes were forced through the apical foramen into the periapical tissues [55].

6.2.2 Characteristics of an Ideal Root Canal Filling

An ideal root canal filling three-dimensionally fills the entire root canal system as close to the cemento-dentinal junction as possible. Indeed, on the basis of microscopic analysis and clinical tests, it has been reported that optimum filling is achieved when canals are instrumented and filled 0 to 2.0 mm short of the root apex

[56, 57]. Root canal sealers, most of which have been shown to be biocompatible or tolerated by the tissues in their set state, are used in conjunction with a core filling material to establish an adequate seal. Radiographically, the root canal filling should have the appearance of a dense, three-dimensional filling that extends up to 0–2 mm from the radiographic root apex [2] and should be extended to the terminus of the root canal system without extruding materials into the surrounding tissues [14]. In fact, complete periradicular healing after endodontic treatment may be influenced by not only the effectiveness of the microbial control procedures but also the apical extent of the root filling materials, the composition, the biocompatibility, and the performance of these materials [58, 59].

6.2.3 Contemporary Filling Materials

At the present time, gutta-percha is the most popular core material used for obturation. Gutta-percha is utilized in combination with a root canal sealer that fills the minor irregularities [60] and acts as a lute between gutta-percha and the canal wall [61].

6.2.3.1 Endodontic Sealers

Sealers are used between dentin surfaces and core materials to fill spaces that are created due to the physical inability of the core materials to fill all areas of the canal. Traditionally, desirable characteristics were to adhere to dentin and the core material as well as to have adequate cohesive strength. Various types of sealers have been proposed, including zinc oxide-eugenol, as well as polymer resins, silicon-based materials, calcium hydroxide, glass ionomer, bioglass, and calcium silicate [36]. Newer generation of sealers is being engineered to improve the ability to penetrate into dentinal tubules and bond to, instead of just adhering to, both the dentin and core material surfaces. Various types of delivery systems such as auto-mix syringes have improved not only the efficiency of mixing but also the quality of the mix and ultimately the properties of the set material.

Zinc Oxide-Eugenol Sealers

Zinc oxide-eugenol sealers have a history of successful use in root canal obturation for over 100 years. They are widely used root canal sealers because of their plasticity, slow setting time in the absence of moisture, and small volumetric change on setting. They get resorbed if extruded into the periapical tissue. The zinc oxide-eugenol sealers have antimicrobial activity and popularity among clinicians, especially when used with thermoplasticized obturation technique [62]. However, eugenol is found to leak and is known to induce toxic effect and decrease the transmission in nerve cells. The effect is persistent even after setting. Localized inflammation with zinc oxide-eugenol sealers has been seen, both in soft tissue and in the bone [63].

Polymer Resin Sealers

Epoxy resin sealer exhibits reduced solubility [64] and disintegration [65] and microretention to root dentine with higher bond strength than other root canal sealers [66, 67] as well as adequate dimensional stability [68]. However, these sealers have shown no bioactive properties [69] or osteogenic potential [70]. Some studies reported that epoxy resin-based sealers showed toxicity and mutagenicity before setting and decreasing with time [71], but other authors [72–74] found no cytotoxic effect and moreover aged specimens appeared to induce cellular proliferation. New resin sealers have been designed to improve the adhesion of the sealer to dentine, both in combination with a dentine primer and without it [72–74]. For these new resin sealers, various studies reported toxic effects that did not decrease with time [65, 73, 75, 76].

Silicon-Based Sealers

These materials have been developed as root canal sealers, and laboratory and clinical data are promising [65, 73, 75–78]. Some of them contain gutta-percha powder. In different studies, silicone-based sealers, both fresh and aged, demonstrated slight cytotoxic effects [75, 79, 80].

Calcium Hydroxide-Based Sealers

They promote hard tissue formation but tend to dissolve over time and may thus compromise the endodontic seal [75, 79–82].

Glass-Ionomer Sealers

They might exhibit long-term adhesion to dentin, which would be an obvious advantage over zinc oxide-eugenol-type or epoxy resin-type sealer cements [83, 84]. However, it has been reported that pretreatment with phosphoric acid or citric acid should be used in association with glass-ionomer root canal sealers to achieve the most effective removal of the smear layer and to provide better adhesion [83–85].

Bioglass-Based Sealers

In contrast to calcium hydroxide, bioactive glasses not only have antibacterial but also bioactive/remineralizing effects [86]. One most promising field for the application of composite dental materials containing alkaline bioactive glass powders is endodontology. Adding particles of bioactive glasses to endodontic sealers could be a valuable add-on because of Ca/P deposition, bioactivity, and pH increase induction, mainly responsible for the antimicrobial effect of bioactive glasses [87].

Calcium Silicate-Based Sealers

In addition to antibacterial activity [87–89], they show cytocompatibility [90], good sealing ability [91], and good bonding to root canal dentin even under various conditions of dentin moisture [92, 93]. Bioceramic sealers have been recently developed for orthograde root canal obturation as a consequence of the success of some basic calcium silicate materials such as mineral trioxide aggregate (MTA), being today the material of choice for perforation repair, root-end fillings, pulp caps, pulpotomies, and obturation of immature teeth with open apices [94, 95].

These materials have been specifically designed as a nontoxic calcium silicate cement that is easy to use as an endodontic sealer while simultaneously taking advantage of its bioactive characteristics. In addition to its excellent physical and mechanical properties, some of the advantages are the following: they increase the pH value (up to 12.8) during the initial 24 h of the setting process (which is strongly antibacterial); they are hydrophilic, not hydrophobic; they have enhanced biocompatibility; they do not shrink or resorb (which is critical for a sealer-based technique); they are radiopaque; they have excellent sealing ability; they set quickly (3–4 h); they have good handling properties and are easy to use (particle size is so small; it can be used in a syringe to improve the convenience and delivery method).

Additionally, and this is very important in endodontics, bioceramics will not result in a significant inflammatory response if an overfill occurs during the obturation process or in a root repair. A further advantage of the material itself is its ability (during the setting process) to form hydroxyapatite and ultimately create a bond between dentin and the filling material. A significant component of improving this adaptation to the canal wall is the hydrophilic nature of the material [96–98].

Bioceramics are biocompatible, nontoxic, non-shrinking, and usually chemically stable within the biological environment [99]. A further advantage of these materials is their ability to form hydroxyapatite and ultimately create a bond between dentin and the material [100]. The majority of papers show favorable properties for bioceramic materials including biocompatibility, bioactivity, and antimicrobial properties, and they have sealing properties similar to MTA. While in vitro studies are promising, it is not clear if any of these results influence clinical success. Only well-designed, prospective outcome studies can answer this question [96, 98].

6.2.3.2 Core Materials

Gutta-Percha

Gutta-percha is a hydrocarbon polymer, i.e., a trans-1,4-polyisoprene, and is an isomer of natural rubber [101]. It is obtained from the coagulation of latex produced by trees of the Sapotaceae family and mainly derived from *Palaquium gutta bail* [102]. An important characteristic of gutta-percha and of clinical importance is the fact that when it is exposed to air and light over time, it becomes more brittle [103, 104]. Storage of gutta-percha in a refrigerator extends the shelf life of the material.

Brittleness, stiffness, tensile strength, and radiopacity have been shown to depend primarily on the proportions of organic (gutta-percha polymer and wax/resins) and inorganic (zinc oxide and metal sulfates) components [102]. Zinc oxide is also responsible for the antibacterial activity of gutta-percha points [105]. The particular percentages of components vary according to the manufacturer. It is evident that since the cones differ in their composition, they may differ in their physical properties and even in their biological effect [106].

Gutta-percha is a thermoplastic polymer material within which segments of the polymer molecules may be sufficiently aligned and associated to form crystalline segments randomly dispersed among the rest of the disordered, amorphous volume [107, 108]. The crystalline phase appears in two forms: (1) the alpha phase and (2) the beta phase. The forms differ only in the molecular repeat distance and single carbon-bond configuration [8, 109]. Employing X-ray methods, the degree of crystallinity of gutta-percha was reported to be 55–60% [110]. The crystal structure of pure gutta-percha has been reported in detail [107, 108], and it is known that the application of heat or mechanical energy will increase the mobility of the long molecules, perhaps increasing the size of some of the ordered, crystalline segments but, in general, increasing the proportion of the disordered, amorphous volume [111].

Thus, gutta-percha is rigid at room temperature, becomes pliable at 25–30 °C, softens at 60 °C, and melts at 100 °C with partial decomposition [112]. Gutta-percha undergoes phase transitions when heated from beta to alpha phase at around 46 °C. At a range between 54° and 64 °C, the softening point of gutta-percha, an amorphous phase is reached (Goodman 1981). When cooled at an extremely slow rate, the material will recrystallize to the alpha phase. However, this is difficult to achieve, and under normal conditions, the material returns to the beta phase. The phase transformation is important in thermoplastic obturation techniques. Gutta-percha is soluble in chloroform, eucalyptol, halothane, carbon disulfide, benzene, and xylem and less soluble in turpentine. This property of gutta-percha allows it to be removed for post preparation and in the retreatment of non-healing cases.

Any method manipulating gutta-percha using heat or solvent will result in some shrinkage (1–2%) of the material. Shrinkage of the core material is not desirable when attempting to seal a canal. Dental gutta-percha is not in its pure form or even mostly gutta-percha. Its major component is zinc oxide (50–79%), heavy metal salts (1–17%), wax or resin (1–4%), and only 19–22% actual gutta-percha [113]. The variations in content are because of different manufacturers and distributors desiring different handling properties. Some formulations are softer than others. Some clinicians choose the brand of gutta-percha depending on the technique being used. Compaction with spreaders, condensers, or carriers is usually the means used to attempt to compensate for this shrinkage of the core material [114]. In any case, some means of compensation for this shrinkage must be incorporated into the technique being used. Schilder et al. [113] postulated that vertical pressure must be applied in all warm gutta-percha techniques to compensate the volume changes. However, it has to be underlined that this assumption has never been demonstrated. Meyer et al. [115] suggested that methods for the compensation of shrinkage in root canal obturation should be evaluated.

Resilon

Resilon, a synthetic methacrylate-based resin polycaprolactone polymer, has been developed as a gutta-percha substitute to be used with Epiphany (*Pentron Clinical Technologies, Wallingford, CT, USA*) [116], a new methacrylate-based sealer, in an attempt to form an adhesive bond between the sealer, the core material, and the canal dentin walls. Advocates of this technique propose that the bond to the canal wall and to the core material creates a "monoblock" [117]. It is capable of being supplied in standardized ISO sizes and shapes, conforms to the configuration of the various nickel-titanium rotary instruments, and is available in pellet form for injection devices. The manufacturer states that its handling properties are similar to those of gutta-percha, and therefore it can be used with any obturation technique. Resilon contains polymers of polyester, bioactive glass, and radiopaque fillers (bismuth oxychloride and barium sulfate) with a filler content of approximately 65% [116]. It can be softened with heat or dissolved with solvents like chloroform. This characteristic allows the use of various current treatment techniques. Being a resin-based system makes it compatible with current restorative techniques in which cores and posts are being placed with resin-bonding agents [7, 118]. Some studies reported that Resilon may be degraded by pathogenic bacteria [119–121]. These findings suggest that the seal and integrity of root canal fillings obturated with Resilon may be impaired by a microbial insult.

6.2.3.3 Coated Gutta-Percha Points

This process has been developed in an attempt to achieve similar results as those claimed by Resilon, a bond between the canal wall, the core, and the sealer. Two versions of coating gutta-percha are available. In the first one, the surface of gutta-percha cones is coated with a resin (Ultradent, South Jordan, Utah, USA) [119, 121–124]. A bond is formed when the resin sealer contacts the resin-coated gutta-percha cone, and the manufacturer claims that this will inhibit leakage between the solid core and sealer; with this new coated solid core material, the technique calls for the use of EndoRez sealer (Ultradent, South Jordan, Utah), a methacrylate-based material in two components, dual-cure, whose hydrophilic characteristics allow the penetration into the dentin tubules [125]. Another manufacturer has coated gutta-percha cones with glass ionomer (Brasseler USA, Savannah, GA). This system is called Active GP Plus, and cones are designed for use with their glass-ionomer sealer [126].

To date, manufacturers of bioceramic sealers used for orthograde root canal filling are also producing their proprietary coated gutta-percha cones to bond with the correspondent bioceramic sealer in an attempt to achieve a bond between the core and the sealer [96]. Bioceramic sealer when combined with coated cones offers a new obturation technique (Synchronized Hydraulic Condensation) [97, 98]. Some experimental gutta-percha containing bioactive phosphate glasses have been recently developed with significant improvements, particularly in self-adhesiveness to root dentine and the release of alkaline species in an aqueous environment [127–130].

Injectable Materials

The GuttaFlow (Colténe/Whaledent, Altstätten, Switzerland) is an injectable silicone cement. It consists of a matrix of polydimethylsiloxane highly filled with fine powder of gutta-percha (size less than 30 μ). The GuttaFlow and GuttaFlow2, respectively, incorporate nano- and microparticles of Ag (silver) with antibacterial properties. It is applied in the root canal before inserting the cone of gutta-percha, but can be also injected without any core material. The manufacturer emphasizes the insolubility, the biocompatibility, the slight expansion consequent to the setting, the great fluidity, and the ability to be disposed in thin layer [131, 132]. The last version of this material, the GuttaFlow bioseal, is claimed to be a bioactive material that may provide natural repair constituents such as calcium and silicates.

Mineral Trioxide Aggregate (MTA)

MTA is composed of tricalcium silicate, dicalcium silicate, tricalcium aluminate, tetracalcium aluminoferrite, and bismuth oxide [133]. MTA has a proven track record in clinical and laboratory research. Its biocompatibility [73, 134–137] and bioactive properties are recognized [94]. In addition, MTA is a relatively nontoxic material with a high pH, is insoluble in tissue fluids [94, 138], and is capable of depositing a hydroxyapatite-like layer upon exposure to physiologic tissue fluids [139, 140]. Continuous leaching of calcium, phosphate, and hydroxyl ions not only allows MTA to participate in the process of regeneration and remineralization of hard tissues but may also enhance the sealability of MTA apical plugs by deposition of hydroxyapatite crystals into voids and potential spaces between the dentin and root filling material [141].

Many studies have reported successful long-term clinical outcomes associated with MTA apexification procedures [136, 142, 143]. Even if MTA has been already proposed as the material of choice for orthograde root canal filling owing to its advantageous properties [144], disadvantages of traditional MTA for this application include its long setting time [145–147], difficulty in handling due to its sandy consistency [148], potential to discolor teeth and soft tissues, and the presence of potentially toxic elements in its compositions [94].

6.3 Filling the Root Canal System in Three Dimensions

Successful filling of root canals requires the use of materials and techniques capable of densely filling the entire root canal system and providing a fluid tight seal from the apical segment of the canal to the cavosurface margin in order to prevent reinfection. This also implies that an adequate coronal filling or restoration be placed to prevent oral bacterial microleakage. When preparing the root canals to allow for a three-dimensional obturation and an effective sealing of the root canal space to its proper apical extent, the clinician's inability to maintain the original anatomy in terms of working length, shape, and position of the apical foramen and to create an optimal canal geometry with a continuous, progressive, and uniform conical shape with a circular base within the canal can result in procedural errors. These may include a lack of compaction and adaptation of the filling materials and excessive apical extrusion of these materials into the periapical tissue [94, 149, 150].

6.3.1 Techniques for Filling the Root Canal System

6.3.1.1 Single Cone

The single-cone technique consists of matching a master point to the prepared root canal. For this technique, a type of canal preparation is advocated so that the size of the cone and the shape of the preparation are closely matched. The cone is cemented in place with a root canal sealer, which is advocated to fill the spaces. This technique is simple, but does not fill completely root canals that are seldom round throughout their length [36].

6.3.1.2 Chemoplasticized Gutta-Percha

Especially in the past, solvents such as chloroform, eucalyptol, and xylene have been used to chemically soften gutta-percha. Solvents were used to soften the outer surface of the custom cone as if making an impression of the apical portion of the canal. Indeed, chemical solvent use implies many problems. The techniques that make use of solvents have been criticized because they cause the contraction of the material after evaporation of the solvent itself [151]. The techniques using solvents are also inadvisable for the poor stock control and the related risk of extrusion [151–154]. Chloroform was found carcinogenic [152, 154, 155], and although its use has never been surely correlated with the onset of cancer, in the USA it has been deleted from the list of solvents used in dentistry in 1979 [153]. Chloroform has been widely used in the past for the removal of the gutta-percha from the root canals. For this use, in its replacement, alternative solvents are currently preferred [156, 157], i.e., halothane, which compared to chloroform is more volatile and showed equally effective solvent properties [157, 158]. The eucalyptol shows slower action but provides less damage to the tissues [159, 160].

6.3.1.3 Cold Lateral Compaction

Lateral compaction provides for the cold compaction of gutta-percha: a master cone corresponding to the final instrumentation size and length of the canal is coated with sealer, inserted into the canal, and is laterally compacted with a spreader. Additional accessory cones are placed against it and are laterally compacted as well by means of a spreader. This technique provides a good control of the working length. On the other side, the cold compacted gutta-percha shows poor plastic deformability, a modest degree of elastic deformation, which acts negatively, and no ability to flow. The filling obtained is a mass of leaning cones, with a large amount of interposed spaces which are filled by root canal cement. The poor cold formability would require the compression of the material very close to the apical limit, according to Allison et al. [161]. The lateral compaction requires that relatively high forces are applied by the spreader with some risks of root fracture [162].

6.3.1.4 Warm Lateral Compaction

A master cone corresponding to the final instrument size of the canal is coated with sealer, inserted into the canal, heated with a warm spreader, laterally compacted with spreaders, and filled with additional accessory cones. Some devices use vibration in addition to the warm spreader [163].

6.3.1.5 Warm Vertical Compaction

A master cone corresponding to the final instrument size and length of the canal is fitted, coated with sealer, heated, and compacted vertically with pluggers until the apical 4–5 mm segment of the canal is filled. Then the remaining root canal is back-filled using warm pieces of core material or by injection systems.

The warm vertical compaction technique as described by Schilder [8] provides for the introduction in the root canal of a gutta-percha cone coated by a thin layer of endodontic sealer. The gutta-percha is warmed by means of a heat spreader and compacted vertically by pluggers with multiple waves of condensations from the crown to the apex. This technique has the aim to provide a three-dimensional filling of the root canal system with all its complexities. The compaction of the material is important not only to allow its adaptation to the endodontic space, but also, it is claimed by Schilder et al. [113], to compensate for changes in volume of the gutta-percha that always corresponds to a certain degree of contraction.

6.3.1.6 Continuous Wave of Condensation

Continuous wave [164] is essentially a vertical compaction (down-packing) of core material and sealer in the apical portion of the root canal using commercially available heating devices that use pluggers as heat carrier and then backfill the remaining portion of the root canal with thermoplasticized core material using injection devices. The main difference with the classic Schilder technique is that this technique performs the compaction in only one continuous wave of compaction from crown to the apex. A good apical stop is necessary for both these techniques to prevent apical extrusion of the filling.

6.3.1.7 Injection Technique

It provides that preheated, thermoplasticized, injectable core material is injected directly into the root canal, using specific injection devices [165–167]. Sealer is placed in the canal before injection. As a master cone is not used, it is difficult to control the apical extent of the filling with high risk of under- or overfilled root canal obturations. A cold, flowable matrix that is triturated, GuttaFlow® (Coltene Whaledent, Cuyahoga Falls, OH), consists of gutta-percha added to a resin sealer, RoekoSeal. The material is provided in capsules for trituration. The technique involves injection of the material into the canal and placing a single master cone [168].

6.3.1.8 Thermomechanical Compaction

A cone coated with sealer is placed in the root canal, engaged with a rotary instrument mounted on contra-angle handpiece that frictionally warms, plasticizes, and compacts it into the root canal [169]. The compactors are similar to the Hedström files but have spirals oriented in the opposite direction, and the gutta-percha is heated and simultaneously pushed both apically and laterally. This technique can easily cause extrusion. On the other hand, it can be a good backfilling technique [170].

An alternative technique (MicroSeal) uses thermoplasticized softened core material delivered directly by the mechanically activated condenser into the space created on the side of a master point laterally condensed with a mechanical spreader. It will unify the advantages of the apical control of filling material related to the use of a master point and of the effective filling of the lateral space with a thermoplasticized core material forced into the canal [170–172].

6.3.1.9 Carrier-Based

Carrier-based thermoplasticized warm gutta-percha on a plastic or gutta-percha carrier, heated in an oven, is delivered directly into the canal as a root canal filling [173, 174]. Even if root canal walls are only painted with sealer before the insertion of the obturator, the apical control of the filling material is difficult and extrusions common. Furthermore, plastic carriers are not so easy to be removed in the case of retreatment or post-space preparation.

In the carrier-based sectional technique, a sized and fitted section of gutta-percha with sealer is inserted into the apical 4 mm of the root canal. The remaining portion of the root canal is filled with injectable, thermoplasticized gutta-percha using an injection gun. An example is SimpliFill (Discus Dental, Culver City, CA) [116, 175].

6.3.1.10 Apical Barrier

Apical barriers are important for the obturation of canals with immature roots with open apices, whose endodontic management is challenging for the clinician because of the lack of resistance and retention form associated with a blunderbuss apex. A blunderbuss configuration of the apex makes delivery of root filling materials difficult, potentially leading to overextension and/or overfilling of the root canal. Historically, nonsurgical treatment of immature teeth was achieved by calcium hydroxide apexification to induce physiologic formation of a hard tissue barrier before obturation. However, significant improvements to endodontic biomaterials, placed using proper carriers, have allowed for more convenient and efficacious treatment of these teeth in a single-visit procedure [142, 143, 176]. At this time mineral trioxide aggregate (MTA) is generally considered the material of choice for the obturation of canals with immature roots with open apices because of its ability to act as an osteoconductive apical barrier [138, 140].

6.4 Complications Due to Obturation Procedures

Obturation errors often are a result of inadequate cleaning and shaping or preparation errors. Ledges, blockages, perforations, separated instruments, debris present apically, apical or canal transportation, inaccurate working lengths, and underprepared or overprepared canals are frequent errors encountered during root canal instrumentation that create an unpredictable shape of the root canals and that consequently may negatively influence the quality of root canal obturation. These have all been already discussed in detail in the previous chapter.

Complications during or after the endodontic treatment might be prevented by careful preoperative examination, good-quality radiographs, good instrumentation, irrigation, and obturation techniques. In fact, obturation-related complications may be mainly due to the chemical or physical negative consequence of a gross extrusion of filling materials beyond the apex into the periapical tissues.

6.4.1 Prevention of Extrusion of Filling Materials

Prior to the obturation phase, the clinician must establish the proper shape and size of the root canal. Proper canal shaping should create a continuous tapered shape from the apex to the coronal opening to obtain an apical resistance or retention form. The consequences of compression of gutta-percha within a root canal will differ with the physical composition of the gutta-percha, the temperature, the taper of the canal, and the point of application of the compacting force.

The available commercial [103, 177–179] gutta-percha products vary greatly in their composition [177, 178], although not all have been chemically or physically analyzed [103, 178, 179]. These properties affect the adaptation of the gutta-percha to the endodontic space. Schilder [8] declared that a tapered root canal allows the compaction of the gutta-percha cone and its close fitting to the canal walls, minimizing the risk of producing extrusion. With lateral condensation, cold gutta-percha is used. If gutta-percha is compacted at body temperature, only very small elastic and plastic deformation may occur, and the probability that it would flow into irregular spaces is unrealistic. Alternative techniques described above use warm gutta-percha in different ways, applied [8] or frictional heat plasticizes gutta-percha [169], allowing for better adaptation to canal walls and a higher degree of homogeneity [109, 179, 180]. The compacting of heated amorphous gutta-percha is difficult to control, especially close to the apex [181], both because of the frequent lack of apical constriction [182] and the need to enlarge the apical portion of the canal to obtain mechanical debridement [183].

The main difficulty for the practitioner is to adjust the compaction procedure to the softening of the gutta-percha. A plastic mass of gutta-percha forced to flow will deform on contact with the internal surface of the root canal. Thus, when compacting heated amorphous gutta-percha, the major force is directed toward the apex, and the flowing gutta-percha may extrude, if apical patency has been maintained during instrumentation. Extrusion has been reported to be a complication of thermo-softened techniques [181, 184].

Warm vertical compaction [8] and the "continuous wave technique" [164] offer techniques that use the apical control of the internal placement of a cold point while providing the homogeneous, three-dimensional filling advantages of the thermo-softened techniques. Marlin and Schilder stated [151] that heating and compaction may be performed to a distance of 5–7 mm from the endpoint of the gutta-percha. When using the warm vertical condensation technique, a temperature increase to 40–42 °C usually occurs in the apical gutta-percha, and it should not exceed 45 °C to avoid the volume variations dependent on phase changes [185]. In this condition, from a rheological viewpoint, despite the apical patency being maintained, the compacted gutta-percha has no or reduced risk to extrude. In fact, at the interface between gutta-percha and canal wall, reaction forces can be distinguished: normal reaction forces act perpendicular, and shear reaction forces act parallel (friction) to surfaces in contact. When the applied force exceeds the maximum static friction force, surfaces move relative to each other and dynamic friction force occurs [186]. Dynamic friction depends on force squeezing objects together, and on the nature of materials in contact, and has a direction opposite to the motion or the impending motion. However, these frictional phenomena can develop only if the gutta-percha is not too deformable, i.e., in crystalline state [186]. Only if the cone is in crystalline state, the vertical compaction can force it to fit more apically. Thus, a reversible elastic strain may occur, able to increase the force normal to the canal wall, to compress the gutta-percha against the canal walls and squeeze the endodontic cement, and to fill the lateral canals [186].

An increase of friction also occurs that counteracts the cone motion and thus its extrusion [186]. The apical gutta-percha, at the temperatures recorded and advocated by Marlin and Schilder [151], maintains its more crystalline state and shows low plasticity. If gutta-percha is compacted at those temperatures, only very small elastic and plastic deformation may occur, and the probability that it would flow and extrude is less. Obviously, if plasticized gutta-percha is compacted close to the apex, the probability that it would flow and extrude is very high. In contrast, when using carrier-based obturators, thermomechanical compaction [169], and the injection techniques close to the patent apical foramen, gutta-percha is heated to higher temperatures, increasing the proportion of the amorphous phase as happens with all semicrystalline thermopolymers [111] and thus increasing the risk of extrusion of the softened gutta-percha. Furthermore, attention must be paid when placing the sealer in the canal. Placing the sealer with a lentulo spiral or a syringe or activating it with sonic or ultrasonic instruments may promote extrusion of the material because this technique lacks apical control. Placing the sealer with a file and spinning it counterclockwise do not seem to provide an ideal distribution of the sealer on the root canal walls. Placing the sealer with a master cone and pumping it up and down in the canal seem to be the most predictable technique for the application of sealers in root canals, if a filling technique using a master point will be performed. When placing sealer in general, the clinicians should use particular care if the canal presents an open apex, to avoid extrusion of material.

6.4.2 Complications Due to Extrusion of Filling Materials

Numerous reports and reviews in the literature have described complications caused by overextension of root filling materials into the periapical tissues, the mandibular canal, and the maxillary sinuses. A meta-analysis has shown that warm gutta-percha obturation shows a high rate of overextension, more than cold lateral condensation [56]. Gross overextension of obturation materials usually indicates faulty technique (Fig. 6.3). However, as long as the overextension is not in contact with vital structures, such as the inferior alveolar nerve or sinuses, and the apical terminus is well filled in three dimensions, permanent harm is potentially small, unless the obturation materials contain paraformaldehyde (Fig. 6.4). On the other hand, overextension of the root canal filling material risks serious and possibly permanent consequences, should the maxillary sinus or underlying inferior alveolar nerve be adjacent to the root terminus. It is generally considered that four possible types of factor can cause tissue damage [187, 188]: (a) chemical factors because of the neurotoxic effect from the products used to clean (irrigating solutions, intracanal

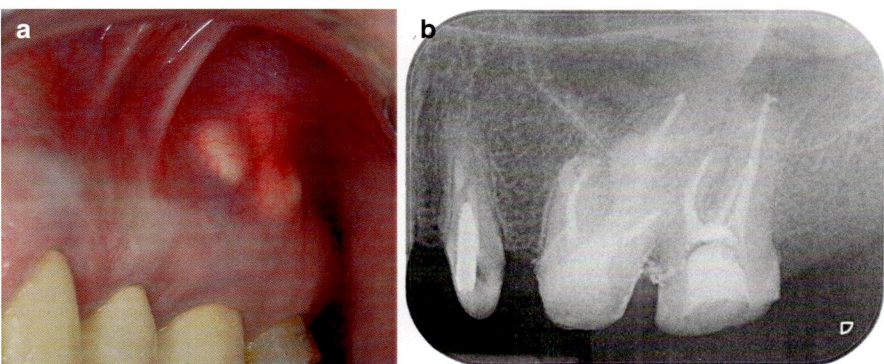

Fig. 6.3 Clinical image (**a**) and radiograph (**b**) of a gross overfilling appearing under the subcutaneous tissues, probably due to the lack of the buccal cortical bone plate. Despite the big amount of filling material extruded, the patient did not complain any pain or discomfort

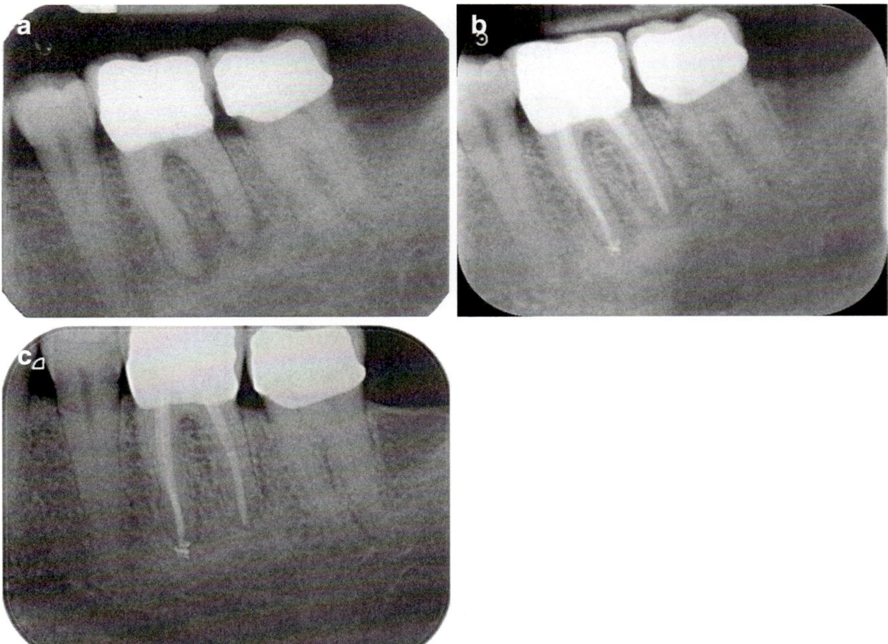

Fig. 6.4 A first left mandibular molar has been endodontically treated due to chronic apical periodontitis (**a**). Despite the overfilling in the mesial root (**b**), complete healing has been obtained at the 2-year control (**c**)

medications, etc.) or fill root canals, (b) mechanical trauma from over-instrumentation, (c) a pressure phenomenon from the presence of core filling material or sealer within the inferior alveolar canal, and (d) tissue overheating because of incorrect warm condensation techniques [189] (Fig. 6.5).

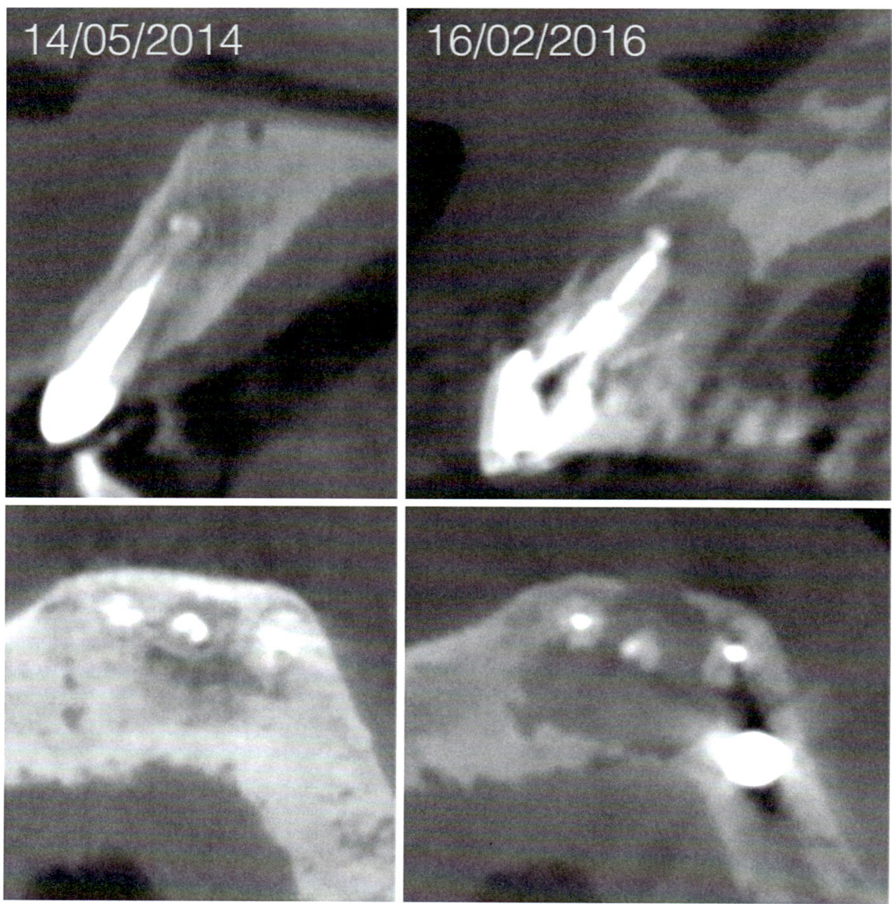

Fig. 6.5 On left, CBCT examination of an upper lateral incisor endodontically treated. It is possible to appreciate the filling material extruded in the periapical bone. At the baseline the patient had no symptoms related with this tooth. On the right, after 20 months the patient presented an acute apical abscess symptom of pain and swelling. A possible association between extrusion of infected material and development of pathology can be hypothesized

6.4.2.1 Anatomical Areas Involved

Maxillary Sinus Damage

The extrusion of root filling materials into the periapical tissues and/or the maxillary sinus has been reported on many occasions in the endodontic literature (Fig. 6.6). The performance of endodontic therapy involving maxillary molars, premolars, and, infrequently, canines has sometimes led to the inadvertent placement of an array of dental materials and instruments into the maxillary sinus. Extrusion of root canal obturation materials into the antrum has been reported with silver points [190],

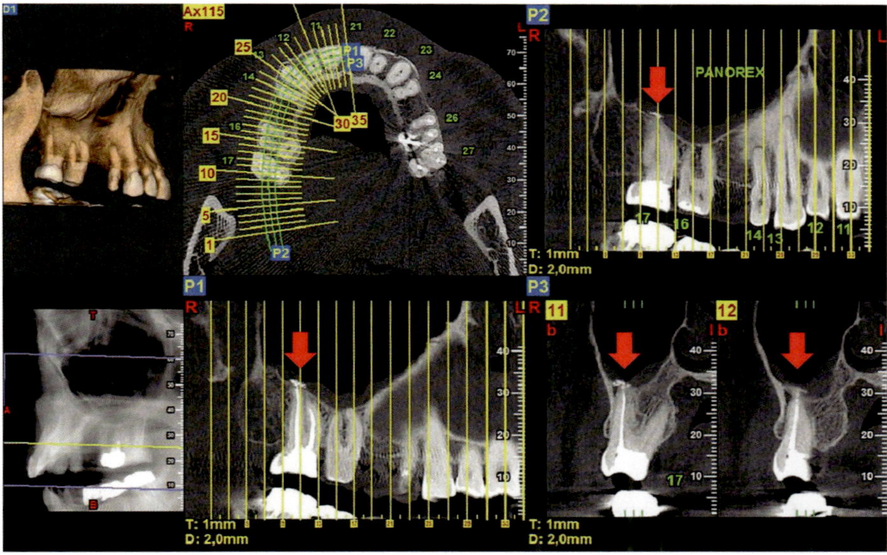

Fig. 6.6 CBCT evaluation of an upper second right molar with extrusion of filling material from the apex of the mesiobuccal root into the maxillary sinus that caused a fibrotic reaction that encapsulated the material

thermoplasticized gutta-percha [190, 191] and gutta-percha points [190–193]. Various root canal pastes and cements, including calcium hydroxide and N2, have been extruded into the sinus [190–198]. Deposition of foreign substances within the maxillary antrum can promote an array of clinical presentations such as sinus pain and pressure, acute and chronic sinusitis, pain on mastication, and tenderness to palpation. However some patients will remain asymptomatic for years after the accidental breaching of the sinus with endodontic obturation substances [199]. The introduction of cone beam computed tomography (CBCT) has provided enhanced endodontic diagnostic utility in such accidents and can be helpful with management of endodontic problems [200], even though few case reports have documented the use of three-dimensional (3D) CBCT for the visualization of extensive thermoplasticized gutta-percha within the maxillary sinus [191]. Extruded gutta-percha has even been reported to have entered into the maxillary sinus and subsequently migrated into the ethmoid sinus, causing sinus tenderness and nasal stuffiness [191, 201, 202]. Using obturators with a core carrier, one challenge is just to control the apical extrusion of material [203, 204] (Fig. 6.7). Bjørndal et al. [202] reported a clinical case of an endodontic overfilling of the palatal root of a maxillary right first molar with a core carrier; the core carrier was impacted in the maxillary sinus for more than 5 years after endodontic treatment, and surgical technique was used for the palatal removal of the core carrier; concomitant with the displacement of the core carrier, the patient developed marked unilateral irritation and blocking of the right nostril; over the years, the patient had undergone several hospitalized treatments targeting the nose region but with no satisfying result.

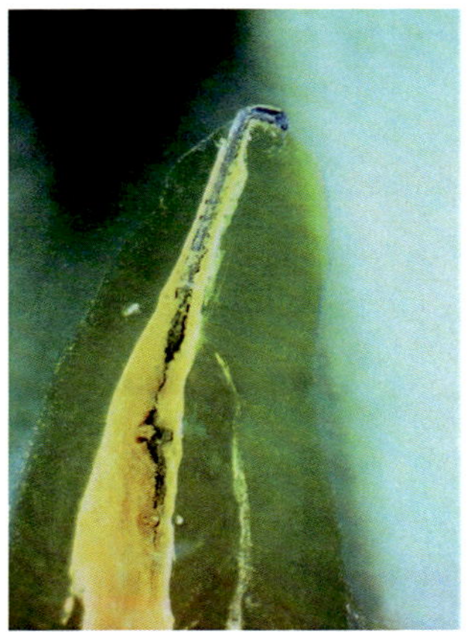

Fig. 6.7 A cleared root of an extracted upper canine showing a possible clinical complication with carrier-based filling techniques: the extrusion of the plastic carrier in the periapical tissues

A case report of extreme overextension of gutta-percha within the maxillary sinus after endodontic retreatment on tooth #14 was provided by Brooks and Kleinman [205]; the mesiobuccal canal had only been filled with thermoplasticized injectable warm gutta-percha, the origin of the extrusion; imaging with three-dimensional cone beam computed tomography was performed for localization of the gutta-percha, the patient underwent a Caldwell-Luc approach for removal of the extruded material, the gutta-percha was successfully removed intact, and the patient had an unremarkable postoperative course; however, the patient continues to have mild tenderness in the sinus region. Several root canal sealers containing zinc have also been implicated with the development of an aspergillosis infection and fungus ball formation within the maxillary sinus [205–208].

Neurological Damage

Endodontic-related paresthesia and anesthesia may result from periapical lesions that inhibit the normal function of nerve as a result of direct mechanical compression, diffusion of toxic metabolic products, and bacterial activity [209]. Overfilling may cause the passage of endodontic materials into the vicinity of the inferior alveolar nerve or its branches, inducing mechanical compression and toxic effects (Fig. 6.8). When the filling materials are either close to or in intimate contact with nerve structures, anesthesia, hypoesthesia, paresthesia, or dysesthesia may occur [210]. Paresthesia is a permanent or episodic sensation of ticking, prickling, or tingling of the lower lip [211]. Numerous case reports have described the occurrence of paresthesia during and after root canal treatment [212].

In mandibular teeth posterior to the mental foramen, extrusion of filling material can be responsible for damage to the inferior alveolar nerve, and labiomandibular paresthesia is the most frequent complication that can occur [187, 188]. Most cases have been reported in connection with mandibular second molars, but cases related to first molars and premolars have also been described [213]. In fact, because of the proximity of the mental foramen, the mental nerve is usually affected by endodontic-related complications in mandibular premolars [214]. Endodontic materials can spread to the periradicular tissues theoretically in four different ways. These include

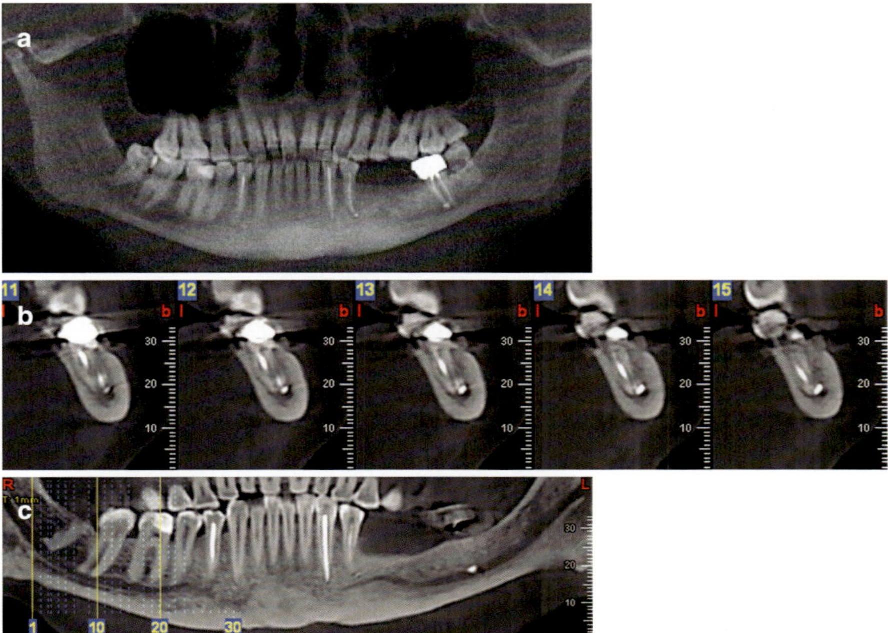

Fig. 6.8 (**a**) A panoramic radiograph, following endodontic treatment of 3.4 and 3.7. (**b**) CBCT exam (coronal slices/cuts) of the 37 revealing filling material extruded in the mandibular canal. (**c**) CBCT sagittal slice/cut through the filling material present into the mandibular canal. (Reprinted with permission by: G. Gambarini, G. Plotino, N. M. Grande, L. Testarelli, M. Prencipe, D. Messineo, L. Fratini, F. D'Ambrosio. Differential diagnosis of endodontic-related inferior alveolar nerve paraesthesia with cone beam computed tomography: a case report. Int Endod J 2011;44:176–181)

migration toward the mandibular nerve bundle, drainage through lymphatic vessels, systemic diffusion within a periapical vein, and progression between the bone and mucosal membrane toward soft tissues [215]. Anatomy of the mandible favors the introduction of endodontic materials into the mandibular canal area and thus the paresthesia to occur. Especially in the posterior area of mandible, the trabecular, vacuole-rich cancellous bone facilitates the diffusion of different materials into the surrounding tissues [188]. This alone is sufficient to cause paresthesia in case of overfill. Periapical infection weakens further the loose trabecular pattern of the bone, which raises the probability of diffusion of endodontic materials and results in paresthesia together with widened apical foramen [216].

Attention should also be paid to the distance between the apices and the mandibular canal. According to one study, this distance varies between 1 and 4 mm in the case of the first mandibular molar; it is less than 1 mm with the second and third mandibular molars [188]. With mandibular premolars, the proximity of mental foramen should always be taken into consideration [214]. Toxic root canal filling materials include sealers and paraformaldehyde-containing pastes [217], but almost all of the endodontic materials are neurotoxic at some level [218]. Neurotoxic materials are able to initiate a host-dependent inflammatory process, which causes damage to cells, ulceration, and hemolysis when in contact with vital tissue [216]. This process might culminate in necrosis of the tissue [217]. Free eugenol, a dissolution product of zinc eugenol, hydrolyzes cell membrane and inhibits cellular respiration [215, 217, 219]. Because of the potential for chemical degeneration of the nerve axons, the use of eugenol-containing pastes is not recommended for endodontic obturation at all [215, 217, 219]. This applies especially when forces are directly connected to the inferior alveolar nerve bundle [220]. In cases of paraformaldehyde paste overfill and introduction to the periradicular tissues, the risk of permanent tissue damage is high. These cases are widely reported in literature. In addition, endodontic-related paresthesia can result from mechanical pressure and ischemia or bacterial toxins involved in periapical pathosis of a nonvital tooth [220–222].

The recovery potential of the nerve depends on the extent of the damage (both mechanical and chemical) and rapidity of cause removal [164, 218, 223]. In some cases a clear overfill with sealer within the mandibular canal can be observed on a radiograph, but the patient is nevertheless free of symptoms [218]. Gutta-percha is traditionally considered as an inert root filling material, and the paresthesia cases involving gutta-percha usually result from overfill of thermoplastic gutta-percha [215]. In these circumstances the resulting paresthesia is of a mechanical or thermal nature. Clinically, the response is often seen as sudden onset of excruciating pain, swelling, and numbness of the affected region. The teeth might be tender to percussion or on palpation, and the opening of the mouth might be limited [216, 217]. It is difficult to ascertain the etiology for paresthesia after treatment with overfill into neurovascular tissue. The clinician must also consider the neurotoxicity of the materials, the possibility of direct mechanical damage due to instrumentation [216, 217, 224, 225], the compression of core materials such as gutta-percha [225, 226], and the possibility of epineural fibrosis resulting in neuroma [227].

In the case of paresthesia or anesthesia in which apical extrusion of endodontic materials is observed, however, because the paresthesia can be of both mechanical and chemical nature, removal of the excess material might not be sufficient if the nerve fibers have already undergone degeneration in a chemical manner. Paresthesia caused by a brief irritation of the nerve, for instance, on overinstrumentation, usually subsides within days. If no signs of healing are seen within 6 months, the chances of healing are considered much lower, although normal sensory function might still return after this [188, 212, 227]. The majority of tissue damage cases are treated by nonsurgical methods such as analgesics, cold packs, corticosteroids, and antibiotics to inhibit secondary infections [228, 229]. Dexamethasone is a corticosteroid that has been widely used in dentistry, and it seems to decrease periapical inflammation caused by a foreign body [220]. Even though care should be taken with the use of corticosteroids, with the correct indications and adequate dosage, the adverse effects seem to be rare [230]. Paresthesia can sometimes result from postoperative infection, in which case antibiotics are the treatment of choice. If the facial nerve has been damaged, physiotherapy might provide additional help [217].

Paresthesia resulting from local infection usually subsides through elimination of infection by root canal treatment, extraction, antibiotics, and/or periapical surgery [231]. The patient must be informed of the nature and possible duration of paresthesia as well as the importance of regular control visits [232]. In some cases surgical exploration is required to remove the foreign material from the periapical area as soon as possible, preferably within 48 h [218]. Surgery is indicated when neurotoxic material migrates along the mandibular nerve bundle, and the nerve must be exposed for debridement [218, 232, 233].

Other possible invasive methods of treatment are extraction of the tooth or incision and drainage [228]. The clinical examination that results in a diagnosis of anesthesia or increasing painful dysesthesia unresponsive to nonsurgical therapy should help guide this decision [234, 235]. It is suggested that the decision to intervene surgically should include the high suspicion of injury resulting in the loss of conduction within the nerve because of suspected chemical toxicity and mechanical compression. The favorable results for long-term spontaneous recovery require thoughtful considerations for taking a "wait-and-observe" approach. When a peripheral nerve is injured, a nonsurgical management that supports spontaneous neurosensory recovery and promotes patient tolerance of the sensory loss is a viable option [234–236]. The most compelling reason to wait is that a majority of injuries are known to recover spontaneously to some degree. Higher levels of recovery can also be expected when the patient is young and healthy. Ørstavik et al. [237] reported that out of 24 patients with paresthesia affecting the mandibular nerve, 14 showed no healing from 3 months to 18 years after the injury; all of the reported cases were lower molars or second premolars. Radiographs are often useful in monitoring the area of tissue damage in relation to hard tissues (e.g., the size and location of lesion or the location of the extruded material in relation to mandibular canal) [188, 189, 212]. It is not always possible to make a precise diagnosis of extrusion into the nerve by showing the contact of the filling material with the alveolar nerves using traditional endodontic radiographs.

One of the major problems is that intraoral radiographs only reveal limited information. The amount of information gained from analogue and digital periapical radiographs is incomplete because the three-dimensional anatomy of the area being radiographed is compressed into a two-dimensional image or shadowgraph [238]. Patel et al. [239] demonstrated CBCT's superior diagnostic accuracy compared with intraoral radiographs [238]. Cone beam computed tomography can be considered an effective radiographic diagnostic device when endodontic-related inferior alveolar nerve or mental foramen paresthesia is suspected, and it is especially useful in the planning of surgical procedures [240–243].

6.4.3 The Management of the Extrusion of Filling Materials and Its Complications

In cases of overextension with the lateral compaction technique or of a thermoplastic core carrier, the filling material can often be teased back through the foramen, provided the sealer has not hardened. If the sealer has hardened, it may still be possible to retrieve the gutta-percha. In cases of overextension, when retraction of the filling material through the apical foramen is difficult, the routine and immediate use of surgical intervention is neither indicated nor justified. In most cases, the periradicular tissues will heal, and the patient will be symptom-free. If, however, the patient exhibits signs or symptoms of periradicular inflammation, surgery may be indicated. Treatment of endodontically related paresthesia remains controversial, varying from a wait-and-see approach [237] to early [244], if not immediate [245], surgical debridement of the inferior alveolar nerve via a number of possible approaches. These include extraction of the tooth and approaching the nerve through the socket [244], decortication of the mandible achieved laterally [245] from an intraoral [246] and extraoral [227] approach, and sagittal splitting of the mandible to expose the nerve within the split [233]. The use of biocompatible materials did not suggest an immediate surgical approach, but rather a wait-and-see approach, even when the maxillary sinus may be involved. It is well known that toxicity tends to reduce and the extruded filling material undergoes resorption over time. In any case, the dangers of any extruded materials during root canal treatment should be highlighted, even if only a limited overfilling occurs, especially in proximity to important anatomical areas.

In conclusion, although proper techniques have been followed, occasionally gutta-percha, resin-bonded filling materials, or root canal sealer may be unintentionally pushed beyond the confines of the root canal system. However, the periradicular tissues generally tolerate these materials. Although sealers may provoke an initial inflammatory response to a greater or lesser degree over a short period, the macrophage scavenger system eliminates the excessive material from the periradicular tissues. In any case, the mere placement of filling material outside the canal system is not a major cause for alarm if the canal space is three-dimensionally obturated. If excessive amounts of materials are extruded, the patient should be informed, and periodic reexaminations are indicated.

6.4.4 Complications Due to Chemical Effects

6.4.4.1 Toxic Effects of Root Canal Filling Materials

Since they are classified as medical devices, root canal sealers and core materials need to meet biocompatibility requirements, which include the evaluation of cytotoxicity potential, in addition to exhibiting proper chemical, physical, and mechanical properties.

During the last three decades, biological properties, or biocompatibility, of a dental material have become increasingly important. Currently, there are mandatory regulatory requirements as well as voluntary standards at national and international levels [247–249]. The European Society of Endodontology guidelines for endodontic therapy state that "the objective of any (endodontic) technique used should be to apply a biocompatible hermetically sealing canal filling that obturates the prepared canal space from pulp chamber just to its apical termination" [250]. An ideal root canal filling material, in addition to have suitable chemical and physical properties, should be biologically compatible and well tolerated by the periapical tissues, avoiding any possible modification and delay of the healing process [251].

The biocompatibility of root canal filling materials has been of concern to dentistry for many decades now because they can come into contact with the connective periapical tissue [252], and the components released from these materials could produce irritation or even degeneration of the surrounding tissues [253]. The periapical tissues can react to the presence of a sealer and a GP point in several ways. It can cause an inflammatory reaction, it can be regarded as a foreign body and encapsulated, and it can be present without causing inflammatory reactions and is not encapsulated, and the sealer can be resorbed over time, with or without an inflammatory reaction.

It has been reported that the extrusion of root filling substances can cause a foreign body reaction leading to the development of periapical lesions that may be refractory to endodontic therapy [229, 254]. Large quantities of excess filling materials in the periapical tissues caused necrosis of bone followed by bone resorption and absorption of the filling materials, despite gutta-percha having a low degree of toxicity when compared with other components used in endodontic obturation [229]. In fact, gutta-percha is the most common component used in root canal filling materials because it is well tolerated from host tissues [255], but other compounds such as zinc oxide-eugenol are capable of inducing cytotoxic effects [178, 256]. On the other side, sealers and components of sealers are recognized by the scientific literature as toxic or highly irritating, especially in their freshly mixed states, and produces an initial acute inflammatory reaction in the connective tissues [178, 257].

However, after setting or curing, some sealers become relatively inert, and it has to be underlined that pastes and sealers will be absorbed more rapidly than solid core materials [258]. If over a relatively short period of time (up to 30 days) a mild inflammation is present and it has diminished over time, a material with otherwise favorable properties can be considered acceptable [259].

Elution of components has been recognized [260], and the inflammatory process as a result of this is the body's response to irritation. Fibrous encapsulation is the body's response to isolate an otherwise biocompatible material. Furthermore, a material, usually small-size particles, can be present in periapical tissues, cause no inflammation, and be present without encapsulation.

Calcium hydroxide sealers. Some studies in rats [261] and dogs reported neurotoxic effects of hydroxide, with partial recovery after various periods of time [262, 263]. A study on human fibroblasts showed early severity cytotoxic effects of calcium hydroxide in the first 48 h with significant reduction in toxicity between the third and fifth day [264].

Paraformaldehyde pastes. Paraformaldehyde paste materials cause mummification and fixation of pulp tissue [265]. In 1959, Sargenti and Richter introduced N2 and subsequently other paraformaldehyde paste formulations, because of their consistent antimicrobial activity when used as root canal filling materials [266]. Thus N2, RC2B, endomethosone, and other paraformaldehyde paste formulations were recommended as the sole filling material. Unfortunately, absorbability and toxicity are serious considerations with paraformaldehyde pastes. A large number of studies reported paresthesia and other complications of the inferior alveolar nerve due to the neurotoxicity of these paraformaldehyde compounds [55, 224, 237, 246, 266–270].

Others have demonstrated the systemic distribution of paraformaldehyde and disintegration products in periapical and periodontal tissues, as well in the blood, regional lymph nodes, kidney, and liver [271]. Moreover several clinical reports of extreme complications have been published [55, 227, 237, 272]. At the present time, the use of N2 or similar type pastes is contraindicated, because of the higher risks associated with these paraformaldehyde-containing endodontic materials.

Polymer and resin sealers. The most commonly known sealers within this category are AH26 and AH26 Plus (Caulk/Dentsply, Milford, DE, USA). The sealer has been reported to be very toxic upon initial mixing [229, 273], due mainly to the formation of a very small amount of formaldehyde as a result of the chemical setting process [229, 273]. However toxicity resolves rapidly within 24 h during the setting process [229]. Diaket (ESPE, Seefeld, Germany) is a polyketone compound adhesive sealer. It has been demonstrated that it is relatively toxic during setting and these effects are persistent [273]. Resorcinol-formalin resin is a paste filling material that is commonly used in Russia, China, and India for the treatment of pulpitis. Although there are many variations of the resin pastes that are used, the main ingredients are resorcinol and formaldehyde [274]. When set, this material creates an almost impenetrable barrier, with loss of the retreatment option [275]. If the paste material is extruded beyond the apical foramen, severe toxic effects may arise. In the event of an overfill into the sinus or neurovascular bundle, irreversible damage may also occur [274].

6.4.4.2 Discoloration

Almost all materials used in modern endodontics may stain teeth. However, for a wide range of materials currently available on the market, there is only scarce or no evidence available on their staining ability.

Endodontic sealers. Parsons et al. [276] assessed coronal discolorations produced by four different sealers (Sealapex, Roth's 801, AH26, and Kerr Pulp Canal Sealer) and reported that all of the experimental teeth revealed coronal discoloration; this effect was attributed to the silver ions that were part of the composition of both materials. A follow-up study published by the same group assessed the penetration depth of the same four sealers into the dentin [277]. All four sealers showed only minimal sealer penetration and no evidence of discoloration of the exposed dentinal surfaces. The findings were assumed to be a result of the smear layer not having been removed, which may prevent the materials from diffusing into the dentin. However, the 2-year set sealers in the endodontic cavity showed marked levels of discoloration compared to fresh mixes.

A recent study assessed the degree of staining in tooth crowns caused by commonly used endodontic sealers via a computer analysis method [278]. Discoloration induced by the root canal sealers AH26, Endofill, Tubuli Seal, zinc oxide-eugenol (ZnOE), Apatite Root Canal Sealer III, gutta-percha, and Cavizol (a filling material containing ZnOE) was assessed on extracted human premolars. After 3, 6, and 9 months, the order of severity of tooth discoloration (from the highest to lowest values) was as follows: amalgam = Endofill > ZOE > Tubli Seal > AH26 > gutta-percha > Apatite Root Sealer III > Cavizol > distilled water. For all groups, the discoloration was most evident in the cervical third of the crown and on the cervical root surface. Elkhazin investigated the discoloration effects of AH Plus, EndoRez, Sealapex, and Kerr Pulp Canal. The teeth were root-filled with gutta-percha with one of the four materials. After 6 and 8 weeks, all four sealers showed significant coronal discoloration, which increased with time [279].

Portland cement-based materials. Mineral trioxide aggregate (MTA) is based on portland cement and was introduced to the field of endodontics in 1993. Owing to its high level of biocompatibility and its good sealing properties, it is regarded as the material of choice in cases of vital pulp therapy (pulp capping, partial pulpotomy) or to seal pathways of communication between the root canal system and the external root surface (perforation, apexification, or retrograde filling) [95, 280]. One of the main drawbacks of MTA is its discoloration potential [94]. The gray-colored formula, which was first introduced to the market, led to visible color changes on the outer surface. When it was used as a pulpotomy agent in primary molars, discoloration occurred in 60% of all cases [281].

To reduce the discoloration potential, the chemical composition of MTA was changed and an improved formulation was later introduced as white MTA. The most significant difference between the two types of MTA is the lack of iron ions in white MTA [282, 283]. However, it has been reported that white MTA may cause discoloration as well [282, 283]. Some authors state that the discoloration induced by MTA may be attributed to bismuth oxide, which is added to improve the radiopacity in both gray and white formulations [282, 283]. Mineral trioxide aggregate (MTA) has been successfully used in perforations of the root canal. Bortoluzzi et al. [284] reported a clinical case of a root perforation sealed with gray MTA that resulted in discoloration of the marginal gingiva. Treatment consisted of replacing gray MTA with white MTA with the aid of a dental operating microscope, producing satisfactory esthetic results.

Resorcinol-formalin resin materials. A deep brownish to red discoloration of the tooth structure given by resorcinol-formalin resin material when set has been clearly reported [275] (Fig. 6.9).

6.4.5 Complications Due to Heat

One of the drawbacks of warm gutta-percha techniques is the elevated temperature on the external root surface. Among possible types of factors that can cause tissue damage, tissue overheating because of incorrect warm condensation techniques should be also considered [188, 218]. In a series of in vitro [285] and in vivo studies on dogs [286], the heat of thermoplasticized gutta-percha was evaluated for its potential injurious effects. Eriksson and Albrektsson [287] concluded that exposure to a temperature of 47° C caused fat cell necrosis and irreversible bone damage in rabbit tibia. Therefore, dental procedures that increase the outer root surface temperature above the accepted critical level (10° C) may result in periodontal tissue

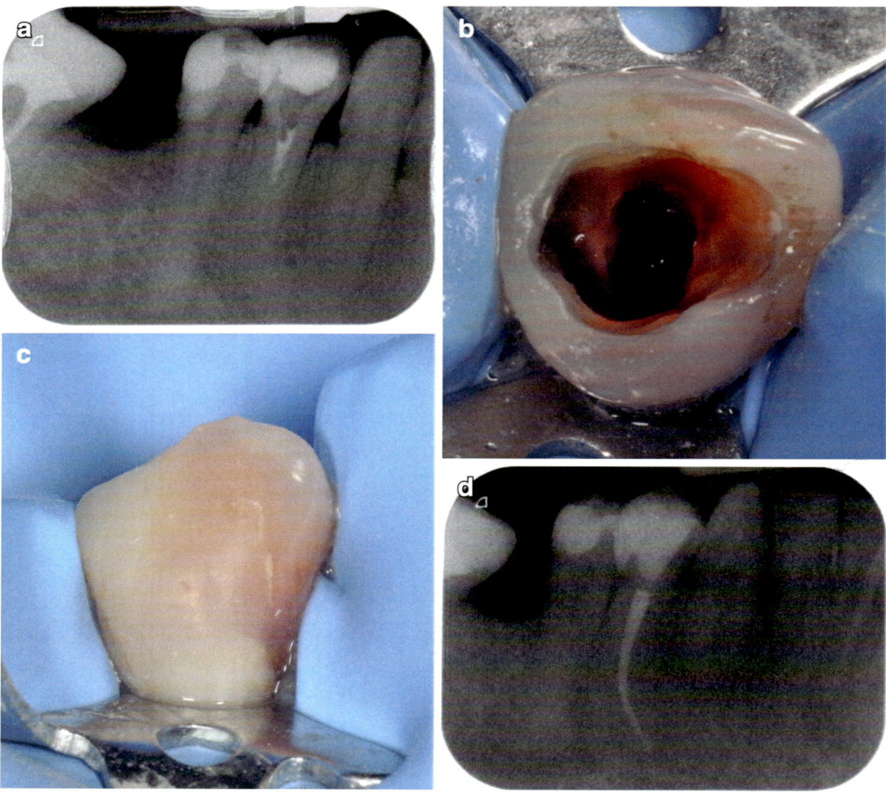

Fig. 6.9 Retreatment of a lower premolar filled with resorcinol-formalin resin "Russian red" material (**a**) which created an important discoloration of the tooth ((**b**), (**c**)). (**d**) Two-years control radiograph

destruction. In particular, the surface temperature of roots with a thin dentinal wall was reported to be increased over this threshold when the canals were filled with thermoplastic gutta-percha techniques [288]. The use of heat and the potential for injurious heat transfer to the dentin and bone has been investigated for several different devices used in endodontics and associated restorative procedures [287, 289–292]. McCullagh et al. [293] studied the pattern of temperature rise on the root surface associated with thermomechanical obturation using the Gutta Condensor. The maximum temperatures recorded would place demands on the surrounding tissues and blood supply to dissipate this heat.

Floren et al. [294] reported that any temperature setting of the System B HeatSource at or above 250° C has the potential to cause the root surface temperature to rise 10 °C. Whether this occurs in vivo or if it is maintained long enough to cause any tissue damage, remains to be determined. On the other side, Romero et al. [295] using the System B measured the temperatures transferred to the outer surface of the root during obturation. The average temperature increase was approximately 1° C at the apex and approximately 2° at the 5 mm mark. The resulting temperature increase appear not to allow for the heat disseminating effect of the PDL. Using the Thermafil Plus system, Behnia and McDonald [296] found temperatures well below the critical level of 10 °C that cause damage to the attachment apparatus. Clinical case reports reporting overfill with heat-softened gutta-percha are increasing in the literature [246, 297]. Lipsky [165] obturated maxillary and mandibular central incisors with the injected gutta-percha heated to 160 °C (Obtura II): temperature changes on the mesial outer surface of the roots resulted in the rises of the root surface temperature by 8.5 °C (no damage) and 22.1 °C (dangerous), respectively.

Only a few investigators and authors have cautioned that ultrasonic energy can be harmful through heat generation [163, 290]. In clinical situations, Bailey et al. [163] using ultrasonic condensation of gutta-percha found that the combination of a high-power setting and a 15 s application of energy induced a temperature rise on the root surface beyond the recognized deleterious threshold of 10° centigrade. Ulusoy et al. [298] reported that the use of System B and Obtura II for filling canals with internal resorptive cavities resulted in surface temperature rise over the critical threshold; however, Soft-Core root filling did not increase the temperature over 10 °C.

6.4.6 Complications Due to Mechanical Damage

Another obturation-related complication may be linked to the use of metal spreaders and pluggers during the lateral and vertical compaction of gutta-percha. These rigid instruments may create root distortions and sometimes dentinal defects, tooth cracks, or fracture, if the elastic coefficient of the root dentin is exceeded, especially when used in curved root canals [299] (Fig. 6.10).

Lateral compaction is commonly used to fill the root canal system, and its use may be associated with increased VRF (vertical root fracture) risk [300, 301], from the spreader design and forces applied during the lateral compaction procedure [302–307]. While doing lateral compaction obturation technique, a metal spreader that reaches the working length or within 0.5 mm should be chosen and fitted in the canal to compact the master cone apically and laterally and subsequently to compact the accessory cones more coronally. The main risk of this technique is to exert excessive apical force or to inadvertently perform oblique lateral movement with the metal spreader that may cause root fracture or dentinal cracks [303, 308] (Fig. 6.11). Recent research suggests that decreased stress on root structure when compacting with NiTi finger spreaders exists, thus potentially decreasing the chance of vertical root fracture [300, 309]. For the same reason, fitting of the root canal pluggers is of importance when a warm vertical or continuous wave of condensation technique is performed. Pluggers must be prefitted to ensure depth of penetration into the apical third of the canal

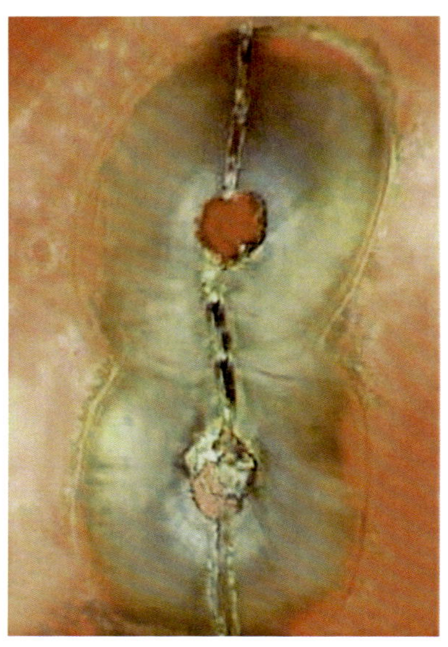

Fig. 6.10 A buccolingual longitudinal vertical root fracture due to excessive vertical forces of condensation to the root canal walls that lead to extraction of an upper first premolar tooth

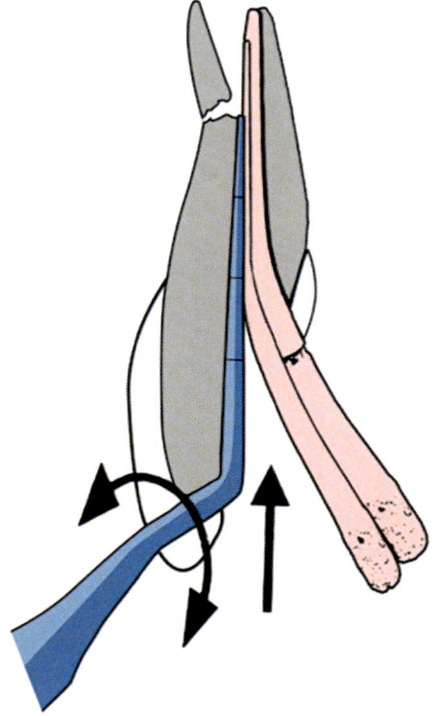

Fig. 6.11 A drawing explaining the possible mechanism of root fracture caused by the incorrect use of spreaders during lateral compaction of gutta-percha technique

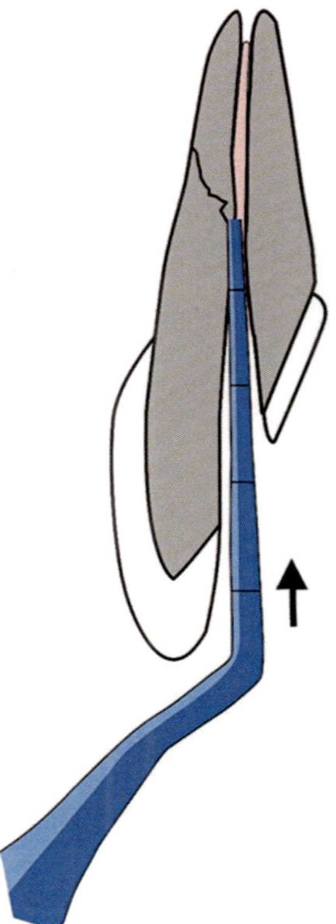

Fig. 6.12 A drawing explaining the possible mechanism of root crack caused by the incorrect use of pluggers during vertical compaction of gutta-percha

without binding on the canal walls (Fig. 6.12). In fact, if binding should occur, there is a chance for tooth fracture by exerting excessive pressures on the root canal walls (Fig. 6.13).

To decrease such damage, certain filling techniques use no compaction force while creating apical sealing similar to that of lateral compaction [300, 310, 311]. The use of NiTi finger spreader during lateral condensation can lead clinicians to reduce the axial force of condensation and consequently the risk of mechanical damage to the root [309, 312–314]. VRFs are a particularly significant clinical problem because they are associated with a poor prognosis for the affected tooth [275, 315] and often lead to tooth extraction [301, 316]. Root fractures may originate from preexisting dentinal defects (e.g., craze lines or incomplete cracks). Diagnosing and locating crack lines are difficult in clinical trials [317], even though cone beam computed tomography has improved VRF diagnosis [194, 250, 318, 319]. Thus, a cautious and rigorous clinical approach to the diagnosis and follow-up of suspected VRFs should be performed [250, 318].

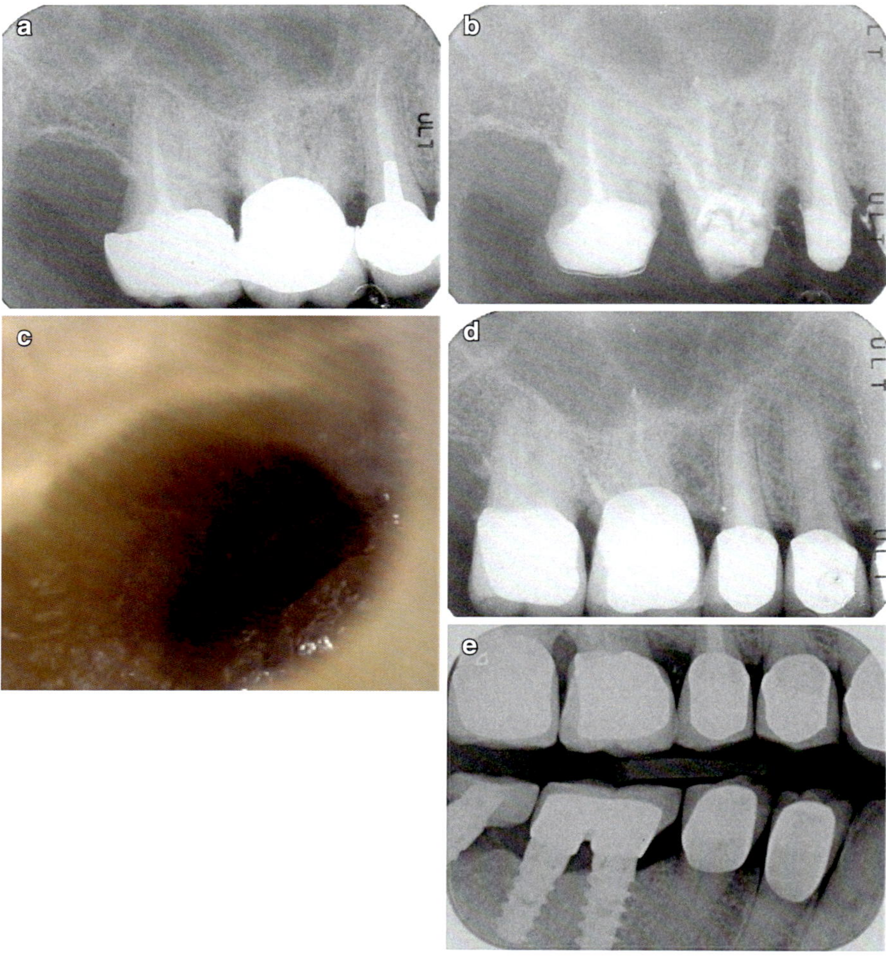

Fig. 6.13 An upper first molar has been retreated due to persistent apical periodontitis in the mesiobuccal root (**a**). A vertical root fracture has been detected after the filling procedures (**b**) causing persistent pain to pressure and probably due to a preexisting dentinal crack (**c**). One-year radiographic control after extraction of the mesiobuccal root and prosthetic restorations (**d**, **e**)

References

1. Kakehashi S, Stanley HR, Fitzgerald RJ. The effects of surgical exposures of dental pulps in germ-free and conventional laboratory rats. Oral Surg Oral Med Oral Pathol. 1965;20:340–9.
2. Quality guidelines for endodontic treatment: consensus report of the European Society of Endodontology. Int Endod J. 2006;39(12):921–930.
3. Siqueira JF Jr, Araujo MC, Garcia PF, Fraga RC, Dantas CJ. Histological evaluation of the effectiveness of five instrumentation techniques for cleaning the apical third of root canals. J Endod. 1997;23(8):499–502.

4. Barrieshi-Nusair KM, Hammad HM. Intracoronal sealing comparison of mineral trioxide aggregate and glass ionomer. Quintessence Int (Berlin, Germany: 1985). 2005;36(7–8):539–45.
5. Jack RM, Goodell GG. In vitro comparison of coronal microleakage between Resilon alone and gutta-percha with a glass-ionomer intraorifice barrier using a fluid filtration model. J Endod. 2008;34(6):718–20.
6. Mavec JC, McClanahan SB, Minah GE, Johnson JD, Blundell RE Jr. Effects of an intracanal glass ionomer barrier on coronal microleakage in teeth with post space. J Endod. 2006;32(2):120–2.
7. Shipper G, Orstavik D, Teixeira FB, Trope M. An evaluation of microbial leakage in roots filled with a thermoplastic synthetic polymer-based root canal filling material (Resilon). J Endod. 2004;30(5):342–7.
8. Schilder H. Filling root canals in three dimensions. Dent Clin N Am. 1967:723–44.
9. Schilder H. Cleaning and shaping the root canal. Dent Clin N Am. 1974;18(2):269–96.
10. Saunders WP, Saunders EM. Coronal leakage as a cause of failure in root-canal therapy: a review. Endod Dent Traumatol. 1994;10(3):105–8.
11. Sundqvist G, Figdor D, Persson S, Sjogren U. Microbiologic analysis of teeth with failed endodontic treatment and the outcome of conservative re-treatment. Oral Surg Oral Med Oral Pathol Oral Radiol Endod. 1998;85(1):86–93.
12. Bergenholtz G, Spangberg L. Controversies in endodontics. Crit Rev Oral Biol Med. 2004;15(2):99–114.
13. Ng YL, Mann V, Gulabivala K. Outcome of secondary root canal treatment: a systematic review of the literature. Int Endod J. 2008;41(12):1026–46.
14. Ng YL, Mann V, Rahbaran S, Lewsey J, Gulabivala K. Outcome of primary root canal treatment: systematic review of the literature - part 1. Effects of study characteristics on probability of success. Int Endod J. 2007;40(12):921–39.
15. Setzer FC, Kim S. Comparison of long-term survival of implants and endodontically treated teeth. J Dent Res. 2014;93(1):19–26.
16. Azim AA, Griggs JA, Huang GT. The Tennessee study: factors affecting treatment outcome and healing time following nonsurgical root canal treatment. Int Endod J. 2016;49(1):6–16.
17. Bernstein SD, Horowitz AJ, Man M, Wu H, Foran D, Vena DA, et al. Outcomes of endodontic therapy in general practice: a study by the practitioners engaged in applied research and learning network. J Am Dent Assoc. 2012;143(5):478–87.
18. Imura N, Pinheiro ET, Gomes BP, Zaia AA, Ferraz CC, Souza-Filho FJ. The outcome of endodontic treatment: a retrospective study of 2000 cases performed by a specialist. J Endod. 2007;33(11):1278–82.
19. Kim S, Jung H, Kim S, Shin SJ, Kim E. The influence of an isthmus on the outcomes of surgically treated molars: a retrospective study. J Endod. 2016;42(7):1029–34.
20. Somma F, Leoni D, Plotino G, Grande NM, Plasschaert A. Root canal morphology of the mesiobuccal root of maxillary first molars: a micro-computed tomographic analysis. Int Endod J. 2009;42(2):165–74.
21. Vertucci FJ. Root canal anatomy of the human permanent teeth. Oral Surg Oral Med Oral Pathol. 1984;58(5):589–99.
22. Bystrom A, Sundqvist G. Bacteriologic evaluation of the efficacy of mechanical root canal instrumentation in endodontic therapy. Scand J Dent Res. 1981;89(4):321–8.
23. Pataky L, Ivanyi I, Grigar A, Fazekas A. Antimicrobial efficacy of various root canal preparation techniques: an in vitro comparative study. J Endod. 2002;28(8):603–5.
24. Zandi H, Rodrigues RC, Kristoffersen AK, Enersen M, Mdala I, Orstavik D, et al. Antibacterial effectiveness of 2 root canal Irrigants in root-filled teeth with infection: a randomized clinical trial. J Endod. 2016;42(9):1307–13.
25. Fedorowicz Z, Nasser M, Sequeira-Byron P, de Souza RF, Carter B, Heft M. Irrigants for non-surgical root canal treatment in mature permanent teeth. Cochrane Database Syst Rev. 2012;12(9):Cd008948.
26. Goncalves LS, Rodrigues RC, Andrade Junior CV, Soares RG, Vettore MV. The effect of sodium hypochlorite and Chlorhexidine as Irrigant solutions for root canal disinfection: a systematic review of clinical trials. J Endod. 2016;42(4):527–32.

27. Orstavik D, Kerekes K, Molven O. Effects of extensive apical reaming and calcium hydroxide dressing on bacterial infection during treatment of apical periodontitis: a pilot study. Int Endod J. 1991;24(1):1–7.
28. Siqueira JF Jr, Lima KC, Magalhaes FA, Lopes HP, de Uzeda M. Mechanical reduction of the bacterial population in the root canal by three instrumentation techniques. J Endod. 1999;25(5):332–5.
29. Clark-Holke D, Drake D, Walton R, Rivera E, Guthmiller JM. Bacterial penetration through canals of endodontically treated teeth in the presence or absence of the smear layer. J Dent. 2003;31(4):275–81.
30. Siqueira JF Jr, Rocas IN. Clinical implications and microbiology of bacterial persistence after treatment procedures. J Endod. 2008;34(11):1291–1301.e1293.
31. Taylor JK, Jeansonne BG, Lemon RR. Coronal leakage: effects of smear layer, obturation technique, and sealer. J Endod. 1997;23(8):508–12.
32. Violich DR, Chandler NP. The smear layer in endodontics—a review. Int Endod J. 2010;43(1):2–15.
33. White RR, Goldman M, Lin PS. The influence of the smeared layer upon dentinal tubule penetration by plastic filling materials. J Endod. 1984;10(12):558–62.
34. Oksan T, Aktener BO, Sen BH, Tezel H. The penetration of root canal sealers into dentinal tubules. A scanning electron microscopic study. Int Endod J. 1993;26(5):301–5.
35. White RR, Goldman M, Lin PS. The influence of the smeared layer upon dentinal tubule penetration by endodontic filling materials. Part II. J Endod. 1987;13(8):369–74.
36. American Association of Endodontists. Colleagues for excellence. Obturation of Root Canal Systems. 2009.
37. Grossman LI. Root canal therapy. Philadelphia: Lea & Febiger; 1940.
38. Koch CRET, B.L.T. A history of dentistry. Fort Wayne, IN: National Art; 1909.
39. Grossman LI. Endodontics 1776–1976: a bicentennial history against the background of general dentistry. J Am Dent Assoc. 1976;93(1):78–87.
40. Perry SG. Preparing and filling the roots of teeth. Dental Cosmos. 1883;25:1.
41. Keane HC. A century of service to dentistry. Philadelphia: SS White Dental; 1944.
42. Weinberger BW. An introduction to the history of dentistry. St. Louis, MO: Mosby; 1948.
43. Callahan JR. Rosin solution for the sealing of the dental tubuli as an adjuvant in the filling of root canals. J Allied Dent Soc. 1914;9:110.
44. Cohen SB, History RC. In: Company CM, editor. Pathways of the pulp. St. Louis, MO: Elsevier; 1980. p. 687–701.
45. Brady JM, del Rio CE. Corrosion of endodontic silver cones in humans: a scanning electron microscope and X-ray microprobe study. J Endod. 1975;1(6):205–10.
46. Goldberg F. Relation between corroded silver points and endodontic failures. J Endod. 1981;7(5):224–7.
47. Seltzer S, Green DB, Weiner N, DeRenzis F. A scanning electron microscope examination of silver cones removed from endodontically treated teeth. Oral Surg Oral Med Oral Pathol. 1972;33(4):589–605.
48. Sargenti A. Endodontic course for the general practitioner. 3rd ed. Bruxelles, Belgium: EES; 1965.
49. Sargenti A. The endodontic debate ends? CDS Rev. 1977;70(1):28–9.
50. Sargenti A. The Sargenti N-2 method. Dent Surv. 1978;54(10):55–8.
51. Oswald RJ, Cohn SA. Systemic distribution of lead from root canal fillings. J Endod. 1975;1(2):59–63.
52. Block RM, Lewis RD, Hirsch J, Coffey J, Langeland K. Systemic distribution of N2 paste containing 14C paraformaldehyde following root canal therapy in dogs. Oral Surg Oral Med Oral Pathol. 1980;50(4):350–60.
53. Cohler CM, Newton CW, Patterson SS, Kafrawy AH. Studies of Sargenti's technique of endodontic treatment: short-term response in monkeys. J Endod. 1980;6(3):473–8.
54. Gutmann JL. Adaptation of injected thermoplasticized gutta-percha in the absence of the dentinal smear layer. Int Endod J. 1993;26(2):87–92.

55. Kleier DJ, Averbach RE. Painful dysesthesia of the inferior alveolar nerve following use of a paraformaldehyde-containing root canal sealer. Endod Dent Traumatol. 1988;4(1):46–8.
56. Peng L, Ye L, Tan H, Zhou X. Outcome of root canal obturation by warm gutta-percha versus cold lateral condensation: a meta-analysis. J Endod. 2007;33(2):106–9.
57. Schaeffer MA, White RR, Walton RE. Determining the optimal obturation length: a meta-analysis of literature. J Endod. 2005;31(4):271–4.
58. Chugal NM, Clive JM, Spangberg LS. A prognostic model for assessment of the outcome of endodontic treatment: effect of biologic and diagnostic variables. Oral Surg Oral Med Oral Pathol Oral Radiol Endod. 2001;91(3):342–52.
59. Ray HA, Trope M. Periapical status of endodontically treated teeth in relation to the technical quality of the root filling and the coronal restoration. Int Endod J. 1995;28(1):12–8.
60. Hata G, Kawazoe S, Toda T, Weine FS. Sealing ability of Thermafil with and without sealer. J Endod. 1992;18(7):322–6.
61. Najar AL, Saquy PC, Vansan LP, Sousa-Neto MD. Adhesion of a glass-ionomer root canal sealer to human dentine. Aust Endod J. 2003;29(1):20–2.
62. Gutmann JL, Rakusin H. Perspectives on root canal obturation with thermoplasticized injectable gutta-percha. Int Endod J. 1987;20(6):261–70.
63. Yesilsoy C, Koren LZ, Morse DR, Kobayashi C. A comparative tissue toxicity evaluation of established and newer root canal sealers. Oral Surg Oral Med Oral Pathol. 1988;65(4):459–67.
64. Carvalho-Junior JR, Guimaraes LF, Correr-Sobrinho L, Pecora JD, Sousa-Neto MD. Evaluation of solubility, disintegration, and dimensional alterations of a glass ionomer root canal sealer. Braz Dent J. 2003;14(2):114–8.
65. Versiani MA, Carvalho-Junior JR, Padilha MI, Lacey S, Pascon EA, Sousa-Neto MD. A comparative study of physicochemical properties of AH plus and epiphany root canal sealants. Int Endod J. 2006;39(6):464–71.
66. Ersahan S, Aydin C. Dislocation resistance of iRoot SP, a calcium silicate-based sealer, from radicular dentine. J Endod. 2010;36(12):2000–2.
67. Tagger M, Tagger E, Tjan AH, Bakland LK. Measurement of adhesion of endodontic sealers to dentin. J Endod. 2002;28(5):351–4.
68. Zhou HM, Shen Y, Zheng W, Li L, Zheng YF, Haapasalo M. Physical properties of 5 root canal sealers. J Endod. 2013;39(10):1281–6.
69. Borges RP, Sousa-Neto MD, Versiani MA, Rached-Junior FA, De-Deus G, Miranda CE, et al. Changes in the surface of four calcium silicate-containing endodontic materials and an epoxy resin-based sealer after a solubility test. Int Endod J. 2012;45(5):419–28.
70. Kim TG, Lee YH, Lee NH, Bhattarai G, Lee IK, Yun BS, et al. The antioxidant property of pachymic acid improves bone disturbance against AH plus-induced inflammation in MC-3T3 E1 cells. J Endod. 2013;39(4):461–6.
71. Schweikl H, Schmalz G, Federlin M. Mutagenicity of the root canal sealer AHPlus in the Ames test. Clin Oral Investig. 1998;2(3):125–9.
72. Camps J, About I. Cytotoxicity testing of endodontic sealers: a new method. J Endod. 2003;29(9):583–6.
73. Eldeniz AU, Mustafa K, Orstavik D, Dahl JE. Cytotoxicity of new resin-, calcium hydroxide- and silicone-based root canal sealers on fibroblasts derived from human gingiva and L929 cell lines. Int Endod J. 2007;40(5):329–37.
74. Leyhausen G, Heil J, Reifferscheid G, Waldmann P, Geurtsen W. Genotoxicity and cytotoxicity of the epoxy resin-based root canal sealer AH plus. J Endod. 1999;25(2):109–13.
75. Bouillaguet S, Wataha JC, Lockwood PE, Galgano C, Golay A, Krejci I. Cytotoxicity and sealing properties of four classes of endodontic sealers evaluated by succinic dehydrogenase activity and confocal laser scanning microscopy. Eur J Oral Sci. 2004;112(2):182–7.
76. Fujisawa S, Atsumi T. Cytotoxicities of a 4-META/MMA-TBBO resin against human pulp fibroblasts. Dent Mater J. 2004;23(2):106–8.
77. Huumonen S, Lenander-Lumikari M, Sigurdsson A, Orstavik D. Healing of apical periodontitis after endodontic treatment: a comparison between a silicone-based and a zinc oxide-eugenol-based sealer. Int Endod J. 2003;36(4):296–301.

78. Wu MK, Tigos E, Wesselink PR. An 18-month longitudinal study on a new silicon-based sealer, RSA RoekoSeal: a leakage study in vitro. Oral Surg Oral Med Oral Pathol Oral Radiol Endod. 2002;94(4):499–502.
79. Miletic I, Anic I, Karlovic Z, Marsan T, Pezelj-Ribaric S, Osmak M. Cytotoxic effect of four root filling materials. Endod Dent Traumatol. 2000;16(6):287–90.
80. Schwarze T, Leyhausen G, Geurtsen W. Long-term cytocompatibility of various endodontic sealers using a new root canal model. J Endod. 2002;28(11):749–53.
81. Hovland EJ, Dumsha TC. Leakage evaluation in vitro of the root canal sealer cement Sealapex. Int Endod J. 1985;18(3):179–82.
82. Huang FM, Tai KW, Chou MY, Chang YC. Cytotoxicity of resin-, zinc oxide-eugenol-, and calcium hydroxide-based root canal sealers on human periodontal ligament cells and permanent V79 cells. Int Endod J. 2002;35(2):153–8.
83. Aboush YE, Jenkins CB. An evaluation of the bonding of glass-ionomer restoratives to dentine and enamel. Br Dent J. 1986;161(5):179–84.
84. Powis DR, Folleras T, Merson SA, Wilson AD. Improved adhesion of a glass ionomer cement to dentin and enamel. J Dent Res. 1982;61(12):1416–22.
85. Timpawat S, Harnirattisai C, Senawongs P. Adhesion of a glass-ionomer root canal sealer to the root canal wall. J Endod. 2001;27(3):168–71.
86. Vollenweider M, Brunner TJ, Knecht S, Grass RN, Zehnder M, Imfeld T, et al. Remineralization of human dentin using ultrafine bioactive glass particles. Acta Biomater. 2007;3(6):936–43.
87. Gubler M, Brunner TJ, Zehnder M, Waltimo T, Sener B, Stark WJ. Do bioactive glasses convey a disinfecting mechanism beyond a mere increase in pH? Int Endod J. 2008;41(8):670–8.
88. Wang Z, Shen Y, Haapasalo M. Dentin extends the antibacterial effect of endodontic sealers against enterococcus faecalis biofilms. J Endod. 2014;40(4):505–8.
89. Zhang H, Shen Y, Ruse ND, Haapasalo M. Antibacterial activity of endodontic sealers by modified direct contact test against enterococcus faecalis. J Endod. 2009;35(7):1051–5.
90. Zhang W, Li Z, Peng B. Ex vivo cytotoxicity of a new calcium silicate-based canal filling material. Int Endod J. 2010;43(9):769–74.
91. Zhang W, Li Z, Peng B. Assessment of a new root canal sealer's apical sealing ability. Oral Surg Oral Med Oral Pathol Oral Radiol Endod. 2009;107(6):e79–82.
92. Ersahan S, Aydin C. Solubility and apical sealing characteristics of a new calcium silicate-based root canal sealer in comparison to calcium hydroxide-, methacrylate resin- and epoxy resin-based sealers. Acta Odontol Scand. 2013;71(3–4):857–62.
93. Nagas E, Uyanik MO, Eymirli A, Cehreli ZC, Vallittu PK, Lassila LV, et al. Dentin moisture conditions affect the adhesion of root canal sealers. J Endod. 2012;38(2):240–4.
94. Parirokh M, Torabinejad M. Mineral trioxide aggregate: a comprehensive literature review--part III: clinical applications, drawbacks, and mechanism of action. J Endod. 2010;36(3):400–13.
95. Torabinejad M, Parirokh M. Mineral trioxide aggregate: a comprehensive literature review—part II: leakage and biocompatibility investigations. J Endod. 2010;36(2):190–202.
96. Wang Z. Bioceramic materials in endodontics. Endod Top. 2015;32(1):3–30.
97. Haapasalo M, Parhar M, Huang X, Wei X, Lin J, Shen Y. Clinical use of bioceramic materials. Endod Top. 2015;32(1):97–117.
98. Koch K, Brave D, Nasseh AA. A review of bioceramic technology in endodontics. Roots. 2012;4:6–12.
99. Camilleri J, Pitt Ford TR. Mineral trioxide aggregate: a review of the constituents and biological properties of the material. Int Endod J. 2006;39(10):747–54.
100. Reyes-Carmona JF, Felippe MS, Felippe WT. Biomineralization ability and interaction of mineral trioxide aggregate and white portland cement with dentin in a phosphate-containing fluid. J Endod. 2009;35(5):731–6.
101. Schilder H, Goodman A, Aldrich W. The thermomechanical properties of gutta-percha. I. The compressibility of gutta-percha. Oral Surg Oral Med Oral Pathol. 1974;37(6):946–53.

102. Marciano J, Michailesco P, Abadie MJ. Stereochemical structure characterization of dental gutta-percha. J Endod. 1993;19(1):31–4.
103. Friedman CE, Sandrik JL, Heuer MA, Rapp GW. Composition and physical properties of gutta-percha endodontic filling materials. J Endod. 1977;3(8):304–8.
104. Wong M, Peters DD, Lorton L, Bernier WE. Comparison of gutta-percha filling techniques: three chloroform--gutta-percha filling techniques, part 2. J Endod. 1982;8(1):4–9.
105. Moorer WR, Genet JM. Antibacterial activity of gutta-percha cones attributed to the zinc oxide component. Oral Surg Oral Med Oral Pathol. 1982;53(5):508–17.
106. Tagger M, Gold A. Flow of various brands of Gutta-percha cones under in vitro thermomechanical compaction. J Endod. 1988;14(3):115–20.
107. Bunn CW. Molecular structure and rubber-like elasticity: I. The crystal structures of b gutta-percha, rubber and polychloroprene. Proc Math Phys Eng Sci. 1941;180:40–66.
108. Fisher D. Crystal structures of gutta-percha. Proc R Soc Lond A Biol Sci. 1952;66:7–16.
109. Schilder H, Goodman A, Aldrich W. The thermomechanical properties of gutta-percha. 3. Determination of phase transition temperatures for gutta-percha. Oral Surg Oral Med Oral Pathol. 1974;38(1):109–14.
110. Goppel JMA, J.J. The degree of crystallization in frozen row rubber and stretched vulcanized rubber. Appl Sci Res. 1948;1:310–9.
111. Smith TL. Strength and related properties of elastomeric block copolymers. IBM J Res Dev. 1977;21:154–67.
112. Budavari S, O'Neil MJ, Smith A, Heckelman PE, Kinneary J. The Merck index. 12th ed. Whitehouse Station, NJ: Merck; 1996.
113. Schilder H, Goodman A, Aldrich W. The thermomechanical properties of gutta-percha. Part V. Volume changes in bulk gutta-percha as a function of temperature and its relationship to molecular phase transformation. Oral Surg Oral Med Oral Pathol. 1985;59(3):285–96.
114. Mc ED. Physical properties of root canal filling materials. J Am Dent Assoc. 1955;50(4):433–40.
115. Meyer KM, Kollmar F, Schirrmeister JF, Schneider F, Hellwig E. Analysis of shrinkage of different gutta-percha types using optical measurement methods. Schweiz Monatsschr Zahnmed. 2006;116(4):356–61.
116. Shipper G, Trope M. In vitro microbial leakage of endodontically treated teeth using new and standard obturation techniques. J Endod. 2004;30(3):154–8.
117. Tay FR, Pashley DH. Monoblocks in root canals: a hypothetical or a tangible goal. J Endod. 2007;33(4):391–8.
118. Oliet S, Sorin SM. Effect of aging on the mechanical properties of hand-rolled gutta-percha endodontic cones. Oral Surg Oral Med Oral Pathol. 1977;43(6):954–62.
119. Hiraishi N, Yau JY, Loushine RJ, Armstrong SR, Weller RN, King NM, et al. Susceptibility of a polycaprolactone-based root canal-filling material to degradation. III. Turbidimetric evaluation of enzymatic hydrolysis. J Endod. 2007;33(8):952–6.
120. Tay FR, Pashley DH, Yiu CK, Yau JY, Yiu-fai M, Loushine RJ, et al. Susceptibility of a polycaprolactone-based root canal filling material to degradation. II. Gravimetric evaluation of enzymatic hydrolysis. J Endod. 2005;31(10):737–41.
121. Whatley JD, Spolnik KJ, Vail MM, Adams BH, Huang R, Gregory RL, et al. Susceptibility of methacrylate-based root canal filling to degradation by bacteria found in endodontic infections. Quintessence Int (Berlin, Germany: 1985). 2014;45(8):647–52.
122. Doyle MD, Loushine RJ, Agee KA, Gillespie WT, Weller RN, Pashley DH, et al. Improving the performance of EndoRez root canal sealer with a dual-cured two-step self-etch adhesive. I. Adhesive strength to dentin. J Endod. 2006;32(8):766–70.
123. Kardon BP, Kuttler S, Hardigan P, Dorn SO. An in vitro evaluation of the sealing ability of a new root-canal-obturation system. J Endod. 2003;29(10):658–61.
124. Tay FR, Loushine RJ, Monticelli F, Weller RN, Breschi L, Ferrari M, et al. Effectiveness of resin-coated gutta-percha cones and a dual-cured, hydrophilic methacrylate resin-based sealer in obturating root canals. J Endod. 2005;31(9):659–64.

125. Zmener O, Pameijer CH, Serrano SA, Vidueira M, Macchi RL. Significance of moist root canal dentin with the use of methacrylate-based endodontic sealers: an in vitro coronal dye leakage study. J Endod. 2008;34(1):76–9.
126. Nikhil V, Singh V, Singh S. Relationship between sealing ability of Activ GP and Gutta flow and methods of calcium hydroxide removal. J Conserv Dent. 2012;15(1):41–5.
127. Alani A, Knowles JC, Chrzanowski W, Ng YL, Gulabivala K. Ion release characteristics, precipitate formation and sealing ability of a phosphate glass-polycaprolactone-based composite for use as a root canal obturation material. Dent Mater. 2009;25(3):400–10.
128. Carvalho CN, Martinelli JR, Bauer J, Haapasalo M, Shen Y, Bradaschia-Correa V, et al. Micropush-out dentine bond strength of a new gutta-percha and niobium phosphate glass composite. Int Endod J. 2015;48(5):451–9.
129. Marending M, Bubenhofer SB, Sener B, De-Deus G. Primary assessment of a self-adhesive gutta-percha material. Int Endod J. 2013;46(4):317–22.
130. Mohn D, Zehnder M, Imfeld T, Stark WJ. Radio-opaque nanosized bioactive glass for potential root canal application: evaluation of radiopacity, bioactivity and alkaline capacity. Int Endod J. 2010;43(3):210–7.
131. De-Deus G, Brandao MC, Fidel RA, Fidel SR. The sealing ability of GuttaFlow in oval-shaped canals: an ex vivo study using a polymicrobial leakage model. Int Endod J. 2007;40(10):794–9.
132. Elayouti A, Achleithner C, Lost C, Weiger R. Homogeneity and adaptation of a new gutta-percha paste to root canal walls. J Endod. 2005;31(9):687–90.
133. Camilleri J. Composition and setting reaction. In: Camilleri J, editor. Mineral trioxide aggregate in dentistry: from preparation to application. New York: Springer; 2014.
134. Koh ET, McDonald F, Pitt Ford TR, Torabinejad M. Cellular response to mineral trioxide aggregate. J Endod. 1998;24(8):543–7.
135. Koh ET, Torabinejad M, Pitt Ford TR, Brady K, McDonald F. Mineral trioxide aggregate stimulates a biological response in human osteoblasts. J Biomed Mater Res. 1997;37(3):432–9.
136. Mente J, Geletneky B, Ohle M, Koch MJ, Friedrich Ding PG, Wolff D, et al. Mineral trioxide aggregate or calcium hydroxide direct pulp capping: an analysis of the clinical treatment outcome. J Endod. 2010;36(5):806–13.
137. Nair PN, Duncan HF, Pitt Ford TR, Luder HU. Histological, ultrastructural and quantitative investigations on the response of healthy human pulps to experimental capping with mineral trioxide aggregate: a randomized controlled trial. Int Endod J. 2008;41(2):128–50.
138. Torabinejad M, Pitt Ford TR. Root end filling materials: a review. Endod Dent Traumatol. 1996;12(4):161–78.
139. Baek SH, Plenk H Jr, Kim S. Periapical tissue responses and cementum regeneration with amalgam, SuperEBA, and MTA as root-end filling materials. J Endod. 2005;31(6):444–9.
140. Sarkar NK, Caicedo R, Ritwik P, Moiseyeva R, Kawashima I. Physicochemical basis of the biologic properties of mineral trioxide aggregate. J Endod. 2005;31(2):97–100.
141. Martin RL, Monticelli F, Brackett WW, Loushine RJ, Rockman RA, Ferrari M, et al. Sealing properties of mineral trioxide aggregate orthograde apical plugs and root fillings in an in vitro apexification model. J Endod. 2007;33(3):272–5.
142. Holden DT, Schwartz SA, Kirkpatrick TC, Schindler WG. Clinical outcomes of artificial root-end barriers with mineral trioxide aggregate in teeth with immature apices. J Endod. 2008;34(7):812–7.
143. Witherspoon DE, Small JC, Regan JD, Nunn M. Retrospective analysis of open apex teeth obturated with mineral trioxide aggregate. J Endod. 2008;34(10):1171–6.
144. Giovarruscio M, Uccioli U, Malentacca A, Koller G, Foschi F, Mannocci F. A technique for placement of apical MTA plugs using modified Thermafil carriers for the filling of canals with wide apices. Int Endod J. 2013;46(1):88–97.
145. Ber BS, Hatton JF, Stewart GP. Chemical modification of proroot mta to improve handling characteristics and decrease setting time. J Endod. 2007;33(10):1231–4.
146. Bortoluzzi EA, Broon NJ, Bramante CM, Felippe WT, Tanomaru Filho M, Esberard RM. The influence of calcium chloride on the setting time, solubility, disintegration, and

pH of mineral trioxide aggregate and white Portland cement with a radiopacifier. J Endod. 2009;35(4):550–4.
147. Torabinejad M, Hong CU, McDonald F, Pitt Ford TR. Physical and chemical properties of a new root-end filling material. J Endod. 1995;21(7):349–53.
148. Johnson BR. Considerations in the selection of a root-end filling material. Oral Surg Oral Med Oral Pathol Oral Radiol Endod. 1999;87(4):398–404.
149. Allison DA, Weber CR, Walton RE. The influence of the method of canal preparation on the quality of apical and coronal obturation. J Endod. 1979;5(10):298–304.
150. Peters OA. Current challenges and concepts in the preparation of root canal systems: a review. J Endod. 2004;30(8):559–67.
151. Marlin J, Schilder H. Physical properties of gutta-percha when subjected to heat and vertical condensation. Oral Surg Oral Med Oral Pathol. 1973;36(6):872–9.
152. Administration FDA. Memorandum to state drug officials. Washington, D.C.: Government Printing Office; 1974.
153. Council on Dental Therapeutics. Accepted dental therapeutics. 37th ed. Bethesda, MA: American Dental Associatio; 1979.
154. IARC. Monographs on the evaluation of carcinogenic risk to humans. Int Agency Res Cancer Suppl. 1987;7:152–4.
155. Allard U, Andersson L. Exposure of dental personnel to chloroform in root-filling procedures. Endod Dent Traumatol. 1992;8(4):155–9.
156. Wennberg A, Orstavik D. Evaluation of alternatives to chloroform in endodontic practice. Endod Dent Traumatol. 1989;5(5):234–7.
157. Wourms DJ, Campbell AD, Hicks ML, Pelleu GB Jr. Alternative solvents to chloroform for gutta-percha removal. J Endod. 1990;16(5):224–6.
158. Hunter KR, Doblecki W, Pelleu GB Jr. Halothane and eucalyptol as alternatives to chloroform for softening gutta-percha. J Endod. 1991;17(7):310–1.
159. Grossman LI, Lally ET. Assessment of irritation potential of essential oils for root canal cement. J Endod. 1982;8(5):208–12.
160. Morse DR, Martell B, Pike CG, Fantasia J, Esposito JV, Furst ML. A comparative tissue toxicity evaluation of Gutta-percha root canal sealers. Part I Six-hour findings. J Endod. 1984;10(6):246–9.
161. Allison DA, Michelich RJ, Walton RE. The influence of master cone adaptation on the quality of the apical seal. J Endod. 1981;7(2):61–5.
162. Blum JY, Esber S, Micallef JP. Analysis of forces developed during obturations. Comparison of three gutta-percha techniques. J Endod. 1997;23(5):340–5.
163. Bailey GC, Cunnington SA, Ng YL, Gulabivala K, Setchell DJ. Ultrasonic condensation of gutta-percha: the effect of power setting and activation time on temperature rise at the root surface—an in vitro study. Int Endod J. 2004;37(7):447–54.
164. Buchanan LS. The continuous wave of obturation technique: 'centered' condensation of warm gutta percha in 12 seconds. Dent Today. 1996;15(1):60–2. 64–67
165. Lipski M. Root surface temperature rises in vitro during root canal obturation with thermoplasticized gutta-percha on a carrier or by injection. J Endod. 2004;30(6):441–3.
166. Yee FS, Marlin J, Krakow AA, Gron P. Three-dimensional obturation of the root canal using injection-molded, thermoplasticized dental gutta-percha. J Endod. 1977;3(5):168–74.
167. Tanomaru-Filho M, Pinto RV, Bosso R, Nascimento CA, Berbert FL, Guerreiro-Tanomaru JM. Evaluation of the thermoplasticity of gutta-percha and Resilon(R) using the Obtura II system at different temperature settings. Int Endod J. 2011;44(8):764–8.
168. Kontakiotis EG, Tzanetakis GN, Loizides AL. A 12-month longitudinal in vitro leakage study on a new silicon-based root canal filling material (Gutta-flow). Oral Surg Oral Med Oral Pathol Oral Radiol Endod. 2007;103(6):854–9.
169. Mc SJ. Self-study course for the Thermatic condensation of Gutta-Percha. Toledo, OH: Ransomand Randolph; 1980.
170. Venturi M. Evaluation of canal filling after using two warm vertical gutta-percha compaction techniques in vivo: a preliminary study. Int Endod J. 2006;39(7):538–46.

171. Gencoglu N, Yildirim T, Garip Y, Karagenc B, Yilmaz H. Effectiveness of different gutta-percha techniques when filling experimental internal resorptive cavities. Int Endod J. 2008;41(10):836–42.
172. Ordinola-Zapata R, Bramante CM, de Moraes IG, Bernardineli N, Garcia RB, Gutmann JL. Analysis of the gutta-percha filled area in C-shaped mandibular molars obturated with a modified MicroSeal technique. Int Endod J. 2009;42(3):186–97.
173. Chu CH, Lo EC, Cheung GS. Outcome of root canal treatment using Thermafil and cold lateral condensation filling techniques. Int Endod J. 2005;38(3):179–85.
174. Gandolfi MG, Parrilli AP, Fini M, Prati C, Dummer PM. 3D micro-CT analysis of the interface voids associated with Thermafil root fillings used with AH plus or a flowable MTA sealer. Int Endod J. 2013;46(3):253–63.
175. Gopikrishna V, Parameswaren A. Coronal sealing ability of three sectional obturation techniques--SimpliFill, Thermafil and warm vertical compaction--compared with cold lateral condensation and post space preparation. Aust Endod J. 2006;32(3):95–100.
176. Mente J, Leo M, Panagidis D, Ohle M, Schneider S, Lorenzo Bermejo J, et al. Treatment outcome of mineral trioxide aggregate in open apex teeth. J Endod. 2013;39(1):20–6.
177. Combe EC, Cohen BD, Cummings K. Alpha- and beta-forms of gutta-percha in products for root canal filling. Int Endod J. 2001;34(6):447–51.
178. Gurgel-Filho ED, Andrade Feitosa JP, Teixeira FB, Monteiro de Paula RC, Araujo Silva JB, Souza-Filho FJ. Chemical and X-ray analyses of five brands of dental gutta-percha cone. Int Endod J. 2003;36(4):302–7.
179. Marciano J, Michailesco PM. Dental gutta-percha: chemical composition, X-ray identification, enthalpic studies, and clinical implications. J Endod. 1989;15(4):149–53.
180. Camps JJ, Pertot WJ, Escavy JY, Pravaz M. Young's modulus of warm and cold gutta-percha. Endod Dent Traumatol. 1996;12(2):50–3.
181. Clinton K, Van Himel T. Comparison of a warm gutta-percha obturation technique and lateral condensation. J Endod. 2001;27(11):692–5.
182. Dummer PM, McGinn JH, Rees DG. The position and topography of the apical canal constriction and apical foramen. Int Endod J. 1984;17(4):192–8.
183. Aminoshariae A, Kulild JC. Master apical file size—smaller or larger: a systematic review of healing outcomes. Int Endod J. 2015;48(7):639–47.
184. Gilhooly RM, Hayes SJ, Bryant ST, Dummer PM. Comparison of lateral condensation and thermomechanically compacted warm alpha-phase gutta-percha with a single cone for obturating curved root canals. Oral Surg Oral Med Oral Pathol Oral Radiol Endod. 2001;91(1):89–94.
185. Goodman A, Schilder H, Aldrich W. The thermomechanical properties of gutta-percha. Part IV. A thermal profile of the warm gutta-percha packing procedure. Oral Surg Oral Med Oral Pathol. 1981;51(5):544–51.
186. Venturi M, Di Lenarda R, Breschi L. An ex vivo comparison of three different gutta-percha cones when compacted at different temperatures: rheological considerations in relation to the filling of lateral canals. Int Endod J. 2006;39(8):648–56.
187. Pogrel MA. Permanent nerve damage from inferior alveolar nerve blocks--an update to include articaine. J Calif Dent Assoc. 2007;35(4):271–3.
188. Tilotta-Yasukawa F, Millot S, El Haddioui A, Bravetti P, Gaudy JF. Labiomandibular paresthesia caused by endodontic treatment: an anatomic and clinical study. Oral Surg Oral Med Oral Pathol Oral Radiol Endod. 2006;102(4):e47–59.
189. Gambarini G, Plotino G, Grande NM, Testarelli L, Prencipe M, Messineo D, et al. Differential diagnosis of endodontic-related inferior alveolar nerve paraesthesia with cone beam computed tomography: a case report. Int Endod J. 2011;44(2):176–81.
190. Dodd RB, Dodds RN, Hocomb JB. An endodontically induced maxillary sinusitis. J Endod. 1984;10(10):504–6.
191. Yamaguchi K, Matsunaga T, Hayashi Y. Gross extrusion of endodontic obturation materials into the maxillary sinus: a case report. Oral Surg Oral Med Oral Pathol Oral Radiol Endod. 2007;104(1):131–4.

192. Kaplowitz GJ. Penetration of the maxillary sinus by overextended gutta percha cones. Report of two cases. Clin Prev Dent. 1985;7(2):28–30.
193. Liston PN, Walters RF. Foreign bodies in the maxillary antrum: a case report. Aust Dent J. 2002;47(4):344–6.
194. Costa F, Robiony M, Toro C, Sembronio S, Politi M. Endoscopically assisted procedure for removal of a foreign body from the maxillary sinus and contemporary endodontic surgical treatment of the tooth. Head Face Med. 2006;2:37.
195. Fava LR. Calcium hydroxide paste in the maxillary sinus: a case report. Int Endod J. 1993;26(5):306–10.
196. Horre R, Schumacher G, Marklein G, Kromer B, Wardelmann E, Gilges S, et al. Case report. Maxillary sinus infection due to Emericella nidulans. Mycoses. 2002;45(9–10):402–5.
197. Orlay HG. Overfilling in root canal treatment. Two accidents with N2. Brit Dental J. 1966;120(8):376.
198. Yaltirik M, Kocak Berberoglu H, Koray M, Dulger O, Yildirim S, Aydil BA. Orbital pain and headache secondary to overfilling of a root canal. J Endod. 2003;29(11):771–2.
199. Haidar Z. Facial pain of uncommon origin. Oral Surg Oral Med Oral Pathol. 1987;63(6):748–9.
200. Patel S, Dawood A, Ford TP, Whaites E. The potential applications of cone beam computed tomography in the management of endodontic problems. Int Endod J. 2007;40(10):818–30.
201. Batur YB, Ersev H. Five-year follow-up of a root canal filling material in the maxillary sinus: a case report. Oral Surg Oral Med Oral Pathol Oral Radiol Endod. 2008;106(4):e54–6.
202. Ishikawa M, Mizuno T, Yamazaki Y, Satoh T, Notani K, Fukuda H. Migration of gutta-percha point from a root canal into the ethmoid sinus. Br J Oral Maxillofac Surg. 2004;42(1):58–60.
203. Bjorndal L, Amaloo C, Markvart M, Rud V, Qvortrup K, Stavnsbjerg C, et al. Maxillary sinus impaction of a Core carrier causing sustained apical periodontitis, sinusitis, and nasal stenosis: a 3-year follow-up. J Endod. 2016;42(12):1851–8.
204. Gutmann JL, Saunders WP, Saunders EM, Nguyen L. A assessment of the plastic Thermafil obturation technique. Part 1. Radiographic evaluation of adaptation and placement. Int Endod J. 1993;26(3):173–8.
205. Brooks JK, Kleinman JW. Retrieval of extensive gutta-percha extruded into the maxillary sinus: use of 3-dimensional cone-beam computed tomography. J Endod. 2013;39(9):1189–93.
206. Khongkhunthian P, Reichart PA. Aspergillosis of the maxillary sinus as a complication of overfilling root canal material into the sinus: report of two cases. J Endod. 2001;27(7):476–8.
207. Legent F, Billet J, Beauvillain C, Bonnet J, Miegeville M. The role of dental canal fillings in the development of Aspergillus sinusitis. A report of 85 cases. Arch Otorhinolaryngol. 1989;246(5):318–20.
208. Mensi M, Piccioni M, Marsili F, Nicolai P, Sapelli PL, Latronico N. Risk of maxillary fungus ball in patients with endodontic treatment on maxillary teeth: a case-control study. Oral Surg Oral Med Oral Pathol Oral Radiol Endod. 2007;103(3):433–6.
209. Ahonen M, Tjaderhane L. Endodontic-related paresthesia: a case report and literature review. J Endod. 2011;37(10):1460–4.
210. Escoda-Francoli J, Canalda-Sahli C, Soler A, Figueiredo R, Gay-Escoda C. Inferior alveolar nerve damage because of overextended endodontic material: a problem of sealer cement biocompatibility? J Endod. 2007;33(12):1484–9.
211. Di Lenarda R, Cadenaro M, Stacchi C. Paresthesia of the mental nerve induced by periapical infection: a case report. Oral Surg Oral Med Oral Pathol Oral Radiol Endod. 2000;90(6):746–9.
212. Giuliani M, Lajolo C, Deli G, Silveri C. Inferior alveolar nerve paresthesia caused by endodontic pathosis: a case report and review of the literature. Oral Surg Oral Med Oral Pathol Oral Radiol Endod. 2001;92(6):670–4.
213. Knowles KI, Jergenson MA, Howard JH. Paresthesia associated with endodontic treatment of mandibular premolars. J Endod. 2003;29(11):768–70.
214. Ngeow WC. Is there a "safety zone" in the mandibular premolar region where damage to the mental nerve can be avoided if periapical extrusion occurs? Canad Dental Assoc J. 2010;76:a61.

215. Poveda R, Bagan JV, Fernandez JM, Sanchis JM. Mental nerve paresthesia associated with endodontic paste within the mandibular canal: report of a case. Oral Surg Oral Med Oral Pathol Oral Radiol Endod. 2006;102(5):e46–9.
216. Pelka M, Petschelt A. Permanent mimic musculature and nerve damage caused by sodium hypochlorite: a case report. Oral Surg Oral Med Oral Pathol Oral Radiol Endod. 2008;106(3):e80–3.
217. Kruse A, Hellmich N, Luebbers HT, Gratz KW. Neurological deficit of the facial nerve after root canal treatment. Oral Surg Oral Med Oral Pathol Oral Radiol Endod. 2009;108(2):e46–8.
218. Pogrel MA. Damage to the inferior alveolar nerve as the result of root canal therapy. J Am Dent Assoc. 2007;138(1):65–9.
219. Hume WR. Effect of eugenol on respiration and division in human pulp, mouse fibroblasts, and liver cells in vitro. J Dent Res. 1984;63(11):1262–5.
220. Morse DR. Endodontic-related inferior alveolar nerve and mental foramen paresthesia. Compend Contin Educ Dent (Jamesburg, NJ: 1995). 1997;18(10):963–8. 970–963, 976–968 passim; quiz 998
221. Cohenca N, Rotstein I. Mental nerve paresthesia associated with a non-vital tooth. Endod Dent Traumatol. 1996;12(6):298–300.
222. Jerjes W, Swinson B, Banu B, Al Khawalde M, Hopper C. Paraesthesia of the lip and chin area resolved by endodontic treatment: a case report and review of literature. Br Dent J. 2005;198(12):743–5.
223. Ozkan BT, Celik S, Durmus E. Paresthesia of the mental nerve stem from periapical infection of mandibular canine tooth: a case report. Oral Surg Oral Med Oral Pathol Oral Radiol Endod. 2008;105(5):e28–31.
224. Forman GH, Rood JP. Successful retrieval of endodontic material from the inferior alveolar nerve. J Dent. 1977;5(1):47–50.
225. Nitzan DW, Stabholz A, Azaz B. Concepts of accidental overfilling and overinstrumentation in the mandibular canal during root canal treatment. J Endod. 1983;9(2):81–5.
226. Fanibunda K, Whitworth J, Steele J. The management of thermomechanically compacted gutta percha extrusion in the inferior dental canal. Br Dent J. 1998;184(7):330–2.
227. LaBanc JP, Epker BN. Serious inferior alveolar nerve dysesthesia after endodontic procedure: report of three cases. J Am Dent Assoc. 1984;108(4):605–7.
228. Farren ST, Sadoff RS, Penna KJ. Sodium hypochlorite chemical burn. Case report. N Y State Dent J. 2008;74(1):61–2.
229. Spangberg LS, Barbosa SV, Lavigne GD. AH 26 releases formaldehyde. J Endod. 1993;19(12):596–8.
230. Dan AE, Thygesen TH, Pinholt EM. Corticosteroid administration in oral and orthognathic surgery: a systematic review of the literature and meta-analysis. J Oral Maxillofac Surg. 2010;68(9):2207–20.
231. Yeler H, Ozec I, Kilic E. Infection-related inferior alveolar and mental nerve paresthesia: case reports. Quintessence Int (Berlin, Germany: 1985). 2004;35(4):313–6.
232. Blanas N, Kienle F, Sandor GK. Inferior alveolar nerve injury caused by thermoplastic gutta-percha overextension. J Can Dent Assoc. 2004;70(6):384–7.
233. Scolozzi P, Lombardi T, Jaques B. Successful inferior alveolar nerve decompression for dysesthesia following endodontic treatment: report of 4 cases treated by mandibular sagittal osteotomy. Oral Surg Oral Med Oral Pathol Oral Radiol Endod. 2004;97(5):625–31.
234. Donoff RB. Surgical management of inferior alveolar nerve injuries (part I): the case for early repair. J Oral Maxillofac Surg. 1995;53(11):1327–9.
235. Fleisher KE, Stevens MR. Diagnosis and management of inferior alveolar nerve injury. Compend Contin Educ Dent (Jamesburg, NJ: 1995). 1995;16(10):1028. 1031–1022, 1034–1040
236. Gregg JM. Surgical management of inferior alveolar nerve injuries (part II): the case for delayed management. J Oral Maxillofac Surg. 1995;53(11):1330–3.
237. Orstavik D, Brodin P, Aas E. Paraesthesia following endodontic treatment: survey of the literature and report of a case. Int Endod J. 1983;16(4):167–72.

238. Patel S, Dawood A, Wilson R, Horner K, Mannocci F. The detection and management of root resorption lesions using intraoral radiography and cone beam computed tomography - an in vivo investigation. Int Endod J. 2009;42(9):831–8.
239. Patel S, Horner K. The use of cone beam computed tomography in endodontics. Int Endod J. 2009;42(9):755–6.
240. Bornstein MM, Wiest R, Balsiger R, Reichart PA. Anterior Stafne's bone cavity mimicking a periapical lesion of endodontic origin: report of two cases. J Endod. 2009;35(11):1598–602.
241. de Paula-Silva FW, Wu MK, Leonardo MR, da Silva LA, Wesselink PR. Accuracy of periapical radiography and cone-beam computed tomography scans in diagnosing apical periodontitis using histopathological findings as a gold standard. J Endod. 2009;35(7):1009–12.
242. Rodrigues CD, Villar-Neto MJ, Sobral AP, Da Silveira MM, Silva LB, Estrela C. Lymphangioma mimicking apical periodontitis. J Endod. 2011;37(1):91–6.
243. Simon JH, Enciso R, Malfaz JM, Roges R, Bailey-Perry M, Patel A. Differential diagnosis of large periapical lesions using cone-beam computed tomography measurements and biopsy. J Endod. 2006;32(9):833–7.
244. Yaltirik M, Ozbas H, Erisen R. Surgical management of overfilling of the root canal: a case report. Quintessence Int (Berlin, Germany: 1985). 2002;33(9):670–2.
245. Grotz KA, Al-Nawas B, de Aguiar EG, Schulz A, Wagner W. Treatment of injuries to the inferior alveolar nerve after endodontic procedures. Clin Oral Investig. 1998;2(2):73–6.
246. Fanibunda KB. Adverse response to endodontic material containing paraformaldehyde. Br Dent J. 1984;157(7):231–5.
247. (ISO) IOfS. Dentistry - Preclinical evaluation of biocompatibility of medical devices used in dentistry - Test methods for dental materials. ISO 7405 1997.
248. (ISO) IOfS. International Standard. Biological Evaluation of Medical Devices - Part 12: Sample Preparation and Reference Materials. Second Edition. ISO 10993–12 2002.
249. (ANSI/ADA) ANSIADA. Specification No. 41: Recommended standard practices for biological evaluation of dental materials. ADA41-2005D.
250. Consensus report of the European Society of Endodontology on quality guidelines for endodontic treatment. Int Endod J 1994;27(3):115–24.
251. Gambarini G, Romeo U, Tucci E, Gerosa R, Nocca G, Lupi A, et al. Cytotoxicity of epiphany SE endodontic sealer: a comparative in vitro study. Med Sci Monit. 2009;15(4):Pi15–8.
252. Geurtsen W, Leyhausen G. Biological aspects of root canal filling materials--histocompatibility, cytotoxicity, and mutagenicity. Clin Oral Investig. 1997;1(1):5–11.
253. Tepel J, Darwisch el Sawaf M, Hoppe W. Reaction of inflamed periapical tissue to intracanal medicaments and root canal sealers. Endod Dent Traumatol. 1994;10(5):233–8.
254. Nair PN, Sjogren U, Krey G, Sundqvist G. Therapy-resistant foreign body giant cell granuloma at the periapex of a root-filled human tooth. J Endod. 1990;16(12):589–95.
255. Pascon EA, Spangberg LS. In vitro cytotoxicity of root canal filling materials: 1. Gutta-percha. J Endod. 1990;16(9):429–33.
256. Scotti R, Tiozzo R, Parisi C, Croce MA, Baldissara P. Biocompatibility of various root canal filling materials ex vivo. Int Endod J. 2008;41(8):651–7.
257. Langeland K. Root canal sealants and pastes. Dent Clin N Am. 1974;18(2):309–27.
258. Branstetter J, von Fraunhofer JA. The physical properties and sealing action of endodontic sealer cements: a review of the literature. J Endod. 1982;8(7):312–6.
259. Zmener O. Tissue response to a new methacrylate-based root canal sealer: preliminary observations in the subcutaneous connective tissue of rats. J Endod. 2004;30(5):348–51.
260. Ferracane JL, Condon JR. Rate of elution of leachable components from composite. Dent Mater. 1990;6(4):282–7.
261. Boiesen J, Brodin P. Neurotoxic effect of two root canal sealers with calcium hydroxide on rat phrenic nerve in vitro. Endod Dent Traumatol. 1991;7(6):242–5.
262. Serper A, Ucer O, Onur R, Etikan I. Comparative neurotoxic effects of root canal filling materials on rat sciatic nerve. J Endod. 1998;24(9):592–4.
263. Kawakami T, Nakamura C, Eda S. Effects of the penetration of a root canal filling material into the mandibular canal. 1. Tissue reaction to the material. Endod Dent Traumatol. 1991;7(1):36–41.

264. Briseno BM, Willershausen B. Root canal sealer cytotoxicity with human gingival fibroblasts. III. Calcium hydroxide-based sealers. J Endod. 1992;18(3):110–3.
265. Seidler B. Irrationalized endodontics: N2 and us too. J Am Dent Assoc. 1974;89(6):1318–31.
266. Sargenti A. Rationalised root canal treatment and the use of cortico-steroids. J Br Endod Soc. 1967;1(1):11–2.
267. Montgomery S. Paresthesia following endodontic treatment. J Endod. 1976;2(11):345–7.
268. Kaufman AY, Rosenberg L. Paresthesia caused by Endomethasone. J Endod. 1980;6(4):529–31.
269. Brodin P. Neurotoxic and analgesic effects of root canal cements and pulp-protecting dental materials. Endod Dent Traumatol. 1988;4(1):1–11.
270. Allard KU. Paraesthesia--a consequence of a controversial root-filling material? A case report. Int Endod J. 1986;19(4):205–8.
271. Block RM, Lewis RD, Hirsch J, Coffey J, Langeland K. Systemic distribution of 14C-labeled paraformaldehyde incorporated within Formocresol following pulpotomies in dogs. J Endod. 1983;9(5):176–89.
272. Rowe AH. Damage to the inferior dental nerve during or following endodontic treatment. Br Dent J. 1983;155(9):306–7.
273. Briseno BM, Willershausen B. Root canal sealer cytotoxicity on human gingival fibroblasts: 2. Silicone- and resin-based sealers. J Endod. 1991;17(11):537–40.
274. Schwandt NW, Gound TG. Resorcinol-formaldehyde resin "Russian red" endodontic therapy. J Endod. 2003;29(7):435–7.
275. Vranas RN, Hartwell GR, Moon PC. The effect of endodontic solutions on resorcinol-formalin paste. J Endod. 2003;29(1):69–72.
276. Parsons JR, Walton RE, Ricks-Williamson L. In vitro longitudinal assessment of coronal discoloration from endodontic sealers. J Endod. 2001;27(11):699–702.
277. Davis MC, Walton RE, Rivera EM. Sealer distribution in coronal dentin. J Endod. 2002;28(6):464–6.
278. Partovi M, Al-Havvaz AH, Soleimani B. In vitro computer analysis of crown discolouration from commonly used endodontic sealers. Aust Endod J. 2006;32(3):116–9.
279. Elkhazin M. Analysis of coronal discoloration from common obturation materials. An in vitro spectrophotometry study. Saarbruecken: Lambert Academic Publishing; 2011.
280. Bakland LK. Management of traumatically injured pulps in immature teeth using MTA. J Calif Dent Assoc. 2000;28(11):855–8.
281. Naik S, Hegde AH. Mineral trioxide aggregate as a pulpotomy agent in primary molars: an in vivo study. J Indian Soc Pedod Prev Dent. 2005;23(1):13–6.
282. Maroto M, Barberia E, Planells P, Garcia GF. Dentin bridge formation after mineral trioxide aggregate (MTA) pulpotomies in primary teeth. Am J Dent. 2005;18(3):151–4.
283. Song JS, Mante FK, Romanow WJ, Kim S. Chemical analysis of powder and set forms of Portland cement, gray ProRoot MTA, white ProRoot MTA, and gray MTA-angelus. Oral Surg Oral Med Oral Pathol Oral Radiol Endod. 2006;102(6):809–15.
284. Bortoluzzi EA, Araujo GS, Guerreiro Tanomaru JM, Tanomaru-Filho M. Marginal gingiva discoloration by gray MTA: a case report. J Endod. 2007;33(3):325–7.
285. Gutmann JL, Creel DC, Bowles WH. Evaluation of heat transfer during root canal obturation with thermoplasticized gutta-percha. Part I. In vitro heat levels during extrusion. J Endod. 1987;13(8):378–83.
286. Gutmann JL, Rakusin H, Powe R, Bowles WH. Evaluation of heat transfer during root canal obturation with thermoplasticized gutta-percha. Part II. In vivo response to heat levels generated. J Endod. 1987;13(9):441–8.
287. Eriksson AR, Albrektsson T. Temperature threshold levels for heat-induced bone tissue injury: a vital-microscopic study in the rabbit. J Prosthet Dent. 1983;50(1):101–7.
288. Lipski M. In vitro infrared thermographic assessment of root surface temperatures generated by high-temperature thermoplasticized injectable gutta-percha obturation technique. J Endod. 2006;32(5):438–41.
289. Sweatman TL, Baumgartner JC, Sakaguchi RL. Radicular temperatures associated with thermoplasticized gutta-percha. J Endod. 2001;27(8):512–5.

290. Satterthwaite JD, Stokes AN, Frankel NT. Potential for temperature change during application of ultrasonic vibration to intra-radicular posts. Eur J Prosthodont Restor Dent. 2003;11(2):51–6.
291. Kreisler M, Al-Haj H, D'Hoedt B. Intrapulpal temperature changes during root surface irradiation with an 809-nm GaAlAs laser. Oral Surg Oral Med Oral Pathol Oral Radiol Endod. 2002;93(6):730–5.
292. Atrizadeh F, Kennedy J, Zander H. Ankylosis of teeth following thermal injury. J Periodontal Res. 1971;6(3):159–67.
293. McCullagh JJ, Biagioni PA, Lamey PJ, Hussey DL. Thermographic assessment of root canal obturation using thermomechanical compaction. Int Endod J. 1997;30(3):191–5.
294. Floren JW, Weller RN, Pashley DH, Kimbrough WF. Changes in root surface temperatures with in vitro use of the system B HeatSource. J Endod. 1999;25(9):593–5.
295. Romero AD, Green DB, Wucherpfennig AL. Heat transfer to the periodontal ligament during root obturation procedures using an in vitro model. J Endod. 2000;26(2):85–7.
296. Behnia A, McDonald NJ. In vitro infrared thermographic assessment of root surface temperatures generated by the thermafil plus system. J Endod. 2001;27(3):203–5.
297. Blanas N, Kienle F, Sandor GK. Injury to the inferior alveolar nerve due to thermoplastic gutta percha. J Oral Maxillofac Surg. 2002;60(5):574–6.
298. Ulusoy OI, Yilmazoglu MZ, Gorgul G. Effect of several thermoplastic canal filling techniques on surface temperature rise on roots with simulated internal resorption cavities: an infrared thermographic analysis. Int Endod J. 2015;48(2):171–6.
299. Rivera EM, Walton RE. Longitudinal tooth fractures: findings that contribute to complex endodontic diagnoses. Endod Top. 2007;16(1):82–111.
300. Wilcox LR, Roskelley C, Sutton T. The relationship of root canal enlargement to finger-spreader induced vertical root fracture. J Endod. 1997;23(8):533–4.
301. Meister F Jr, Lommel TJ, Gerstein H. Diagnosis and possible causes of vertical root fractures. Oral Surg Oral Med Oral Pathol. 1980;49(3):243–53.
302. Saw LH, Messer HH. Root strains associated with different obturation techniques. J Endod. 1995;21(6):314–20.
303. Pitts DL, Matheny HE, Nicholls JI. An in vitro study of spreader loads required to cause vertical root fracture during lateral condensation. J Endod. 1983;9(12):544–50.
304. Hammad M, Qualtrough A, Silikas N. Effect of new obturating materials on vertical root fracture resistance of endodontically treated teeth. J Endod. 2007;33(6):732–6.
305. Gharai SR, Thorpe JR, Strother JM, McClanahan SB. Comparison of generated forces and apical microleakage using nickel-titanium and stainless steel finger spreaders in curved canals. J Endod. 2005;31(3):198–200.
306. Dang DA, Walton RE. Vertical root fracture and root distortion: effect of spreader design. J Endod. 1989;15(7):294–301.
307. Blum JY, Cathala C, Machtou P, Micallef JP. Analysis of the endogrammes developed during obturations on extracted teeth using system B. J Endod. 2001;27(11):661–5.
308. Doyon GE, Dumsha T, von Fraunhofer JA. Fracture resistance of human root dentin exposed to intracanal calcium hydroxide. J Endod. 2005;31(12):895–7.
309. Berry KA, Loushine RJ, Primack PD, Runyan DA. Nickel-titanium versus stainless-steel finger spreaders in curved canals. J Endod. 1998;24(11):752–4.
310. Tidswell HE, Saunders EM, Saunders WP. Assessment of coronal leakage in teeth root filled with gutta-percha and a glass of ionomer root canal sealer. Int Endod J. 1994;27(4):208–12.
311. Dalat DM, Spangberg LS. Comparison of apical leakage in root canals obturated with various gutta percha techniques using a dye vacuum tracing method. J Endod. 1994;20(7):315–9.
312. Lopes HP, Neves MA, Elias CN, Moreira EJ, Siqueira JF Jr. Comparison of some physical properties of finger spreaders made of stainless steel or nickel-titanium alloys. Clin Oral Investig. 2011;15(5):661–5.
313. Shahi S, Shakouie S, Rahimi S, Yavari HR, Mohammadi N, Abdolrahimi M. Comparison of apical microleakage using Ni-Ti with stainless steel finger spreaders. Iranian Endod J. 2009;4(4):149–51.

314. Wilson BL, Baumgartner JC. Comparison of spreader penetration during lateral compaction of .04 and .02 tapered gutta-percha. J Endod. 2003;29(12):828–31.
315. Onnink PA, Davis RD, Wayman BE. An in vitro comparison of incomplete root fractures associated with three obturation techniques. J Endod. 1994;20(1):32–7.
316. Toure B, Faye B, Kane AW, Lo CM, Niang B, Boucher Y. Analysis of reasons for extraction of endodontically treated teeth: a prospective study. J Endod. 2011;37(11):1512–5.
317. Seo DG, Yi YA, Shin SJ, Park JW. Analysis of factors associated with cracked teeth. J Endod. 2012;38(3):288–92.
318. Ozer SY. Detection of vertical root fractures by using cone beam computed tomography with variable voxel sizes in an in vitro model. J Endod. 2011;37(1):75–9.
319. Edlund M, Nair MK, Nair UP. Detection of vertical root fractures by using cone-beam computed tomography: a clinical study. J Endod. 2011;37(6):768–72.

Part III

Miscellaneous

Complications Due to Medicaments

7

Zuhair Alkhatib and Rashid El Abed

7.1 Introduction

Medicament uses in root canal system are of so many varieties and have effects on both pulpal tissues and microbial flora not just inside the root canal system but the periodontium as well. That is why when choosing any medicament, the clinician must make the right choice. Choose a medicament which has an effect on the microorganisms, as this is the most important factor in root canal failures and it should have the least effect on the tissues surrounding the root. The medicament should be confined in the root canal system during its use, and care should be taken not to expel it beyond the root apex into the periapical tissues. In case this happens, damage to the periapical tissues ensues leading to inflammation, swelling and probably tooth loss.

In this chapter we will discuss the most common intracanal irrigation solutions and interim medicament use by endodontist referring to literature and case reports of those with scientifically based evidence.

7.2 Sodium Hypochlorite (NaOCl)

Successful root canal therapy can be achieved by using mechanical instrumentation in combination with chemical irrigation and intracanal medication. One technique by itself cannot achieve the cleaning and shaping of the complexed root canal system [1, 2].

The practice of irrigants in root canal therapy (RCT) is imperative to its success, with the emphasis on cleaning and over shaping of the root canal system [3].

Z. Alkhatib, B.D.S., M.S. (✉) • R. El Abed
MBR University of Medicine and Health Sciences, Dubai, UAE
e-mail: zzk321@gmail.com

P. Jain (ed.), *Common Complications in Endodontics*,
https://doi.org/10.1007/978-3-319-60997-3_7

The ideal irrigating solution should have the ability to dissolve organic and inorganic tissues, as well as have an antimicrobial action, zero toxicity, low surface tension and lubricating action. Nevertheless, till date, no irrigating solution fulfils all the above-mentioned requirements [4]. Sodium hypochlorite is the most common irrigant used in modern endodontics. It was first recognized as an antibacterial agent in 1843 when hand washing with hypochlorite solution between patients produced unusually low rates of infection transmission between patients. It was first recorded as an endodontic irrigant in 1920 and is now used routinely worldwide [5]. Its beneficial properties are:

1. Antimicrobial activity
2. Ability to dissolve organic matter
3. Bleaching
4. Lubricating action
5. Low surface tension

The concentration of the irrigants is still a matter of debate and remains controversial; many authors recommend a 5.25% concentration of sodium hypochlorite; others prefer a lower concentration of 3% or even 0.5%. Until now, no other irrigating solution has matched the efficacy of NaOCl. Although it confers many advantageous properties, care must be taken when using and handling NaOCl as it is caustic to the vital tissues and related injuries are a recognized risk [6, 7].

7.2.1 Complications

Literature has shown that potential complications can occur with sodium hypochlorite in clinical practice. They are described below [3–5]:

7.2.1.1 Due to Accidental Spillage

1. *Damage to clothing*: Probably, most common complication during root canal irrigation. Even spillage of minute quantities of this agent on clothing will lead to rapid, irreparable bleaching.
2. *Damage to the eye*: Contact between the patient's/operator's eyes and irrigant solution results in immediate pain, profuse watering, intense burning and erythema. Loss of epithelial cells in the outer layer of the cornea may occur.
3. *Damage to skin*: NaOCl may cause hypersensitivity or dermatitis when in contact with unprotected skin.
4. *Damage to oral mucosa*: When in contact with the oral mucosa, due to its caustic action, the patient develops discomfort (bad taste), a burning sensation and/or wounds (whenever the reaction is prolonged). If it is swallowed, NaOCl might cause a feeling of suffocation and gagging in addition to seriously affecting the tissues and causing necrosis, swelling, haemorrhagic congestion, erosion and/or ulceration.

7.2.1.2 Arising from Hypochlorite Extrusion Beyond the Root Apex

Sodium hypochlorite extrusion beyond the apex, also known as 'a hypochlorite accident', is a well-known complication that seldom occurs during the biomechanical preparation phase of the root canal therapy. The cytotoxic activity is a well-known shortcoming of NaOCl that may cause acute injurious effects when/if it reaches the periapical tissues. Once in contact with the vital tissues, NaOCl quickly oxidizes surrounding tissues leading to rapid haemolysis and ulceration, inhibition of neutrophil migration and destruction of endothelial and fibroblast cells [7].

Such phenomena may cause the following:

1. *Chemical burns and tissue necrosis*: Given the widespread use of hypochlorite, this complication is fortunately very rare indeed. Chemical burn with a localized or extensive tissue necrosis may happen due to a severe acute inflammatory reaction of the tissues. This leads to rapid tissue swelling both intra-orally (within the surrounding mucosa) and extra-orally (within the skin and subcutaneous tissues). The swelling may be oedematous, haemorrhagic or both and may extend beyond the region that might be expected with an acute infection of the affected tooth. Involvement of the maxillary sinus will lead to acute sinusitis. Associated bleeding into the interstitial tissues may result in bruising and ecchymosis of the surrounding mucosa and possibly the facial skin and may include the formation of a haematoma (Fig. 7.1).

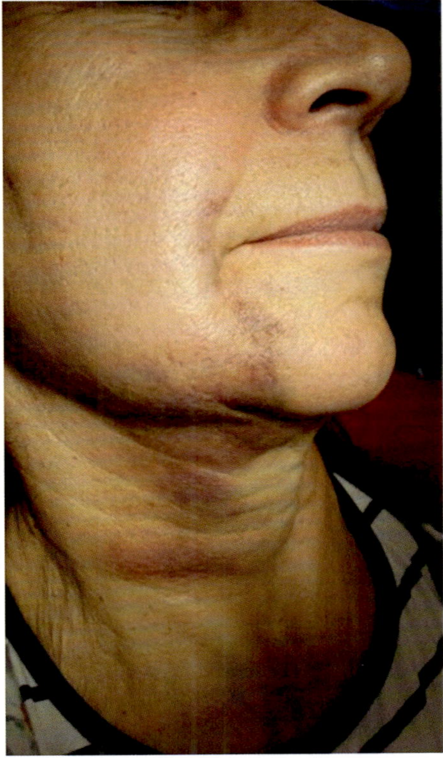

Fig. 7.1 NaOCl extrusion (Courtesy of Dr. Daniel OTT)

2. *Neurological complications*: Paraesthesia and anaesthesia affecting the mental, inferior dental and infraorbital branches of the trigeminal nerve following inadvertent extrusion of sodium hypochlorite beyond the root canal system have been described in the literature. However, further research is required in this area.
3. *Upper airway obstruction*: The use of sodium hypochlorite for root canal irrigation without adequate isolation of the tooth can lead to leakage of the solution into the oral cavity and ingestion or inhalation by the patient. This could result in throat irritation, and in severe cases, the upper airway could be compromised. In a systematic review done by Guivarc'h et al. (2017) [8], two patients presented with life-threatening airway obstruction caused by massive swelling in the submental and sublingual spaces with elevation of the floor of the mouth after extrusion of the solution through the root canals of mandibular teeth [9, 10]. Indicators of the severity of these extrusions included difficulties in swallowing followed by respiratory distress. Emergency hospitalization in an intensive care unit was required in these situations.

7.2.2 Probable Aetiological Factors

1. Wide apical foramina
2. If the apical constriction is destroyed probably during root canal instrumentation or by resorption
3. Extreme pressure during irrigation
4. Binding of the irrigation needle tip in the root canal with no release for the irrigant to leave the root canal coronally may result in contact of large volumes of the irrigant to the apical tissues
5. Perforations

7.2.3 Signs and Symptoms of NaOCl Complications

1. Strong taste of chlorine.
2. Burning sensation: When these extrusions involved the maxillary sinus, the first sign noticed is the irrigant flowing from the nostrils along with the taste of NaOCl in the throat. A burning sensation in the maxillary sinus rather than severe pain was usually present, with little or no bleeding from the canal and no evidence of immediate swelling [8].
3. Severe pain.
4. Tissue necrosis: Mucosal and bone necrosis as a result of the chemical burn caused by NaOCl, sometimes accompanied by a purulent discharge.
5. Paraesthesia: Contact with NaOCl is highly toxic to vital tissues, including nerves. Consequently, neurologic signs such as sensory and/or motor defects after extrusion can be expected [5].
6. Haematoma.
7. Ulcer and haemorrhage (Fig. 7.2).

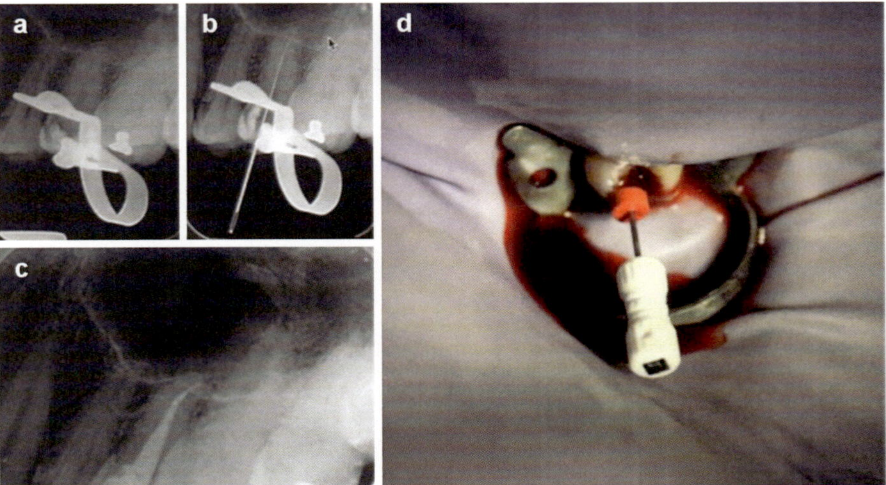

Fig. 7.2 NaOCl accident showing haemorrhage (Courtesy of Dr. Frank Diemer)

8. Swelling: Occurs very commonly with sodium hypochlorite extrusion, it appears within a few minutes up to a few hours after the accident. Swelling is usually large and diffuse (similar to cellulitis), extending intra- and extra-orally well beyond the site of the affected tooth. It may sometimes result in difficulties opening the ipsilateral eye [11–13, 108].
9. Ophthalmologic symptoms: It may present as eye pain, blurring of vision, diplopia or right corneal patchy colouration. These constellations of signs/symptoms have been described in the literature as emanating from a maxillary central incisor [12] and canine [13].

7.2.4 Management of NaOCl Extrusion

Despite careful consideration during RCT, if faced with a suspected NaOCl-related extrusion injury, a thorough clinical and radiological assessment is recommended to determine the degree and extent of the injury. This information should assist the clinician to instigate the appropriate management plan to minimize any detrimental effects and to improve the final outcome [14, 109].

Guidelines for the management of NaOCl extrusions [14]:

The guidelines presented have been developed through clinical experience in the management of such injuries in a secondary care environment, as well as through reviewing relevant literature. Researchers have proposed to categorize extrusion injuries as mild, moderate and severe according to a patient's signs and symptoms. Each category has been subdivided into immediate, early and late management to optimize the care provided. Although the patients are initially categorized as mild, moderate or severe according to their degree of the injury, they can be recategorized if their signs and symptoms do change.

Table 7.1 Factors to be assessed during examination

Extra-oral examination	Intra-oral examination
Facial symmetry	Ecchymosis/haematoma
Ecchymosis/haematoma	Oedema/swelling
Oedema/swelling	Ulceration
Neurovascular deficit	Necrosis
Sensory	Neurovascular deficit
Motor	Sensory
Dysphagia	Teeth
Dyspnoea	

Table 7.2 Summary of findings from history and examination and their associated grading

Symptoms	Grade of injury		
Pain (visual pain score)	Mild	Moderate	Severe
	0–3	4–6	7+
Swelling	<30%	30–50%	>50%
Ecchymosis	Localized	Diffuse	Diffuse
Other	No ulceration	Intraoral ulceration	Intraoral ulceration
	No necrosis		Intraoral necrosis
			Airway compromised
			Neurovascular deficit
Pathway	GDP/endodontist	OMFS	OMFS

According to the guidelines, a clear and concise history would identify patients with a high possibility of extrusion injury. Recent history of root canal therapy and rapid onset of signs and symptoms have been recognized as cardinal features of extrusion injury [15]. Systematic approach is recommended to assess extra-oral and intra-oral tissues (Table 7.1).

The importance of a comprehensive history and examination is vital when seeking advice or when referring to secondary care in order to assess the severity of sodium hypochlorite extrusion injury. This information will allow the severity of the injury at presentation to be categorized by assessing these factors as mild, moderate and severe. Although there are many factors a patient may present with, an emphasis on the degree of pain, swelling and ecchymosis are the main factors which are used to determine the grading of such injuries (Table 7.2) [14].

7.2.5 Treatment

The treatment is recommended in two modalities:

1. Relative to severity of injury

7.3 Relative to the Time of Injury and Includes Immediate, Early and Late Treatment (Appendix 7.1)

7.3.1 Prevention

The best treatment of a NaOCl accident is to prevent it from happening. Patient safety is paramount when considering intracanal fluid dynamics, including irrigant delivery rate, agitation and exchange, and needle design; pressure gradient management, wall shear stress and cleaning efficacy; and, ultimately, treatment outcome. Different preventive measures have been recommended in the literature to minimize potential complications associated with the use of NaOCl [5, 15]. These include:

(a) Replacing NaOCl with another irrigant
(b) Using a lower concentration of NaOCl
(c) Placing the needle passively and avoiding wedging of the needle into the root canal
(d) Irrigation needle placed 1–3 mm short of working length.
(e) Using a side-vented needle for root canal irrigation (Fig. 7.3)
(f) Avoiding the use of excessive pressure during irrigation
(g) Plastic bib to protect patient's clothing
(h) Provision of protective eyewear for patient, operator and dental assistant
(i) The use of a sealed rubber dam for isolation of the tooth under treatment

Sodium hypochlorite (NaOCl), the widely used irrigant in endodontics, has many complications following its inadvertent use. However, NaOCl accidents are rare in endodontic practice. Nevertheless, the patient should be notified of potential

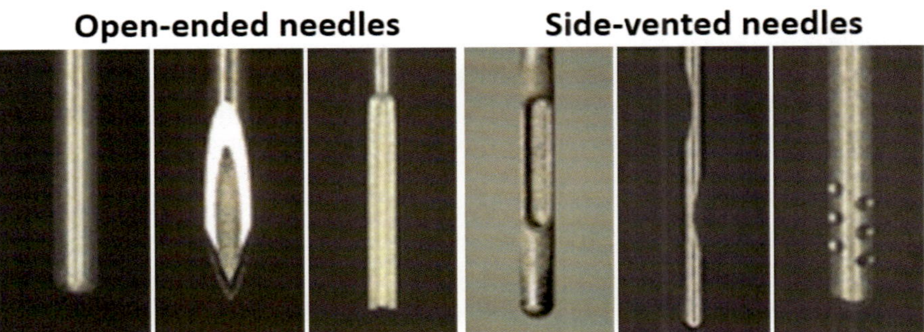

Fig. 7.3 Open-end needles vs. side-vent needles

accidents and the evolution of the case, with appropriate follow-up and, whenever necessary, hospital care.

The extrusion of NaOCl during root canal therapy into the periradicular tissues is a rare occurrence; nevertheless, the consequence of which can be potentially serious and can cause significant morbidity to the patient. Prior to root canal treatment, the assessment of teeth is important to identify any factors which may predispose extrusion injuries, so that adequate preventive measures can be undertaken. As there is currently little in the way of protocols or guidelines to manage such injuries, the clear guidelines to manage hypochlorite extrusion injuries presented in Appendix 7.1 aim to assist practitioners in the assessment of patients following hypochlorite injuries, with the aim to grade the severity of these injuries into mild, moderate and severe. The presented guidelines also aim to help develop standards for future management of sodium hypochlorite extrusion injuries [14].

7.4 Air Emphysema

Emphysema is derived from a Greek word *whick* which means to 'blow in'. This condition refers to trapped air and may occur when the root canal is dried with compressed air, which may be expressed through the apical constriction into the periapical tissues. Air emphysema is usually uncommon but may lead to subcutaneous emphysema, also known as tissue emphysema of the head, neck and thorax due to the introduction of air into the fascial planes of the connective tissue. Using compressed air in endodontics [16], periodontics [17], oral surgery [18] and operative procedures [19] can cause emphysema. It is a possible complication of both nonsurgical and surgical endodontic treatments [20]. When the condition is caused by surgery, it is called surgical emphysema [21]. Surgical emphysema may occur during root treatment, and reports in the literature [22] indicate that the complication occurs most commonly as a result of overzealous irrigation with hydrogen peroxide or drying root canals with compressed air blasts.

Sometimes, spread of larger amounts of air into deeper fascia may cause more serious complications, including accumulation of air in the retropharyngeal space, pneumomediastinum and pneumopericardium [23]. Its occurrence with a dental procedure was first reported more than 100 years ago when Turnbull extracted the premolar of a musician who blew his bugle immediately after extraction. Air enters into anatomical spaces through the root canal space [5]. But it can sometimes pass through the dentoalveolar membrane [24]. Following its introduction into the soft tissues, air remains in the subcutaneous connective tissue and does not spread to deep anatomic spaces in the majority of the cases [25].

However, emphysema can also involve deeper structures as the tissue planes commonly connect [26]. The potential avenues of travel for compressed air involve the superficial area, parotid area, submandibular, sublingual, tonsillar, masticatory and the parapharyngeal region [20].

The apices of the first, second and third molars directly communicate with the sublingual and submandibular spaces. These spaces, in turn, communicate with the parapharyngeal and retropharyngeal spaces, where accumulation of air may lead to airway compromise [27]. The retropharyngeal space ('danger space') is the main route of communication from the mouth to the mediastinum.

Secondarily, it can escape along the path of introduction, such as a patent root canal, and be released into the dental operatory air, causing no damage [28]. From Rickle's [29] post-mortem study, it is obvious that one definite risk of air emphysema during endodontic treatment is introduction of air into the cardiovascular system. In large volume, this can cause heart failure [30].

Air emphysema during endodontic treatment may also be misdiagnosed as infection because of similar location and size of swelling. In fact, such accidents may develop into an infection from microbes forced into the spaces created by the air blast [30].

7.4.1 Hydrogen Peroxide as Endodontic Irrigant Causing Air Emphysema

Hydrogen peroxide (H_2O_2) has been widely used for irrigation of the root canal system, although it is less effective in killing microorganisms. Hydrogen peroxide is a colourless liquid and has been used in dentistry in concentrations varying from 1 to 30%. H_2O_2 degrades to form water and oxygen.

Hydrogen peroxide has been implicated, along with compressed air, in the aetiology of subcutaneous emphysema [31, 32]. It has been used as a canal irrigant and disinfectant during routine root canal therapy [33]. When hydrogen peroxide comes into contact with blood or tissue proteins, it very rapidly undergoes effervescence and liberates oxygen [34]. This gaseous expansion may drive debris or simply gas through the apical foramen or into the adjacent bone if an inadvertent perforation of the canal wall were present [20]. Kaufman et al. [31] presented a case of delayed onset of emphysema subsequent to hydrogen peroxide irrigation.

It is active against viruses, bacteria, bacterial spores and yeasts [35] via the production of hydroxyl free radicals which attack proteins and DNA [36].

It has been shown that sodium hypochlorite (NaOCl) combined with H_2O_2 is no more effective against *E. faecalis* than NaOCl alone [31]; however, chlorhexidine (CHX) combined with H_2O_2 was a better antimicrobial agent than either one on their own [37]. The current evidence does not support the use of H_2O_2 over other irrigants, and it has not been shown to reduce bacterial load in canals significantly [38]. There is the rare but potential danger of effervescence with H_2O_2, and seepage into the tissues may lead to air emphysema [39].

Probable aetiological factors

1. Using compressed air to dry the root canal system instead of paper points.
2. Exhaust of air from a high-speed drill directed towards the tissue and not evacuated to the rear of the handpiece during apical surgery [40].

3. While opening the access cavity for endodontic treatment, subcutaneous emphysema can be caused by the use of an air-driven high-speed handpiece and compressed air syringe [41].
4. Injection of hydrogen peroxide beyond the apex [31, 32].
5. Wedging of irrigation needle in the canal [20].
6. Excessive pressure of syringe used during irrigation.
7. Technical errors, such as the enlargement of the perforation which increases the chances of injuring the periodontal tissues and entering air into the tissue spaces.
8. Iatrogenic widening of the apical constriction.
9. It can be caused by invasion of compressed air into soft tissues through the disrupted intraoral barrier (dentoalveolar membrane or root canal) during tooth extraction (particularly of the third mandibular molars) [42], restorative dentistry, dental implant surgery and root canal or periodontal treatment [23].
10. Many cases of air entering tissues are complicated by inflammation and infection, perhaps from canal debris and/or microorganisms or perhaps from opportunist microbes from other sources within the body that find the inflated space [30].

7.4.2 Signs and Symptoms

The typical symptoms of sudden, severe pain are accompanied by a rapid swelling and erythema in the region of the treated tooth [20]. The area will rapidly swell and examination of the swelling will reveal a mild tenderness [43] (Fig. 7.4). Crepitus [28] is evident along with oedema, erythema and lymphadenopathy [23]. Patient

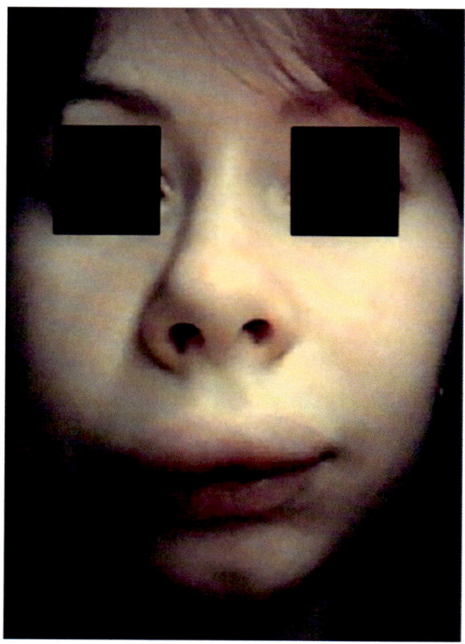

Fig. 7.4 Courtesy of Dr. Tara McMahon

may experience mild fever and local discomfort. Radiographic findings such as dark area of air and bubble accumulation are visible on CT scan and MRI images [44].

If the air pocket breaks through into the neck region, there is a sudden swelling of the neck, the voice sounds brassy and the patient has difficulty breathing and swallowing (dyspnoea) [25]. If it breaks through into the mediastinum, a crunching noise is heard on auscultation.

7.4.3 Management

No standard therapy for further management of the complication has been described in the literature. Few recommendations are:

1. Intervention depends on the nature and severity of the incident. In many cases, no intervention or only a minimal amount is necessary.
2. In mild to moderate cases, the treatment consists of observation and reassurance of the patient [45]. The patient should be informed that healing will take some days, or even weeks, and that symptoms in most cases will resolve completely.
3. To reduce the acute pain, local anaesthesia may be helpful along with the prescription of analgesics.
4. Initially, the swelling should be treated by cold compresses. After 24 h, these should be replaced by warm compresses and warm mouth rinses to stimulate local microcirculation [46].
5. Antibiotics are recommended only in cases where there is a high risk of infection spread; they are not necessary in minor cases.
6. When the acute symptoms have resolved or diminished, endodontic treatment may be completed. The use of a mild no irritating irrigation solution (sterile saline, chlorhexidine gluconate) is recommended in such cases.
7. In the majority of cases, there is no need or indication for extraction or surgical treatment of the involved tooth.
8. Dental extraction may be necessary depending on severity of the case.
9. It has also been reported that administration of 100% oxygen via a non-breather mask can hasten resolution of the emphysema, because oxygen, which replaces the air, is more readily absorbed [27].
10. In cases where the emphysema extends towards the neck or the mediastinum, hospitalization of the patient is necessary for a more complete control and continuous follow-up [25].

7.4.4 Prevention

A well-fitted rubber dam should be used [25]. Perforations may cause seepage of the irrigant into the tissues. Therefore, care must be taken to avoid that. Avoid wedging the irrigating needle into the root canal [46] by using a side-vented irrigation needle (Fig. 7.5). During irrigation, a low and constant pressure should be used and

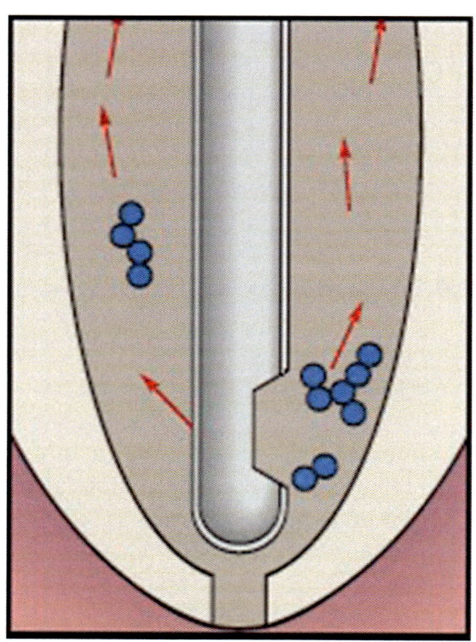

Fig. 7.5 Side-vented irrigation needle

the clinician must ensure that excess irrigant leaves the root canal coronally via the access cavity. However, it has been shown that contact between the periapical tissues and the irrigant cannot be avoided completely.

It is not recommended to use compressed air to dry the root canal system. Use a handpiece that exhausts the spent air out at the back of the handpiece rather than into the operating field. This can be achieved by using remote exhaust handpieces or electric motor-driven handpieces [41].

Use paper points to dry the canal [20], or a vacuum system, and avoid the use of hydrogen peroxide while irrigating canals [23]. Ultrasonic or sonic instruments should be used for root-end cavity preparations. Early recognition may be of extreme importance to prevent possible secondary infections and cardiopulmonary complications [47].

Air emphysema is usually an uncommon complication occurring during a routine endodontic treatment but occurring most commonly due to iatrogenic error by the clinician. Thus, concentration at all times could avoid emergency dental situations like this. The irrigating and local anaesthetic needles should be colour-coded to avoid confusion and mishaps.

7.5 Sodium Hypochlorite Mix with Chlorohexidine

Bacteria in the root canal system provokes and causes periapical inflammatory lesions [48]. The main aim of root canal treatment is to eliminate bacteria from the infected root canal and to prevent reinfection. Biomechanical cleaning and shaping of the root canal greatly decreases the number of bacteria [49]. Nevertheless, because of the anatomical complexity of the root canal system, organic/inorganic residues and bacteria cannot be completely removed and often persist [50]. Various irrigants have been used during the canal preparation to minimize the residual debris, necrotic tissue and bacteria, as well as to remove smear layer formed by the mechanical preparation of the dentin [49, 51, 52].

7.5.1 Concern with Sodium Hypochlorite (NaOCl)

As mentioned before, due to its broad-spectrum antimicrobial action and tissue-dissolving properties, sodium hypochlorite (NaOCl) at various concentrations is the most common endodontic irrigant used [53–55].

Despite its germicidal abilities, NaOCl in high concentration is cytotoxic and can cause necrosis of periapical tissues [54, 56, 57]. NaOCl is not a substantive microbial agent [58]. These troubles have led clinicians and researchers to explore alternative irrigants.

7.5.2 Concern with Chlorhexidine Gluconate (CHX)

Chlorhexidine gluconate (CHX) is a broad-spectrum antimicrobial agent that has been advocated as an effective medication in endodontic treatment [59, 60, 110]. When used as an endodontic irrigant, CHX has an antimicrobial efficacy comparable to that of NaOCl but lacks the cytotoxic effects [59, 61]. CHX has also been shown to have antimicrobial substantivity in root dentin [61–63, 110].

A drawback of CHX is that it lacks the ability to dissolve organic matter. For this reason, CHX is often used in conjunction with NaOCl [54].

7.5.3 NaOCl and CHX Interaction

A combination of NaOCl and CHX has been advocated to enhance their antimicrobial properties. Kuruvilla [54] suggested that the antimicrobial effect of 2.5% NaOCl and 0.2% CHX used in combination was better than that of either component. Zehnder [2] proposed an irrigation regimen in which NaOCl is used throughout instrumentation followed by EDTA, while CHX would be used as a final irrigant. If hypochlorite is still present in the canal, a precipitate was observed when the medications interacted [2, 64] (Fig. 7.6). This precipitate contains the cytotoxin para-chloroaniline (PCA) which can coat the canal surface and significantly occludes the dentinal tubules in the coronal and middle thirds of the canal [65, 66]. The obliteration of dentinal tubules was not found to be significant at the apical third. This might be due to the fact that the apical third is more difficult to irrigate [65].

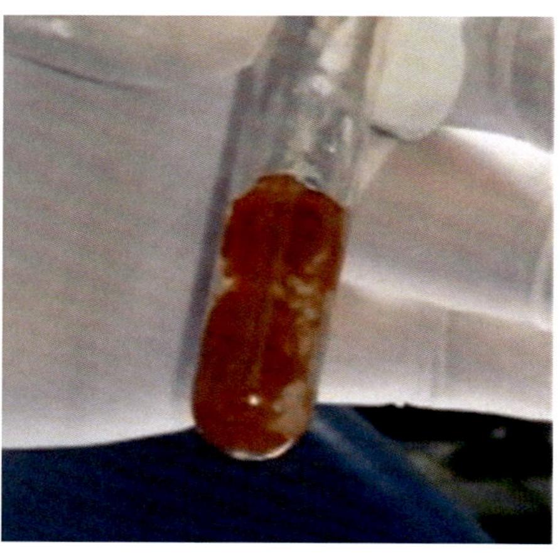

Fig. 7.6 NaOCL and CHX precipitate

Table 7.3 Endodontic irrigation timeline

NaOCl	17% EDTA	NaOCl rinse	Rinse out	2% CHX
During endodontic instrumentation	2 min		Saline or water	

7.5.4 PCA Toxicity

It is known that PCA and its degradation product are toxic and carcinogenic, so potential leaching of PCA into the surrounding tissues is a concern [65]. Short-term exposure of humans to PCA results in cyanosis, which is a manifestation of methaemoglobin formation [67]. In 1991, it was reported that PCA to be carcinogenic in rats due to increased sarcomas in the spleen. Furthermore in male mice, there was an increase in hepatocellular carcinomas and haemangiosarcomas of the spleen [67].

7.6 Prevention

The interaction between NaOCl and CHX can be minimized or prevented using saline or distilled water as intermediate flushes [68]. Also using EDTA alone would be convenient; however, EDTA also produces a precipitate in the presence of CHX [65].

A sequence of irrigation to avoid any interaction between all these chemicals can be seen in Table 7.3.

7.7 Calcium Hydroxide

Calcium hydroxide [$Ca(OH)_2$] has been used in dentistry for many years. Its use in root canal therapy as an intracanal medication has been associated with periradicular healing [69], and thus, the routine use of $Ca(OH)_2$ as an interim intracanal medicament became widespread. $Ca(OH)_2$ is an effective intracanal antibacterial dressing, mainly as a result of its high pH and its destructive effect on bacterial cell walls and protein structures [70]. It has been demonstrated that treatment with $Ca(OH)_2$ as an interim dressing in the presence of large and chronic periapical lesions can create an environment more favourable to healing and encourage osseous repair [71]. $Ca(OH)_2$ is a formless, thin, granular powder with strong basic properties and a density of 2.1. It can dissolve only slightly in water and is insoluble in alcohol. Due to its lack of radiopacity, it is not easily seen radiographically. This is the main reason that radiopaque materials (barium sulphate [BaSO4] and bismuth and other compounds containing iodine and bromine) are added to the paste, thereby allowing identification of lateral and accessory canals, resorptive defects, fractures and other structures [72, 73]. Nevertheless, in apexification cases, it has been recommended that a $Ca(OH)_2$ mixture without the addition of a radiopaque be used because $Ca(OH)_2$ washout is evaluated by its relative radiodensity in the canal in follow-up appointments [74].

7.7.1 Aetiological Factors

During root canal treatment, temporary dressing material may unintentionally escape through the apex of the tooth, resulting in a series of complications including hypaesthesia or paraesthesia of the inferior alveolar nerve [75, 76]. Such complications occur mainly by excess filling material causing direct pressure or by exerting a neurotoxic effect on the neurovascular bundle [75]. The material causes changes in the surrounding bone and affects the inferior alveolar nerve. Extrusion is also evident in case of wide apex of an immature permanent tooth [77]. Complications can occur due to binding of the $Ca(OH)_2$ syringe in the root canal deep enough to create pressure higher than arterial blood pressure, thereby allowing the paste to travel upstream. It should be mentioned that the $Ca(OH)_2$ paste particles are small enough to permeate into capillaries [78] and subsequently obstruct the capillaries mechanically or induce crystallization in the blood, blocking circulation. The extruded medicament may also obstruct the blood circulation by producing thrombi.

7.7.2 Signs and Symptoms

Although it has been considered as a safe agent [78], calcium hydroxide has a very low solubility at body temperature and will remain in the tissue for some time. Calcium hydroxide has been shown to cause irreversible damage to nerve tissue when exposed for less than 1 h in several experimental models [79–81] leading to reduction in nerve activity. The effect is possibly caused by the excess of calcium and hydroxide ions leading to a destabilization of the nerve membrane potential [79]. Some previous studies have indicated that no or only mild problems occur if calcium hydroxide is displaced through the apical foramen providing there is no contact with soft tissue [82–84].

A few reports dealt with the negative side effects of $Ca(OH)_2$ including bone necrosis and continuing inflammatory response in repaired mechanical perforations, the neurotoxic effect of root canal sealers, cytotoxicity on cell cultures, damaged epithelium with or without a cellular atypia when applied on hamster cheek pouches and cellular damage following early $Ca(OH)_2$ dressing of avulsed teeth [84]. Few authors have also reported the deleterious effects if the material is extruded under high pressure during endodontic treatment [78, 85, 86]. Calcium hydroxide paste can result in necrosis and degenerative changes in animal models by intense inflammatory responses [87, 88]. Its pH is around 12 [85], and it has very low solubility at body temperature and will remain in the tissue for considerable time [86] and therefore cannot be considered biocompatible [85] (Fig. 7.7).

De Bruyne et al. [84] reported gingival necrosis after extrusion of $Ca(OH)_2$ paste through a root perforation of maxillary central incisor. They treated the necrotic gingival zone with rinses of hydrogen peroxide 3% and chlorhexidine 2% and daily application (twice daily) of chlorhexidine digluconate 10 mg/g gel and concluded that as long as $Ca(OH)_2$ does not come into direct contact with surrounding soft tissues, problems either do not occur or are of a mild transient nature. Sharma et al. [89] described two severe cases of iatrogenic extrusion of $Ca(OH)_2$ on upper and lower molar teeth. They observed extensive necrosis in the scalp, skin and mucosa in the first case and infraorbital nerve paraesthesia and palatal mucosal necrosis in the second case. Both patients reported severe pain immediately after $Ca(OH)_2$ injection. A computerized tomography (CT) scan with three-dimensional (3-D) reconstruction in second case confirmed the intravascular distribution of the material. Authors explained that an exposure of $Ca(OH)_2$ to blood resulted in crystalline precipitation and the consequent ischaemic tissue necrosis. The patient underwent thrombolytic, steroid and antibiotic therapies to maintain tissue reperfusion, limit inflammatory responses and prevent infections, respectively [89]. A case of lower molar with extrusion of $Ca(OH)_2$ was described by some authors [78]. Patient had severe local pain and paleness, and later during 90 min, the right half of the face and palate became increasingly painful. Facial nerve paralysis and trigeminal paraesthesia developed in all branches of the right side. Vision in the right eye became blurry, cyanotic part of the palate became necrotic [78, 90], and the underlying bone was sequestered. Angiography showed a number of vascular occlusions of vessels of the right external carotid artery while laser Doppler showed severe ischaemia. Case was treated by tissue plasminogen activator and prostacyclin analogue for 4 weeks.

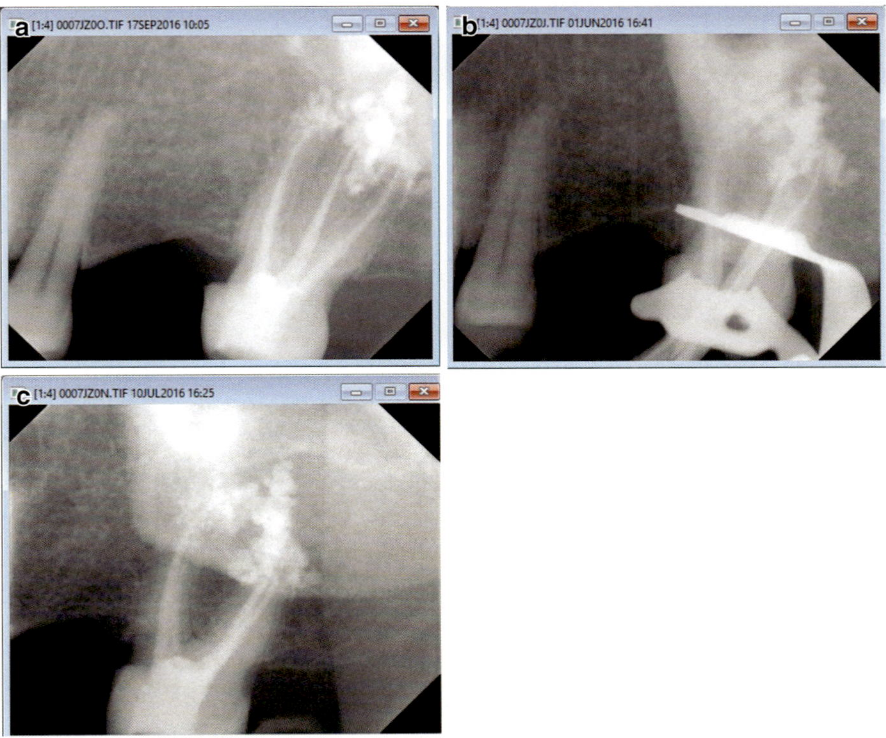

Fig. 7.7 (**a**) $Ca(OH)_2$ beyond the apex. (**b**) After 1 month patient was symptomless. (**c**) 3 months follow-up

$Ca(OH)_2$ if extruded beyond the apex may cause inflammatory resorption and necrotize the buccal mucosa while discharging the material from the site [91] This is presented without pain and can be treated by careful curettage of the lesion [91]. Patient may present with diffuse swelling at the lower buccal mandibular border in case $Ca(OH)_2$ is extruded from a lower premolar tooth, and the offending tooth will be tender to percussion [86, 90] and mobile. It may also show manifestation of paraesthesia in the lower lip [86]. This can be treated with nonsteroidal anti-inflammatory drugs [90] and antibiotic clindamycin [86] and surgical removal of the displaced material [89, 91, 92].

7.7.3 Prevention

Careful application of calcium hydroxide paste into root canals can help avoid the complications. It is important to remove any displaced material early when symptoms develop [86].

Possible complications with premixed calcium hydroxide dressings applied with pressure insertion systems (lentulo spiral or applicator tips) in root canals should be reconsidered especially in paediatric dentistry [92]. Caution should be taken when using premixed, pressure syringe $Ca(OH)_2$ system in root canal therapy, especially if there is no apical stop in the root apex. We would recommend alternative techniques for applying calcium hydroxide to prevent harmful side effects [90].

Instrumentation may develop a traumatic communication facilitating the passage of fluids into the artery. Preparing the canal atraumatically will reduce the likelihood of extruded endodontic material into the periradicular region. The lentulo spiral is the most effective device in delivering $Ca(OH)_2$ paste to working length. Syringe systems are considered less exact for carrying the filling material [93]. Moreover, there is greater risk of calcium hydroxide extrusion when using pressure syringe systems.

7.7.4 Treatment

Treatment modalities differ from case to case. There is no standardized method of treatment in the literature. The most important is to relief the patient's anxiety, reassure him and treat the case according to the signs and symptoms at that specific time. It is important to remove any displaced material before the symptoms progress [86]. If the case is severe, it is always recommended to refer to hospital or oral maxillofacial surgeon. Follow-up by taking periapical radiograph every 3 months is recommended. In most cases after approximately 6 months later, clinical and radiographic evaluations reveal no signs and symptoms and no lesions in periapical radiograph [86, 90, 92].

7.8 Gutta-Percha Solvents

Dental materials are frequently placed in direct contact with live tissues and endodontic materials are not an exception [94]. Endodontic retreatment is often the preferred course of action for failed root canal therapy [95–99]. Gutta-percha (GP) has been the most frequent root canal obturation material for more than 100 years [96, 97, 99] which is simple enough to remove in case of endodontic failure. There are several methods for GP removal: thermal, mechanical and chemical solvent [97, 99]. Chloroform is one of these inorganic solvents widely used for GP softening or dissolving [97]. With less solving ability, xylol is another GP solvent followed by essential oils such as eucalyptol and orange oil [100, 101].

The efficiency, safety and benefit of chloroform as a solvent for softening GP during endodontic treatment have already been proven [98]. In an attempt to assess the antimicrobial effect of chloroform on *Enterococcus faecalis*, Edgar et al. assumed that chloroform reduced bacteria to non-cultivable levels [98]. However, side effects from exposure to chloroform have also been recorded [94]. Furthermore, studies have addressed that chloroform is possibly carcinogenic to humans [99, 102]. Chloroform is classified as a group 2B carcinogen by the *International Agency for Research on Cancer*, which points out the materials that lack adequate evidence of carcinogenicity in humans, but there is sufficient evidence of their carcinogenicity in animals [97].

7.8.1 Toxicity

Chloroform is able to bind to cell membrane and readily penetrate the cells leading to lethal cell injury [102]. Vajrabhaya et al. found that the percentage of cells viability after contact with chloroform was around 5–6% [97]. Their results provided enough information to dentists to warn of any GP solvent discharge through apical foramen [97].

7.8.2 Prevention

The best way to prevent is not to use. Chloroform is hardly used now in developed countries and is banned in others. Some researchers suggest removing the GP in two steps, first to remove the upper part with the solvent then the rest to be removed with files [103]. Use in this way prevents overflow of chloroform out of the canal. By dissolving rather than softening, chloroform leaves residues on the canal and pulp chamber walls and due to fast evaporative action, it needs to be refreshed. On the other hand, xylol proves to be a more efficient and biologically safer solvent [104, 105] in controlling and removing softened rather than the liquefied GP. Cytotoxicity data have shown that chloroform was able to produce cellular death in dose-related fashion, the strongest effect being observed at higher concentrations [102].

Using the available root canal retreatment NiTi rotary systems, which make the retreatment procedure easier and faster, enough heat is generated by the rotating which melts the gutta-percha and, subsequently, then can be washed out. Various nickel titanium rotary instruments have been developed to facilitate cleaning and shaping of root canals and removing gutta-percha remnants from the root canal wall. They also maintain the canal shape, do not cause any canal deformation and have a shorter working time [106, 107].

7.9 Iatrogenic Injury of Oral Mucosa Due to Formaldehyde-Containing Medications

Formaldehyde-containing medications have been used for root canal treatment for many years [111]. Various compounds containing arsenic and paraformaldehyde were used in the past when effective anaesthesia could not be obtained [112].

It was introduced to treat nonvital permanent teeth in the USA by Buckley in 1904 [113]. In 1930, Sweet introduced the formocresol pulpotomy technique. Formocresol has subsequently become a popular pulpotomy medicament for primary teeth.

Formocresol acts through the aldehyde group of formaldehyde, forming bonds with the side groups of the amino acids of both the bacterial proteins and those of the remaining pulp tissue. It is therefore both a bactericidal and devitalizing agent. It kills off and converts bacteria and pulp tissue into inert compounds [114]. Improper use of formocresol can cause necrosis of soft and hard tissues in the oral cavity and swelling.

7.9.1 Formocresol Toxicity

Concerns about the safety of formocresol have been appearing in the literature for more than 20 years. Formaldehyde, a primary component in formocresol, is a hazardous substance [113]. The National Institute for Occupational Safety and Health in the USA states if formaldehyde exposure occurs at a concentration of 20 ppb (parts per billion) or higher, it is instantly dangerous to health and life [115], [116].

Numerous researchers have supported the mutagenicity (genotoxicity), carcinogenicity and toxicity of formaldehyde [117–119]. Clinicians are advised that using formocresol is not recommended by the *American Association of Endodontists* and the *American Academy of Pediatric Dentistry*. Improper handling of formocresol without proper isolation measures (rubber dam) or the use of excess mount of formocresol in cotton pellet can damage the oral tissue which is considered as an iatrogenic error.

Wesley et al. [120] recommended that formocresol be applied to a sterile cotton pellet and squeezed dry in sterile gauze before being placed into the pulp chamber. Improper handling of materials can also be a harmful event for the dentist and dental assistant. Accidental use of formocresol as eye drops may create irreversible damage to the conjunctiva [121].

7.9.2 Signs and Symptoms

The clinical presentation depends on the nature, duration of exposure and its chemical nature. Chemically induced oral ulcerations can affect any site inside the oral cavity, but most commonly affects the labial and buccal mucosa [122].

The typical clinical feature of such chemical injury usually manifests as, superficial white, wrinkled appearance. As the duration of exposure increases, the necrosis proceeds, and the affected epithelium becomes separated from the underlying tissue and appears as desquamated [123]. Removal of the necrotic epithelium reveals red bleeding connective tissue that subsequently gets covered by a yellowish fibrinopurulent membrane. Histopathological examination of such tissue shows features of coagulative necrosis [124]. The diagnosis of a chemical burn depends on the correlation of presenting clinical history, signs, the chronological events related to the suspected agent and onset of ulceration [122]. Histopathological investigations should be considered only in case of failure in establishing the cause.

Cambruzzi and Greenfield [125] described a case in which overmedication of a canal system with formocresol resulted in crystal bone loss. They postulated that the formocresol vapour may have penetrated a dentinal wall that was excessively thinned.

Murdoch-Kinch et al. [126] reported a case where chemical injury to the oral mucosa resulted in obstructive sialadenitis of the submandibular glands.

7.9.3 Management

Treatment of oral ulcerations due to chemical injury primarily requires identification and removal of the responsible agent. No standard therapy for further management of the complication has been described in the literature. Ulcers in the oral cavity usually heal up within 2 weeks without scarring; only palliative and symptomatic treatment should be considered.

Avoidance of plaque accumulation with gentle oral hygiene measures along with anaesthetic mouth wash helps in these cases [122]. A soft diet and avoiding spicy or hot foods is also recommended. The application of topical corticosteroid such as Orabase (triamcinolone—Kenalog Orabase) provides provisional relief due to its well-known action of anti-inflammatory, antipruritic and antiallergic actions. The Orabase form also provides a protective covering which may serve to temporarily reduce the pain associated with oral irritation.

Antibiotic therapy should be considered only in very extensive cases [121].

Extensive injury involving supporting bone loss might result in the extraction of the offending tooth. If the injury involves the salivary gland duct, patient may experience transient obstructive sialadenitis [126], and the scarring of salivary gland duct may result in permanent obstruction and chronic sialadenitis which will then require surgical intervention.

7.9.4 Prevention

The importance of a well-fitted rubber dam cannot be emphasized enough. Formocresol solution should be applied to a sterile cotton pellet and squeezed dry in a sterile gauze before being placed into the pulp chamber. Any poor or defective restorations/perforation may cause seepage of the formocresol into the tissues. Therefore, care must be taken to avoid that to occur. Dentist, dental assistant and patient should wear eye protection at all time to prevent accidental contact of the material with the eye.

Conclusion

To conclude, all the medicaments and irrigating solutions discussed in the chapter are effective antibacterial agents, but, when in contact with vital tissues, they become a potential irritant causing tissue destruction. Therefore, to prevent this, injudicious use should be avoided, sealed rubber dam isolation during treatment should be practised, Luer lock needle for irrigation should be used, wedging of needle into the canal should be avoided and most importantly excessive pressure during irrigation should be avoided.

Acknowledgements We would like to extend our thankfulness to the postgraduate students in Hamdan Bin Mohammed College of Dental Medicine, Dubai, UAE, for their hard work in helping to put this chapter together, wishing them all the best in their future endodontic profession.

Dr. Reem Mahmoud
Dr. Dana Alraeesi
Dr. Nausheen Aga
Dr. Hessa Fezai
Dr. Maamoun Ataya

Appendix 7.1

Mild	Moderate	Severe
Mix by GDP/endodontist	Refer to OMFS/hospital	Refer to OMFS/ hospital
• Pain 0–3 • Swelling <30% • Bruising localized • No ulceration/necrosis	• Pain 4–6 • Swelling 30–5% • Bruising diffuse • Intra-oral ulceration	• Pain 7+ • Swelling >50% • Bruising diffuse oral • Ulcerations/necrosis • Airway obstruction • Neurovascular deficit
Immediate Mx • Irrigation with saline/ sterile water • Analgesia (OTC) Nonsteroidal anti-inflammatory • Cold compress • Investigations to identify perforation or root pathology • Radiographs – IO LCPA – EO DPT	Immediate Mx • Treatment as for mild injury • Analgesia (opioids) • Ref to OMFS • Investigations to identify perforation or root pathology • Radiographs – IO LCPA – EO DPT • CBCT	Immediate Mx • Treatment as for moderate injury • IV antibiotics • IV steroids • Investigations – MRI – CT
Early Mx • Warm towel compress • Regular review	Early Mx • Treatment as for mild injury • Antibiotics if there is any evidence of infection	Early Mx • Treatment as for moderate injury • Incision and drainage of any collection

Mild	Moderate	Severe
Mix by GDP/endodontist	Refer to OMFS/hospital	Refer to OMFS/ hospital
• Extraction of tooth (if required)	• Debridement of necrotic tissue	• Definitive airway (tracheostomy) if airway is compromised (emergency case)
Late Mx	Late Mx	Late Mx
• Complete RCT with a different irrigant	• Complete RCT with a different irrigant • Lipodystrophy – Fillers – Implants – Coleman fat transfer • Reviewed by OMFS	• Lipodystrophy – Fillers – Implants • Coleman fat transfer • Medical management of neuropathic pain • Damage to motor nerves requiring advice from speech and language therapy, physiotherapy due to lip incompetence and poor oral seal • Surgery

References

1. Peters OA, Laib A, Gohring TN, Barbakow F. Changes in root canal geometry after preparation assessed by high-resolution computed tomography. J Endod. 2001;27:1–6.
2. Zehnder M. Root canal irrigants. J Endod. 2006;32:389–98.
3. Harrison JW. Irrigation of the root canal system. Den Clinics North Am. 1984;28:797–808.
4. FPV F. Accidents with sodium hypochlorite in endodontics: a literature review of clinical cases. Dental Press Endod. 2014;4(3):57–70.
5. Spencer HR, Ike V, Brennan PA. Review: the use of sodium hypochlorite in endodontics-potential complications and their management. Br Dent J. 2007;202:555–9.
6. Hülsmann M, Hahn W. Complications during root canal irrigation—literature review and case reports. Int Endod J. 2000;33:186–93.
7. Pashley EL, Birdsong NL, Bowman K, et al. Cytotoxic effects of NaOCl on vital tissue. J Endod. 1985;11:525–8.
8. Guivarc'h M, et al. Sodium hypochlorite accident: a systematic review. JOE. 2017;43(1):16–24.
9. Bowden JR, Ethunandan M, Brennan PA. Life-threatening airway obstruction secondary to hypochlorite extrusion during root canal treatment. Oral Surg Oral Med Oral Pathol Oral Radiol Endod. 2006;101:402–4.
10. Al-Sebaei MO, Halabi OA, El-Hakim IE. Sodium hypochlorite accident resulting in life-threatening airway obstruction during root canal treatment: a case report. Clin Cosmet Investig Dent. 2015;7:41–4.
11. Balto H, Al-Nazhan S. Accidental injection of sodium hypochlorite beyond the root apex. Saudi Dent J. 2002;14:36–8.
12. de Sermeño RF, da Silva LA, Herrera H, et al. Tissue damage after sodium hypochlorite extrusion during root canal treatment. Oral Surg Oral Med Oral Pathol Oral Radiol Endod. 2009;108:46–9.
13. Tegginmani VS, Chawla V, Kahate MM, et al. Hypochlorite accident—a case report. Endodontology. 2011;23:89–94.
14. Farook SA, Shah V, Lenouvel D, Sheikh O, Sadiq Z, Cascarini L. Guidelines for management of sodium hypochlorite extrusion injuries. Br Dent J. 2014;217:679–84.

15. Mehdipour O, Kleier DJ, Averbach RE. Anatomy of sodium hypochlorite accidents. Compend Contin Educ Dentist. 2007;28:544–6.
16. Lloyd RE. Surgical emphysema as a complication in endodontics. Br Dent J. 1975;138:393.
17. Snyder MD, Rosenberg ES. Subcutaneous emphysema during periodontal surgery: report of a case. J Periodontol. 1977;48:790–1.
18. Rhymes R. Post extraction subcutaneous emphysema. Oral Surg. 1964;17:271–3.
19. Hayduk S, Bennett CR, Monheim LM. Subcutaneous emphysema after operative dentistry: report of a case. J Am Dent Assoc. 1970;80:1362.
20. Battrum DE, Gutmann JL. Implications, prevention and management of subcutaneous emphysema during endodontic treatment. Endod Dent Traumatol. 1995;11:109–14.
21. Lindsey B. Oxford concise medical dictionary. 6th ed. Oxford, UK: Oxford University Press; 2003.
22. Noordzji JP, Wambach BA, Josephson GD. Subcutaneous cervicofacial and mediastinal emphysema after dental instrumentation. Otolaryngol Head Neck Surg. 2001;124:170–1.
23. Fruhauf J, Weinke R, Pilger U, Kerl H, Mullegger RR. Soft tissue cervicofacial emphysema after dental treatment. Arch Dermatol. 2005;141:1437–40.
24. Smatt Y, Browaeys H, Genay A, Raoul G, Ferri J. Iatrogenic pneumomediastinum and facial emphysema after endodontic treatment. Br J Oral Maxillofac Surg. 2004;42:160–2.
25. Lambrianidis TP. Emphysema. In: Lambrianidis T, editor. Risk management in root canal treatment. Thessaloniki: University Studio Press; 2001. p. 323–36.
26. Chen SC, Lin FY, Chang KJ. Subcutaneous emphysema and pneumomediastinum after dental extraction. Am J Emerg Med. 1999;17:678–80.
27. Josephson GD, Wambach BA, Noordzji JP. Subcutaneous cervicofacial and mediastinal emphysema after dental instrumentation. Otolaryngol Head Neck Surg. 2001;124:170–1.
28. Shovelton DS. Surgical emphysema as a complication of dental operations. Br Dent J. 1957;102:125–9.
29. Rickles NH, Joshi BA. Death from air embolism during root canal therapy. J Am Dent Assoc. 1963;67:397–404.
30. Eleazer PD, Eleazer KR. Air pressures developed beyond the apex from drying root canals with pressurized air. J Endod. 1998;24:833–6.
31. Kaufman A. Facial emphysema caused by hydrogen peroxide irrigation: report of case. J Endod. 1981;7:470–2.
32. Bhat K. Tissue emphysema caused by hydrogen peroxide. Oral Surg Oral Med Oral Pathol. 1974;38:304–8.
33. Grossman LI. Endodontic practice. Philadelphia: Lea & Febiger; 1981. p. 243–5.
34. Seltzer S, Bender I. The dental pulp. Philadelphia: Lippincott; 1984. p. 218–9.
35. Steinberg D, Heling I, Daniel I, Ginsburg I. Antibacterial synergistic effect of chlorhexidine and hydrogen peroxide against Streptococcus Sobrinus, Streptococcus Faecalis, Staphylococcus aureus. J Oral Rehab. 1999;26:151–2.
36. Seal GJ, Ng L-Y, Spratt D, Bhatti M, Gulabivala K. An in vitro comparison of bacterial efficacy of lethal photosensitisation or sodium hypochlorite irrigation on Streptococcus Intermedius biofilms in root canals. Int Endodont J. 2002;35:268–74.
37. Torabinejad M, Khademi AA, Babagoli J, Cho Y, Johnson WB, Bozhilov K, Kim J, Shabahang S. A new solution for the removal of the smear layer. J Endod. 2003;29:170–5.
38. Hulsmann M, Heckendorff M, Lennon A. Chelating agents in root canal treatment: mode of action and indications for their use. Int Endodont J. 2003;36:810–30.
39. Beltz RE, Torabinejad M, Pouresmail MV. Quantitative analysis of the solubilising action of MTAD, sodium hypochlorite and EDTA on bovine pulp and dentine. J Endod. 2003;29:334–7.
40. Tamir MD, Backleh MD, Hamdan MD, Eliashar MD. Cervico-facial emphysema and pneumomediastinum complicating a high-speed drill dental procedure. IMA J. 2005;7:124–5.
41. Kim Y, Kim MR, Kim SJ. Iatrogenic pneumomediastinum with extensive subcutaneous emphysema after endodontic treatment: report of 2 cases. Oral Surg Oral Med Oral Pathol Oral Radiol Endod. 2010;109:e114–9.

42. Horowitz I, Hirshberg A, Freedman A. Pneumomediastinum and subcutaneous emphysema following surgical extraction of mandibular third molars: three case reports. Oral Surg Oral Med Oral Pathol. 1987;63:25–8.
43. Heyman SN, Babayof I. Emphysematous complications in dentistry, 1960-1993: an illustrative case and review of the literature. Quintessence Int. 1995;26:535–43.
44. Mishra L, Patnaik S, Patro S, Debnath N. Iatrogenic subcutaneous Emphysema of Endodontic origin—case report with literature review. J Clin Diagn Res. 2014;8(1):279–81.
45. Karras SC, Sexton JJ. Cervicofacial and mediastinal emphysema as the result of a dental procedure. J Emerg Med. 1996;14:9–13.
46. Crincoli V, Scivetti M, Di Bisceglie MB, Pilolli GP, Gianfranco FG. Unusual case of adverse reaction in the use of sodium hypochlorite during endodontic treatment: a case report. Quintessence Int. 2008;39:e70–3.
47. Kost M. Thoracic complications associated with utilization of the air turbine dental drill. AANA J. 1996;64:288–92.
48. Kakehashi S, Stanley HR, Fitzgerald RJ. The effects of surgical exposures of dental pulps in germ-free and conventional laboratory rats. Oral Surg Oral Med Oral Pathol. 1965;20:340–9.
49. Bystrom A, Sundqvist G. Bacteriologic evaluation of the efficacy of mechanical root canal instrumentation in endodontic therapy. Scand J Dent Res. 1981;89:321–8.
50. Peters OA. Current challenges and concepts in the preparation of root canal systems: a review. J Endod. 2004;30:559–67.
51. Orstavik D, Haapasalo M. Disinfection by endodontic irrigants and dressings of experimentally infected dentinal tubules. Endod Dent Traumatol. 1990;6:142–9.
52. Peters LB, Wesselink PR. Combinations of bacterial species in endodontic infections. Int Endod J. 2002;35:698–702.
53. Gomes BPFA, Ferraz CCR, Vianna ME, Berber VB, Teixeira FB, Souza-Filho FJ. In vitro antimicrobial activity of several concentrations of sodium hypochlorite and chlorhexidine gluconate in the elimination of enterococcus faecalis. Int Endod J. 2001;34:424–8. PubMed: 11556507
54. Kuruvilla JR, Kamath MP. Antimicrobial activity of 2.5% sodium hypochlorite and 0.2% chlorhexidine gluconate separately and combined, as endodontic irrigants. J Endod. 1998;24:472–6. PubMed: 9693573
55. Vianna ME, Gomes BP, Berber VB, Zaia AA, Ferraz CC, de Souza-Filho FJ. In vitro evaluation of the antimicrobial activity of chlorhexidine and sodium hypochlorite. Oral Surg Oral Med Oral Pathol Oral Radio Endod. 2004;97:79–84.
56. Ehrich DG, Brian JD, Walker WA. Sodium hypochlorite accident: inadvertent injection into the maxillary sinus. J Endod. 1993;19:180–2. PubMed: 8326264
57. Jeansonne MJ, White RR. A comparison of 2.0% chlorhexidine gluconate and 5. 25% sodium hypochlorite as antimicrobial endodontic irrigants. J Endod. 1994;20:276–8. PubMed: 7931023
58. Oncag O, Hosgor M, Hilmioglu S, Zekioglu O, Eronat C, Burhanoglu D. Comparison of antibacterial and toxic effects of various root canal irrigants. Int Endod J. 2003;36:423–32. PubMed: 12801290
59. Ohara P, Torabinejad M, Kettering JD. Antibacterial effects of various endodontic irrigants on selected anaerobic bacteria. Endod Dent Traumatol. 1993;9:95–100. PubMed: 8243347
60. Delaney GM, Patterson SS, Miller CH, Newton CW. The effect of chlorhexidine gluconate irrigation on the root canal flora of freshly extracted necrotic teeth. Oral Surg Oral Med Oral Pathol. 1982;53:518–23. PubMed: 6954427
61. White RR, Hays GL, Janer LR. Residual antimicrobial activity after canal irrigation with chlorhexidine. J Endod. 1997;23:229–31. PubMed: 9594771
62. Rosenthal S, Spangberg L, Safavi K. Chlorhexidine substantivity in root canal dentin. Oral Surg Oral Med Oral Pathol Oral Radio Endod. 2004;98:488–92.
63. Komorowski R, Grad H, Wu XY, Friedman S. Antimicrobial substantivity of chlorhexidine-treated bovine root dentin. J Endod. 2000;26:315–7. PubMed: 11199744

64. Vivacqua-Gomes N, Ferraz CC, Gomes BP, Zaia AA, Teixeira FB, Souza-Filho FJ. Influence of irrigants on the coronal microleakage of laterally condensed guttapercha root fillings. Int Endod J. 2002;35:791–5.
65. Basrani BR, Manek S, Sodhi RNS, Fillery E, Manzur A. Interaction between sodium hypochlorite and chlorhexidine gluconate. J Endod. 2007;33:966–9. PubMed: 17878084
66. Burkhardt-Holm P, Oulmi Y, Schroeder A, Storch V, Braunbeck T. Toxicity of 4-chloraniline in early life stages of Zebrafish (Danio Rerio): II. Cytopathology and regeneration of liver and gills after prolonged exposure to waterborne 4 chloraniline. Arch Environ Contam Toxicol. 1999;37:85–102. PubMed: 10341046
67. Chhabra RS, Huff JE, Haseman JK, Elwell MR, Peters AC. Carcinogenicity of p-chloroaniline in rats and mice. Food Chem Toxicol. 1991;29:119–24.
68. Krishnamurthy S, Sudhakaran S. Evaluation and prevention of the precipitate formed on interaction between sodium hypochlorite and chlorhexidine. J Endod. 2010;36(7):1154–7.
69. Sjogren U, Figdor D, Spangberg L, Sundqvist G. The antimicrobial effect of calcium hydroxide as a short-term intracanal dressing. Int Endod J. 1991;24:119–25.
70. Hauman CH, Love RM. Biocompatibility of dental materials used in contemporary endodontic therapy: a review. Part 1. Intracanal drugs and substances. Int Endod J. 2003;36:75–85.
71. De Moor RJ, De Witte AM. Periapical lesions accidentally filled with calcium hydroxide. Int Endod J. 2002;35:946–58.
72. Alacam T, Gorgul G, Omurlu H. Evaluation of diagnostic radiopaque contrast materials used with calcium hydroxide. J Endod. 1990;16:365–8.
73. Smith GN, Woods S. Organic iodine: a substitute for BaSO4 in apexification procedures. J Endod. 1983;9:153–5.
74. Trope M, Chivian N, Sigurdsson A, Vann WF Jr. Traumatic injuries. In: Cohen S, Burns RC, editors. Pathways of the pulp. 8th ed. St. Louis, MO: Mosby, Inc.; 2002. p. 603–49.
75. AHR R. Damage to the inferior dental nerve during or following endodontic treatment. Br Dent J. 1983;153:306–7.
76. Ørstavik D, Brodin P, Aas E. Paraesthesia following endodontic treatment: survey of the literature and report of a case. Int Endod J. 1983;16:167–72.
77. Vernieks AA, Messer LB. Calcium hydroxide induced healing of periapical lesions: a study of 78 non-vital teeth. J Br Endod Soc. 1978;11:61–9.
78. Lindgren P, Eriksson KF, Ringberg A. Severe facial ischemia after endodontic treatment. J Oral Maxillofac Surg. 2002;60(5):576–9.
79. Brodin P, Ørstavik D. Effects of therapeutic and pulp protecting materials on nerve transmission in vitro. Scand J Dent Res. 1982;91:46–50.
80. Boiesen J, Brodin P. Neurotoxic effect of two root canal sealers with calcium hydroxide on rat phrenic nerve in vitro. Endod Dent Traumatol. 1991;7:242–5.
81. Serper A, Üçer O, Onur R, Etikan I. Comparative neurotoxic effects of root canal filling materials on rat sciatic nerve. J Endod. 1998;24(9):592–4.
82. Foreman PC, Barnes IE. A review of calcium hydroxide. Int Endod J. 1990;23:283–97.
83. Maalouf EM, Gutmann JL. Biological perspectives on the nonsurgical endodontic management of periradicular pathosis. Int Endod J. 1994;27:154–62.
84. De Bruyne MAA, De Moor RJG, Raes FM. Necrosis of the gingiva caused by calcium hydroxide: a case report. Int Endod J. 2000;33:67–71.
85. Wilson A. Severe tissue necrosis following intra-arterial injection of endodontic calcium hydroxide: a case series. Oral Surg Oral Med Oral Pathol Oral Radiol Endod. 2008;105(5):666–9.
86. Ahlgren FK, Johannessen AC, Hellem S. Displaced calcium hydroxide paste causing inferior alveolar nerve paraesthesia: report of a case. Oral Surg Oral Med Oral Pathol Oral Radiol Endod. 2003;96(6):734–7.
87. Nelson Filho P, Silva LA, Leonardo MR, Utrilla LS, Figueiredo F. Connective tissue responses to calcium hydroxide-based root canal medicaments. Int Endod J. 1999;32(4):303–11.
88. Shimizu T, Kawakami T, Ochiai T, Kurihara S, Hasegawa H. Histopathological evaluation of subcutaneous tissue reaction in mice to a calcium hydroxide paste developed for root canal fillings. J Int Med Res. 2004;32(4):416–21.

89. Sharma S, Hackett R, Webb R, Macpherson D, Wilson A. Severe tissue necrosis following intra-arterial injection of endodontic calcium hydroxide: a case series. Oral Surg Oral Med Oral Pathol Oral Radiol Endod. 2008;105(5):666–9.
90. Shahravan A, Jalali S, Mozaffari B, Pourdamghan N. Iran. Endod J. 2012;7(2):102–8.
91. Bramante CM, Luna-Cruz SM, Sipert CR, Bernadineli N, Garcia RB, Moraes IG, Vasconcelos BC. Alveolar mucosa necrosis induced by utilisation of calcium hydroxide as root canal dressing. Int Dent J. 2008;58(2):81–5.
92. Sharma DS, Chauhan SP, Kulkarni VK, Bhusari C, Verma R. Accidental periapical extrusion of non-setting calcium hydroxide: unusual bone response and management. J Indian Soc Pedod Prev Dent. 2014;32(1):63–7.
93. Sigurdsson A, Stancill R, Madison S. Intracanal placement of Ca (OH)2: a comparison of techniques. J Endod. 1992;18(8):367–70.
94. Ribeiro DA. Do endodontic compounds induce genetic damage? A comprehensive review. Oral Surg Oral Med Oral Pathol Oral Radiol Endod. 2008;105(2):251–6.
95. Abbasipour F, Akheshteh V, Rastqar A, Khalilkhani H, Asgari S, Janahmadi M. Comparing the effects of mineral trioxide aggregate and calcium enriched mixture on neuronal cells using an electrophysiological approach. Iran Endod J. 2012;7(2):79–87.
96. Barbosa SV, Burkard DH, Spangberg LS. Cytotoxic effects of gutta-percha solvents. J Endod. 1994;20(1):6–8.
97. Vajrabhaya LO, Suwannawong SK, Kamolroongwarakul R, Pewklieng L. Cytotoxicity evaluation of gutta-percha solvents: Chloroform and GP-Solvent (limonene). Oral Surg Oral Med Oral Pathol Oral Radiol Endod. 2004;98(6):756–9.
98. Edgar SW, Marshall JG, Baumgartner JC. The antimicrobial effect of chloroform on enterococcus faecalis after gutta-percha removal. J Endod. 2006;32(12):1185–7.
99. Ribeiro DA, Matsumoto MA, Marques ME, Salvadori DM. Biocompatibility of gutta-percha solvents using in vitro mammalian test-system. Oral Surg Oral Med Oral Pathol Oral Radiol Endod. 2007;103(5):e106–9.
100. Asgary S, Ahmadyar M. One-visit RCT of maxillary incisors with extensive inflammatory root resorption and periradicular lesions: a case report. Iran Endod J. 2011;6(2):95–8.
101. Ribeiro DA, Marques ME, Salvador DM. In vitro cytotoxic and non-genotoxic effects of gutta-percha solvents on mouse lymphoma cells by single cell gel (comet) assay. Braz Dent J. 2006;17(3):228–32.
102. Huang X, Ling J, Wei X, Gu L. Quantitative evaluation of debris extruded apically by using ProTaper universal Tulsa rotary system in endodontic retreatment. J Endod. 2007;33(9):1102–5.
103. Metzger Z, Ben-Amar A. Removal of overextended gutta-percha root canal fillings in endodontic failure cases. J Endod. 1995;21(5):287–8.
104. Martos J, Bassotto AP, Gonzalez-Rodriguez MP, Ferrer-Luque CM. Dissolving efficacy of eucalyptus and orange oil, xylol and chloroform solvents on different root canal sealers. Int Endod J. 2011;44(11):1024–8.
105. Mushtaq M, Masoodi A, Farooq R, Yaqoob KF. The dissolving ability of different organic solvents on three different root canal sealers: in vitro study. Iran Endod J. 2012;7(4):198–202.
106. Bishop K, Dummer PMH. A comparison of stainless steel Flexofiles and nickel-titanium NiTiFlex files during the shaping of simulated canals. Int Endod J. 1997;30(1):25–34.
107. Esposito PT, Cunningham CJ. A comparison of canal preparation with nickel-titanium and stainless steel instruments. J Endod. 1995;21(4):173–6.
108. Gatot A, Arbelle J, Leiberman A, Yanai-Inbar I. Effects of sodium hypochlorite on soft tissues after its inadvertent injection beyond the root apex. J Endod. 1991;17:573–4.
109. Kandian S, Chander S, Bishop K. Management of sodium hypochlorite extrusion beyond the root apex during root canal treatment: a case report. Prim Dent J. 2013;3:72–5.
110. Ercan E, Ozekinci T, Atakul F, Gul K. Antibacterial activity of 2% chlorhexidine gluconate and 5.25% sodium hypochlorite in infected root canal: in vivo study. J Endod. 2004;30:84–7. PubMed: 14977302
111. John V. Cambruzzi, Raymond S. Greenfeld, (1983) Necrosis of crestal bone related to the use of excessive formocresol medication during endodontic treatment. Journal of Endodontics 9 (12):565–567.

112. Ozmeric N. Localized Alveolar Bone Necrosis Following Use Of An Arsenical Paste- a case report: Int Endod J. 2002;35:295–9.
113. Ranly DM. Pulpotomy therapy in primary teeth: New modalities for old rationales. Pediatr Dent 1994;16:403–9.
114. Restorative techniques in paediatric dentistry,. In: Duggal MS, editor. 2 nd ed.; 2002. p. 50–63.
115. Kim S, Liu M, Simchon S, Dorscher-Kim JE. Effects of selected inflammatory mediators in blood flow and vascular permeability in the dental pulp. Proc Finn Dent Soc 1992;88 Suppl 1:387–92.
116. The National Institute for Occupational Safety and Health (NIOSH) Formaldehyde. Available from: http://www.tricornet.com/nioshdbs/idlh/50000.htm [Last accessed 2006 on Mar 13].
117. Daniel Araki Ribeiro, (2008) Do endodontic compounds induce genetic damage? A comprehensive review. Oral Surgery, Oral Medicine, Oral Pathology, Oral Radiology, and Endodontology 105 (2):251–256.
118. Speit G, Merk O. Evaluation of mutagenic effects of formaldehyde in vitro: detection of crosslinks and mutations in mouse lymphoma cells. Mutagenesis2002; 17: 183–187.
119. Luoping Zhang, Craig Steinmaus, David A. Eastmond, Xianjun K. Xin, Martyn T. Smith, (2009) Formaldehyde exposure and leukemia: A new meta-analysis and potential mechanisms. Mutation Research/Reviews in Mutation Research 681 (2-3):150–168.
120. David Joseph Wesley, F.James Marshall, Samuel Rosen, (1970) The quantitation of formocresol as a root canal medicament. Oral Surgery, Oral Medicine, Oral Pathology 29 (4):603–612.
121. Basak S K, Choudhuri Ayon, Basak S, Bakshi P K. Occular injury with Formocresol mistaken for eye drops. Bengal ophthalmic journal 2010; 10:37–39.
122. C. Gilvetti, S. R. Porter, S. Fedele, (2010) Traumatic chemical oral ulceration: a case report and review of the literature. BDJ 208 (7):297–300.
123. Physical and chemical injuries. In: Neville B W, Damm D, Allen C M, Bouquot J. Oral and maxillofacial pathology. 3rd ed. Philadelphia: W B Saunders; 2009:285–329.
124. M. Hulsmann, W. Hahn, (2000) Complications during root canal irrigation - literature review and case reports. International Endodontic Journal 33 (3):186–193
125. Cambreuzzi JV, Greenfield RS. Necrosis of crestal bone related to the use of excessive formooresol medication during endodontic treatment. J Endodon 1983:9:565–7.
126. Carol Anne Murdoch-Kinch, Mark E. Mallatt, Dale A. Miles, (1995) Oral mucosal injury caused by denture cleanser tablets. Oral Surgery, Oral Medicine, Oral Pathology, Oral Radiology, and Endodontology 80 (6):756–758.

8 Strategies to Reduce the Risk of Reinfection in Endodontics

Federico Foschi

8.1 Endodontic Microbiology

The aetiological role of bacteria in endodontic disease is preponderant [1], although reports of a minor contribution of viruses is surfacing [2, 3]. The molecular methods developed at the turning of the millennium induced an exponential growth of the data available to oral and endodontic microbiologist [4].

The aetiology of the endodontic disease does not follow a Koch postulate. Polymicrobial communities in the form of biofilms are eliciting the endodontic disease, manifesting itself as periapical bone resorption, induced by osteoclast-induced resorptive process triggered by an inflammatory cytokine cascade [5].

Noncultural approaches revealed further subspecies of bacteria involved in specific manifestation of the disease: in particular refractory endodontic disease has represented a major *conundrum* for the endodontists and the researchers alike. Many authors described a reduction in the number of species involved in secondary endodontic infections, whereas others reported an increase in the diversity of species: this underestimation was due to the limitation of the cultural approaches. Certain species have been enumerated as potential culprit of refractory endodontic infections, possibly returning on a quasi-Koch hypothesis (*i.e. E. faecalis* as main player in secondary endodontic infections).

Indeed, specialised bacteria are present in the endodontic niche. Factors such as proteolytic enzyme secretion, motility, dormant/starvation state capabilities, strict anaerobiosis, alkalinity resistance and opportunistic features among many others may represent the main characteristics of the true endodontic pathogens [6].

The original version of this chapter was revised. An erratum to this chapter can be found at https://doi.org/10.1007/978-3-319-60997-3_13

F. Foschi, BDS, MSc, PhD, FHEA, FDS RCS.
Department of Endodontics, King's College London, Guy's Hospital, Tower Wing, Fl 22, Great Maze Pond, London, SE1 9RT UK
e-mail: federico.foschi@kcl.ac.uk

P. Jain (ed.), *Common Complications in Endodontics*,
https://doi.org/10.1007/978-3-319-60997-3_8

Table 8.1 Pre-existing factors and parameters affecting the root canal treatment outcome related to endodontic infection eradication and reoccurrence

Poorer prognosis	Better prognosis
Secondary infection	*Primary infection*
Long-standing infection	
Presence of fistulae	No historical or current oral/endodontic communication
Lack of coronal seal/insufficient residual tooth structure	Sufficient tooth structure allowing gap-free restoration
Hairline cracks	
Endo/perio lesion	

In the dimensions of the endodontic infection however, many other aspects may have a negative effect on the prognosis of primary and secondary root canal treatment [7] (Table 8.1).

The duration of an infection has a very important role: long-standing infection are more difficult to be removed. Several studies confirmed that the maturation of biofilms allows an increased resistance to any antibacterial approach [8]. The nature of bacterial contamination and sources may play a major role too.

Several routes and chances of contamination of the root canal system are present:

1. *De novo* infections of the root canal space
   (a) Deep decays (with a prompter effect on younger patients with wider dentinal tubules).
   (b) Coronal leakage (faulty or missing coronal restoration, degradation of the hybrid layer).
   (c) Coronal and radicular micro-crack (craze lines, hairline cracks, microfractures).
   (d) Long-standing periodontal disease (acidic exposure and root surface instrumentation can lead to dentinal tubules exposure and retrograde dentinal infection).
   (e) Presence of fistulae can sustain extra-radicular and retrograde endodontic infections leading to the formation of extra-radicular biofilm, which are proven to be more aggressive and pathogenic.
2. Recurrent endodontic infection
   (a) Incomplete eradication of the microbial communities presents as biofilms in the main root canal lumen and can lead to a re-propagation of the infection with a delayed recolonisation even in the presence of satisfactory root canal filling.
   (b) Incomplete disinfection of inaccessible areas due to inadequate or short time of disinfection.
   (c) Insufficient operative skills and incomplete chemo-debridement and shaping protocols (missed canals).
   (d) Iatrogenic contaminations, a novel concept in endodontics, may help in understanding the endodontic infection stages and its origin: cross-contamination during the handling of non-sterile endodontic consumables can be a significant cause for refractory infections.

8.1.1 Medically Compromised Patients and Relapse of Endodontic Infections

The evidence regarding the contribution of the endodontic infection to systemic pathologies and diseases in endodontic research is still sparse [9–11], whereas conclusive evidence has been reached in the field of periodontology [12]. The host's role in the establishment and evolution of the endodontic pathology, including the potential systemic effects of a low-grade chronic inflammation/infection, is now taken more seriously. The receiving end of the infection has a major role in terms of permissiveness to the spreading of endodontic infections: B and T cell deficiency can lead to increased spreading of endodontic infection [13].

Vice versa the continuous inflammatory stress of an infected root canal system that triggers the immune response may have systemic effects on the host [14]. The main areas of potential association of endodontic infection and systemic diseases include cardiovascular disease (CVD), diabetes mellitus (DM), chronic liver disease, blood disorders and bone mineral density. The linkage between CVD and endodontic pathology may be conceivable, in particular with a hypothesised role of the endodontic inflammatory mediators on the initiation and progression of CVD; however, further studies are required [14].

In terms of DM, the association of an increased disease prevalence and frequency of onset of periapical lesion for type 2 diabetic patients has been confirmed [15]. However, a delayed or hindered healing of periapical lesions following endodontic treatment in diabetic patients has not been proved yet [16, 17]. The risk of bias for these studies is high, and further investigations are required. Little evidence is currently present for chronic liver disease, blood disorders and bone mineral density [14].

Interestingly the fitness level of the patient apparently has little influence on the manifestation of the endodontic disease [18]. Whereas other studies seemed to point towards a certain association of certain gene polymorphisms that lead to an increased susceptibility to endodontic manifestation (periapical resorption presence and extent), however the evidence is still very limited [19].

8.1.2 The Microbiota of Refractory Endodontic Infection

The microbiota of refractory infection is very dissimilar from the primary endodontic infection. The initial formation of periapical lesion can occur with limited bacteria present in the dentino-pulpal complex [5]. Not rarely tubular dentine infection may be sufficient to trigger a cytokine cascade leading to the formation of the periapical lesion [20]. Primary endodontic infection may however mature with time leading to the development of a complex endodontic biofilm [8]. The endodontic niche provides a selective pressure due to the limited oxygen tension. The starvation of bacteria receiving limited amount of serum proteins or alternative metabolite is another reason for the survival and rise of the most resilient and aggressive pathogens among the endodontic biofilm. With cultural methods the most commonly isolated species in primary endodontic infection are

Peptostreptococcus micros, *Fusobacterium necrophorum*, *Fusobacterium nucleatum*, *Prevotella intermedia* and *Porphyromonas gingivalis* [21]. In primary endodontic infection associated with periapical lesion, the microbiota is mixed with both gram-negative and gram-positive, mostly anaerobic microorganisms and including more than three species per canal. In secondary endodontic infection, facultative anaerobes and gram-positive bacteria prevail, and interestingly only one or two species are isolated. In secondary endodontic infection, certain species are cultured more frequently: *Enterococcus faecalis*, *Streptococcus* spp., *P. micros* and *F. necrophorum* [22]. More recent microbiological studies adopting molecular methods that bypassed the limits of cultural approaches revealed a different picture. The association of *E. faecalis* with failed root canal treatments has been noted in several papers [23–27].

A recent study showed that gram-negative anaerobes previously considered related to symptomatic lesions were also present in asymptomatic cases. A novel hypothesis suggests that different compositions of the endodontic microbiota can result in similar disease outcome characteristics [28]. Another established hypothesis is that the root canal treatment per se may have a direct effect on the microbiota creating an imbalance and selecting certain species by modifying the ecology of the root canal space [29]. Current studies are re-evaluating the sole etiopathological role of *E. faecalis* in the development of refractory endodontic infection showing instead the presence of more complex polymicrobial infection [30, 31].

A further concept regards the possible contribution of the clinician in the establishment of secondary infections in the course of the primary treatment. The nosocomial infections, also defined as hospital-acquired infection (HAI), have been reported in different branches of medicine and affect the outcome of surgical and other operative procedures [32, 33]. The usage of non-sterile consumables and the contact with infected environmental surfaces may lead to the transmission into the root canal space of pathogens, that can subsequently establish a secondary infection [34]. In particular *Staphylococcus epidermidis and Propionibacterium acnes* are not present as common commensal in the oral cavity; however, these species have been isolated in endodontic refractory infections [35]. Increasing the asepsis/sterility during endodontic treatment may prevent nosocomial infections.

8.2 Diagnosis of the Refractory Endodontic Infection

The diagnosis of a refractory endodontic infection is important for the clinician to minimise the chances of failure [25]. A truly refractory endodontic infection may not be eradicated even utilising the most advanced non-surgical techniques [36].

The detection of strains specifically associated with persistent/refractory pathology is still not practical in everyday clinical settings. Culturing methods cannot grow non-cultivable and fastidious bacterial strains, often present in endodontic infections.

Molecular methods are still expensive and require a certain turnaround impractical during a single treatment session. The clinician can only rely on the clinical signs of pathology that are usually related to the more established infection.

Clinical examination revealing presence of symptoms and radiographic signs of non-healing or expanding periapical lesion is indicative, by assumption, of presence of a refractory endodontic infection. Clinician rarely confirms clinically the presence of bacteria. Clinical microbiologic sampling is not commonly used. Novel devices based on fluorescence may be utilised chairside to confirm directly the presence of bacteria in failed root canal treatment. Chairside tests have been previously considered in periodontology (e.g. BANA test) [37]. Reports of contemporary usage of anaerobic tests in endodontology are very limited [38].

Refractory infections may have developed due to iatrogenic infection or persistence of bacteria at the time of the primary endodontic treatment or due to secondary recolonisation of the root canal space. Lack of coronal seal is the major reason for the reinfection of the root canal system. Even in the presence of a well-executed root canal free of voids, bacteria can slowly recolonise the root canal space through a percolation phenomenon [39, 40].

The presence of a large periapical lesion is not related to the bacterial load; however, it does reduce the chances of healing independently of the microbiological status. On the other hand, the existence of sinus tract (*fistula*) is associated with more complex biofilms which are proven to be more resilient [41] (Fig. 8.1a, b). *P. acnes* can be isolated in the presence of fistulae. This bacterial strain has been described as an aggressive pathogen that can lead to failure of orthopaedic implants, cardiac valve and other prosthetic surfaces prone to biofilm development [42]. The formation of fistulous tracts also facilitates the infection of the external surface of the roots leading to the formation of extra-radicular biofilm, which are inaccessible by the non-surgical root canal treatment [43, 44].

The development of extra-radicular biofilm is associated also with specific bacterial strains as *Actinomyces actinomycetemcomitans* that may be also related to intra-radicular polymicrobial biofilms [45]. Another important dimension of the endodontic infection is time: long-standing endodontic infections are more resilient and difficult to be eradicated [46]. The maturation of biofilms causes the formation of complex defence mechanisms, including extracellular matrices [47].

If the clinician is aware at the diagnostic phase of the effect of these parameters on the outcome, a more successful treatment can be planned, possibly including a plan for failure, of which the patient should be made aware at the outset (*i.e.* apicoectomy).

Where several detrimental parameters co-exist very large periapical lesion associated with a tooth with minimal residual coronal structure and with a long-standing fistula) a poor prognosis with high chances of failure can be predicted [48]. The patient should be informed of the risks and alternative treatment options. In certain clinical cases, true refractory endodontic affected may only be resolved with the extraction of the affected tooth.

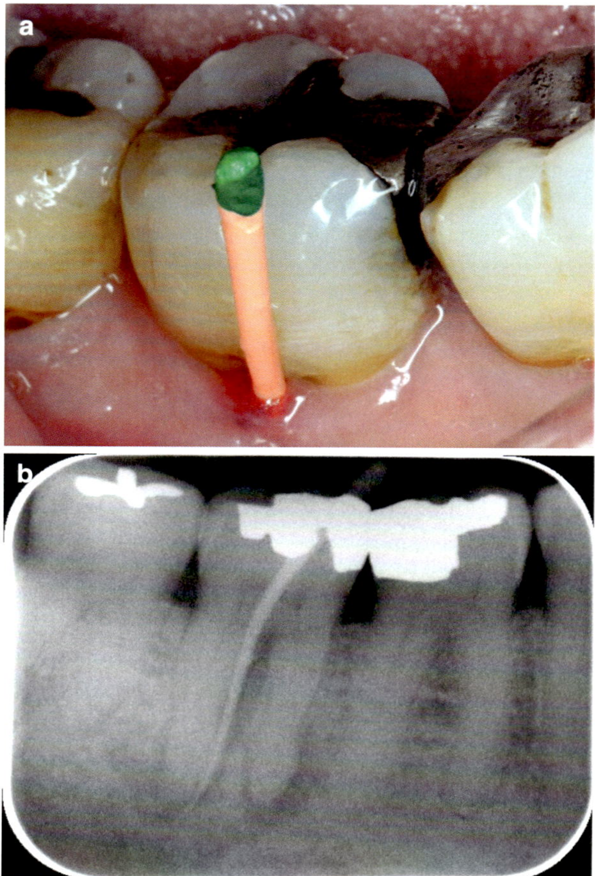

Fig. 8.1 (**a–b**) Clinical photograph (**a**) and long cone periapical X-ray (**b**) showing an intra-radicular fistula. The chances of healing are diminished due to the possibility of oral bacteria to form an extra-radicular biofilm which is inaccessible by orthograde root canal treatment. The presence of hairline crack should be investigated with an operative assessment in the presence of shallow existing restoration which is not impinging on pulp space. Alternative pathway of bacterial contamination of the root canal space should be suspected

8.3 Restorability and Coronal Seal

The amount of remaining tooth structure is related to the provision of a successful restoration that prevents coronal leakage. The presence of marginal gaps in the coronal restorations can lead to a prompt reinfection. The average bacterial cell size of 2 μm allows a prompt passage through failing or deficient restoration. Lack of coronal seal increases the odds of reinfection of the root canal system even in the presence of a satisfactory root canal filling [49].

Limited number of study envisioned an objective restorability index [50, 51]. More recent data revealed that when the residual coronal tooth structure is less than 30%, the outcome of the root canal treatment decreases significantly due to higher chances of reinfection [52].

The main principles to be considered when restoring an endodontically treated tooth are to protect completely the cusps in posterior teeth in order to retain the tooth integrity and to achieve a good peripheral coronal seal. The choice of type of restorative material (amalgam vs. composite) and type of cuspal coverage (onlay vs. full crown) does not affect the longitudinal survival.

Achieving a satisfactory level of coronal seal seems to be independent from the type of restorative material employed and more related to the existing dentinal substratum [53]. The use of resin-based restoration or intracanalar fibre post has been advocated to improve the hermetic seal of the root canal system by clinicians, but no evidence is present in the literature [54]. However, the limited evidence present in literature reveals no superior advantages compared with more traditional coronal and intracanalar restoration [55]. Previous approaches included the use of the Nayyar core technique that requires removing 2–3 mm of sub-orifice gutta-percha to create a dovel space to allow the extension of an amalgam core in these areas [56]. The evidence seems very scarce in terms of type of restoration to achieve the best possible coronal seal [49]. The amount of residual tooth structure is more important than the type of post or restorative material supporting single crowns [57].

Another important parameter to be considered is the time of provision of the final restoration. Historically the tendency to wait for a full healing of the periapical lesion following root canal treatment was a common place [58]. Current approach dictates a prompt finalisation of the coronal restoration. The provision of a good coronal seal is a key aspect of maintaining the periapical health (Fig. 8.2). The final restoration should be provided as soon as practical: the survival of root canal-treated

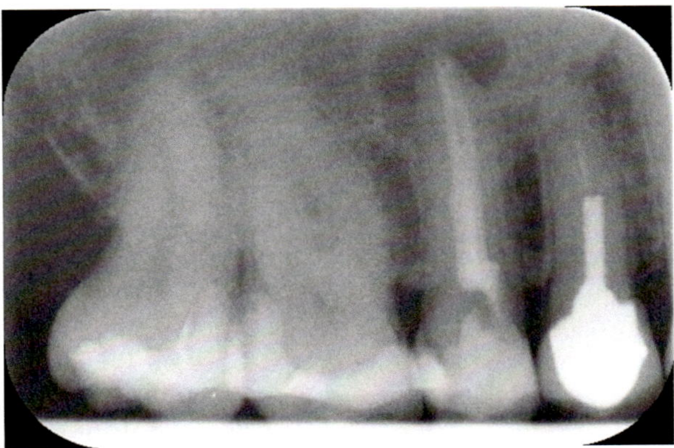

Fig. 8.2 Long cone periapical X-ray showing the co-existence of unsatisfactory root canal filling on the *upper right* first premolar associated with a satisfactory coronal seal. Conversely the *upper right* second premolar has a poor coronal seal in the presence of a well-executed root canal filling. The role of the coronal restoration in maintaining the periapical health should be emphasised

teeth that received a crown within 4 months and after 4 months following RCT was 85 and 68%, respectively. Endodontically treated teeth that received a crown 4 months after RCT were extracted at three times the rate of teeth that received a crown within 4 months after RCT [59]. The presence of symptoms is the only major contraindication to a prompt restoration. Waiting unnecessarily for the completion of the ongoing bone healing process (up to 4 years according to the ESE guidelines) may instead lead to the reoccurrence of the endodontic infection due to loss of the coronal seal.

8.4 Operative Strategies to Eradicate Endodontic Infection

The chemo-debridement of the canal is based on the use of files (stainless steel or NiTi, manual or mechanised) to remove the infected dentine with the concomitant irrigation with adequate disinfectants. The resection of infected dentine operated by the endodontic instruments removes not only the surface of the dentine but also exposes the infected tubules. The subsequent action of the irrigants is based on a direct physical effect creating a shear stress that can detach the biofilm adhering on the root canal wall and on the direct antibacterial effect on the biofilm. Several steps can allow achieving a better outcome of the root canal treatment and minimise the risk of relapse of the endodontic infection (Table 8.2).

To date no objective measurement is available to the clinician to determine the level of disinfection achieved during the chemo-debridement. Even in the case of microbiological sampling with a turnaround of at least 2 weeks for slow-growing fastidious anaerobes, the information provided regards only the bacteria of the main canal lumen. Different areas that are not reached by sampling such as isthmuses, lateral canals, apical deltas and dentinal tubules may contain an unknown amount of bacteria. Many study questioned whether the presence of bacteria in these inaccessible areas may contribute to the reinfection of the root canal system following primary root canal treatment. No clear evidence has been given so far to the clinicians to determine the endpoint of root canal treatment, that is, the required level of cleanliness or maximum acceptable bacterial cells count that does not hinder a successful outcome. Classic study compared the different outcomes depending on the presence of bacteria (positive cultures) prior to obturation; the agreement is that presence of bacteria at the time of obturation has a detrimental effect on the healing of periapical lesions [60–62]. Bacterial entombment, where a well-executed root canal would entrap bacteria within the dentinal tubules and devoid them of any metabolite and substratum to sustain the root canal infection, may not be sufficient to eradicate the infection [63]. Starvation modalities of bacteria can lead to high resistance and a lapse in the reappearance of the infection [64]. Bacteria in a dormant state and starvation may maintain a viable but non-culturable state that may still lead to reinfection of the endodontic niche [47, 65] (Fig. 8.3).

The traditional indications for reaching the clinical endpoint in endodontic treatment are based on subjective or dogmatic approaches. Clinicians referred to

Table 8.2 Operative phases and their significance aimed at maximising the disinfection of the root canal system, preventing nosocomial cross-contamination and reducing the risk of reinfection

Clinical steps	Significance
Rubber dam isolation	Saliva cross-contamination elimination
Disinfection of the operative field	Decontamination of tooth surface to avoid introduction of oral bacteria into the root canal system
Removal of existing restorations (i.e. direct or indirect restorations)	Confirmation of restorability and future coronal seal
Removal of infected dentine	Reduces chances of reinfection of the root canal system
Confirmation of absence of hairline cracks	Prevention of bacterial leakeage
Coronal flare	Creates an irrigation reservoir and maximise the exchange of irrigants
Copious irrigation with NaOCl solution	Enough contact time to reach the infected non-instrumented areas
Patency filing	Closed system vs. open system and removal of vapour lock
Adequate shaping	Apical gauging to remove sufficient infected dentine
Removal of dentinal debris from instruments flutes	Avoids cross-contamination between canals
Activation of irrigants (sonic or ultrasonic)	Increased antibacterial activity
EDTA irrigation	Penultimate rinse to remove smear layer
Final irrigation with NaOCl	Disinfection of the exposed dentinal tubules
Drying the canal with sterile paper points	Avoiding iatrogenic infection
Dressing with CaOH (if used)	Maximisation of the disinfection in the presence of fistulae (debatable) or wide periapical lesions or drainage (pus/exudate) within the canal (weeping tooth syndrome)
Change of gloves at time of obturation	Reduction of environmental cross-contamination
Disinfection of gutta-percha points for 1' in NaOCl	Reduction of nosocomial infection risk
Rapid provision of a final restoration and/or full cuspal coverage	Maximisation of the coronal seal

presence or absence of smell from dentinal shavings as an indicator of persistence or eradication of the infection; others observed the shade of the dentinal shaving collected on the file flutes [66]. More rigorous and dogmatic approaches indicated certain protocols to achieve dentinal cleanliness: it has been recommended to instrument at least three sizes bigger of the first file to bind at the apex to remove sufficient infection at the apical level [67]. Alternatively, protocols dictating a minimal dressing time with CaOH implied that the biofilm could be eradicated after a sufficient time of exposure to an alkaline environment [68]. However, both methods can be easily proved fallacious: tubular infection may infect the dentine to a depth of 1000 μm which is beyond the three sizes increase; on the other hand, bacteria such as *E. faecalis* have been shown to survive in alkaline environment [69, 70].

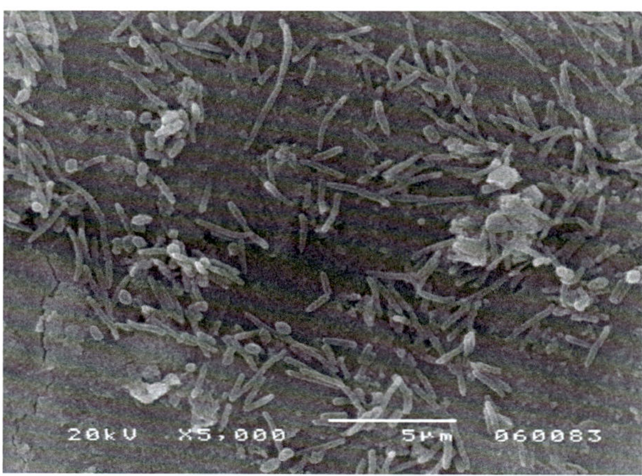

Fig. 8.3 SEM photomicrograph depicting an infected smear layer covering the root canal walls following shaping with insufficient irrigation. The clinical relevance of entombed bacteria is not clear; however, recent studies described the dormant state of bacteria embedded in the smear layer. Refractory endodontic infection may occur due to the recolonisation of the root canal system starting from these sparse bacteria

8.5 Access Cavity and Infection Prevention

The clinician needs to follow certain operative procedure to maximise the level of disinfection of the root canal system. The use of the rubber dam should be considered as the primary means to avoid the relapse of primary endodontic treatment. Despite the evidence that carrying out root canal treatment without rubber dam nullify the attempt to achieve a clean root canal, the adoption by general practitioner is extremely limited (<5%) [71, 72]. Furthermore, in absence of rubber dam, sodium hypochlorite is sparingly used due to potential ingestion [72]. Mastering the placement of the rubber dam is essential. Single tooth isolation with winged clamps and OraSeal (Ultradent, St. Louis, MO, USA) used as an adjuvant to increase the peripheral seal around the tooth to be treated improves significantly the ability to achieve complete sterility of the operative field. In case a sufficient isolation cannot be achieved (often due to the lack of residual coronal tooth structure), the feasibility of the root canal treatment should be questioned unless pre-endodontic restoration cannot be placed to improve seal. Still the provision of pre-endodontic restorations should not override the restorative consideration where a tooth is not restorable if the sound dentine is subgingival [73].

A good practice is to use surface disinfectants once the rubber dam is placed prior to accessing the *endodontium*. This simple step minimises the risk of introduction of further plaque bacteria into the root canal system especially in cases with limited endodontic bacteria load (i.e. irreversible pulpitis).

Following the essential step of a leakage-free rubber dam isolation, a thorough removal of carious infected dentine is recommended, despite minimal invasive approaches recommended in pulp vitality preservation cases say otherwise [74]. A convenient access cavity needs to be considered avoiding key-hole approaches (ninja, truss, calla lily, etc.) that limit the visibility and ability to fully disinfect the root canal system. Subsequently a thorough examination of the pulp chamber under magnification will rule out the presence of hairline cracks or other defects that would lead to a prompt reinfection of the *endodontium* via periodontal space. Hairline cracks visible under magnification can have a width of 40 μm, which are readily accessible by bacteria of 2 μm size [75]. The consensus regarding the management of visible hairline crack within the root canal system is still limited. Zero tolerance to hairline crack present on the floor of the pulp chamber is recommended to increase the outcome of the root canal treatment [76]. Other authors consider problematic only the hairline cracks that reach the canal orifice level, and others would consider unsalvageable only teeth with hairline crack penetrating into the canal below the orifice level [77].

Operatively the main advices are to prevent hairline propagation by taking the tooth off the occlusion (cusp trimming) and/or cement orthodontic bands. Alternatively, an acrylic temporary crown can be considered for similar reasons. The evidence for repair of dentine with bonding and resin composite is limited, and this technique should be avoided. Whereas deep apical root cracks cannot be detected at the diagnostic stage, the presence of deep single-spot (tubular) probing associated with hairline crack should discourage from any attempt to provide root canal treatment [78].

Once the integrity of the pulp chamber is confirmed, all existing canal orifices need to be detected. The overlooking of the endodontic anatomy may lead to prompt failure. The use of CBCT at the treatment planning phase may greatly reduce the occurrence of missed anatomy and iatrogenic errors [79]. In certain clinical condition in elderly patients or with previous history of pulpal irritation, secondary and/or tertiary dentine may have caused a significant reduction of the patency of the canals and size of the pulp chamber [80]. Canals that are not patent macroscopically can still be patent to microorganism that can freely colonise the niche and reach the apex. At this stage it is extremely important to have a good knowledge of the textbook anatomy of each type of tooth. This knowledge should be backed up by the use of high magnification and illumination to fully comprehend the canal orifice position and relationship. Missed canal is still one of the main reasons for root canal treatment failure [81, 82]. On this account, again, minimal access cavities (ninja, truss, calla lily) leaving undercuts and not allowing visual and tactile exploration of the pulp chamber may cause failure to treat the whole root canal system. At this stage the use of ultrasonic tips or of long shank rose-head burs as the gooseneck or Meisinger can aid the task to remove calcifications within the pulp chamber. Pulp stones can be present and obstruct the access to the orifice and leave a false bottom at the furcation level; the virtual space between the furcation floor and pulp stones can be rife with bacteria, and even in the absence of an existing infection, pulp remnants may represent a future substrate for bacteria infecting the root canal space. For these reasons leaving pulp stones in situ may cause future relapse of the endodontic treatment.

8.6 Shaping with Stainless Steel and NiTi Instruments

The next operative stage following initial patency confirmation and manual scouting of the root canal system is the establishment of a coronal flare. With the advent of double flare techniques and modified step back, a great emphasis on avoiding rushing to the apex has been recommended to minimise the extrusion of bacteria and debris through the apex together with the formation of blockages [83]. A premature shaping of the apical third without coronal flare is bound to have limited effectiveness as the irrigant penetration is limited.

Prior to the NiTi revolution, predicting the amount of dentine removed during the shaping was difficult [84]. Stainless steel files have a 2% taper to retain enough flexibility. To achieve a sufficient preparation taper, as per the Schilder's technique, the step back technique was utilised. Depending if stepping back 1 or 0.5 mm, a taper of 5 or 10% would be achieved. The advent of more flexible alloy allows increased tapers that can lead to a predictable and standardised removal of dentine. Still to date no study provided sufficient evidence regarding the effect of different shaping tapers on the success of root canal treatment. The microscopic anatomy of dentinal tubules varies among the different levels of the canal with wider tubules and increased density per square μm at the coronal level with respect to the apical. For these reasons the permeability of dentine to endodontic irrigant may be very efficient independently of an increased removal of dentine dictated by an increased taper instrument. Very few studies analysed the contribution to removal of the infection of instruments independently of the irrigation [85]. Clinically hand or mechanised instruments should never be used without irrigants. The presence of a prematurely enlarged coronal third improves the fluid dynamics of irrigants and increases the volume entering in the root canal system [86]. Nonetheless one of the main limitations of root canal shaping is the difficulty of any type of instrument to contact the full extent of the root canal wall surface [87]. The effect of an incomplete disinfection of the root canal system will have a major effect if larger amount of bacteria is left behind, in particular in the main canal lumen as demonstrated by the cultural studies [60].

Among the different envelopes of movement of hand files, the balanced force together with circumferential and anticurvature filling is the best combination to maximise the contact with the dentinal walls to remove the adhering biofilm. Similarly, in *de novo* cases where the root canal is minimally infected, great care should be paid to remove effectively all the pulpal tissue as this may represent a future *substratum* for bacteria leading to a prompt bacterial regrowth. The collagen component of the ground substance of the pulp and of the dentine can favour the early adhesion of biofilms [88].

Instead mechanised NiTi instrument (both rotary and reciprocating) have a fixed envelope of motions (rotation associated with pecking or with brushing movement or progressive reciprocation associated with pecking or with brushing). Furthermore, the NiTi alloy is characterised with a self-centring ability especially in curved canals. These features lead to the presence of untouched areas of the canal that can reach up to 49% of the total surface [87].

The current mechanised NiTi instrument sequences, usually based on a fewer number of files, are based on a preliminary enlargement of the coronal third of the canal. Even single file techniques recommend to approach the shaping of the root canal in thirds, usually focusing on the coronal third first. The removal of the bulk of infection present within the pulp chamber underneath decays and in the coronal third of the canal can reduce further cross-contamination from the coronal third to the middle and the apical thirds [85]. During mechanised shaping the production of infected dentinal shavings cut from the root canal walls is increased compared with manual filing [89]. The operator will remove the infected dentinal debris from the flutes of the NiTi instruments after each passage. The use of a sponge may facilitate this task. Using different sponges may reduce the chances of cross-contamination between thirds of each individual canal and among different canals. In multi-rooted teeth different levels of contamination and inflammation may be present in each individual canal; for this reason cross-contamination should be avoided with a thorough cleaning of the file after each passage: ten strokes of an "in and out" movement of the file in a dense sponge saturated in NaOCl or chlorhexidine achieve 85–100% cleaning [90].

8.7 Irrigation

The shaping action of endodontic instruments is complemented by the use of irrigation. Its main purposes are the direct eradication of the endodontic biofilm and the removal of organic and inorganic debris produced during the shaping [91]. The selection of the best irrigant solutions and the optimisation of their usage required several trials and errors. One of the important aspects is also the biocompatibility of irrigants to be used in the root canal system. Irrigation efficacy is based on the type of irrigant, the volume, the delivery method and other activation methods, which will be later discussed.

Three main categories of irrigants are used in endodontics: tissue-dissolving agents, antibacterial agents and chelating agents.

Currently, solution combining all activities together, although being developed, did not acquire a widespread use [92]. The irrigant needle allowing the best fluid dynamic of the irrigant within the root canal system is the side-vented ones. Compared to flat or bevelled one, the risk of irrigant extrusion is limited. As previously discussed taper and apical preparation may affect the effectiveness of the irrigants. The creation of a coronal flare increases the volume and exchange rate of the irrigant to the middle and apical third. An increased taper increases shear stress

Table 8.3 Correspondence between irrigation needle gauge and their lumen calibre in mm and the corresponding ISO files considering their external diameter

Gauge size	Diameter of the needle lumen (mm)	Corresponding file (considering the external diameter of the needle)
23	0.6	70
25	0.5	55
27	0.4	45
30	0.3	35

on the root canal walls, still maintaining a limited risk of apical extrusion. The shear stress can detach adhering biofilm allowing their dislodgment and complete removal from the coronal aspect by means of aspirating the irrigant outflowing from the root canal orifice [86, 93].

The gauge of the needle used for irrigation is affecting the level of irrigation within the shaped canal (Table 8.3). Several studies reported the presence of a stagnation plane beyond the tip of irrigation needles under which the exchange of irrigants is limited. Knowing the diameter of the needle allows to determine the exact level reached by the irrigants effectively. To obtain a continuous exchange of irrigants, the side-vented needle should be ideally positioned within 2 mm of the working length [93]. The irrigation needs to be carried out by expressing the plunger of the syringe gently with the index finger and maintaining a continuous in and out movement to avoid locking of the needle.

The main limitations faced by the irrigation are the difficulty in reaching non-instrumented area, in particular, isthmuses, accessory canals and dentinal tubules; the resilience of mature biofilms that are well adhering to the root canal walls; the limited contact time; and volume of delivery [94].

The mainstay of root canal disinfection is sodium hypochlorite (NaOCl). The concentration used clinically ranges between 0.1 and 6%. The overall balance between effectiveness in tissue-dissolving activity, antibacterial potency and risk of periradicular tissue damage favours the selection of mid-range NaOCl concentration as 2% [95, 96]. The chlorhexidine although promising for the broad-spectrum activity has very limited organic matrix dissolving property. Mixing the two irrigants is the cause of concerns and should be avoided [97]. For these reasons the use of 2% NaOCl solution is the main irrigant throughout root canal treatment both in cases of irreversible pulpitis and necrotic infected pulp.

The all-round effect of NaOCl both dissolving pulp remnants and affecting endodontic biofilm makes it the irrigant of choice. The main limitation of NaOCl is the inability to remove the smear layer produced during manual and mechanised instrumentation. The presence of the smear layer on the root canal walls has no clear clinical significance; however, several in vitro studies demonstrated an increased tubular disinfection [98]. For the purpose of removing the smear layer, a penultimate irrigation with 17% EDTA solution is recommended. The EDTA solution should be left *in situ* to soak the root canal space for at least 1 min. No agreement has been fully reached regarding the ideal irrigation

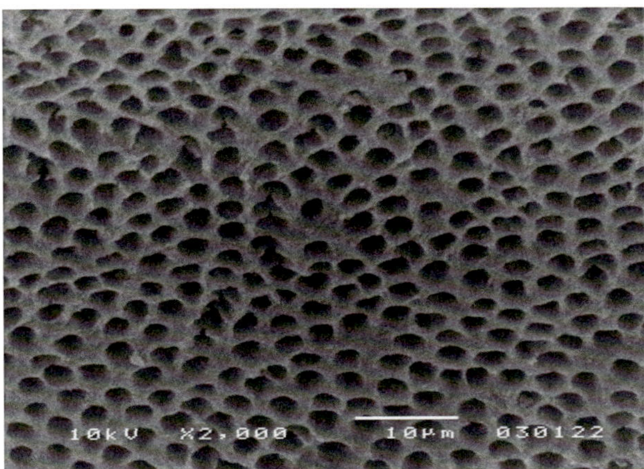

Fig. 8.4 SEM photomicrograph showing the root canal walls completely free from smear layer and fully debrided with no organic and inorganic debris. A strict adherence to the shaping and irrigation protocols is required. In particular, the use of NaOCl irrigant solution followed by a penultimate rinse for 1 min with EDTA solution followed again by NaOCl allows this level of cleanliness

regimen and also depending on the original diagnosis. Primary root canal treatment may require a different approach compared with long-standing infections. Great emphasis has been given to the interactions between different irrigants [99]. The risk of over-chelation and excessive opening of the dentinal tubules has limited effect on the dentine resilience [100]. On the other hand, the efficient removal of infected smear layer and opening of dentinal tubules allow a deeper disinfection of the dentine [88, 101] (Fig. 8.4).

For this reason, after the penultimate rinse with EDTA, the last irrigation is carried out with the NaOCl to complete the tubular disinfection (Fig. 8.5). Deactivation of the NaOCl used as last irrigant is not required. An irrigation protocol can be suggested following the evidence available (Table 8.4). The drying of the canal lumen prior to obturation is to be carried out with sterile paper points. The potential mishaps related to irrigant use are discussed in the relevant chapter.

Following the complete drying of the root canal, the obturation of the root canal system contributes to the prevention of the endodontic reinfection. However as large evidence suggested, the contribution of the type of root canal obturation is less relevant than the previous disinfection procedures and the provision of a good coronal seal. To date no study with high hierarchy of evidence (*i.e.* randomised controlled trial or meta-analysis) demonstrated any difference in endodontic outcome with different types of obturation technique (*i.e.* warm vertical condensation technique vs. cold lateral condensation). Future study will likely focus in analysing the effectiveness of the seal of single cone technique in conjunction with bioceramic sealer.

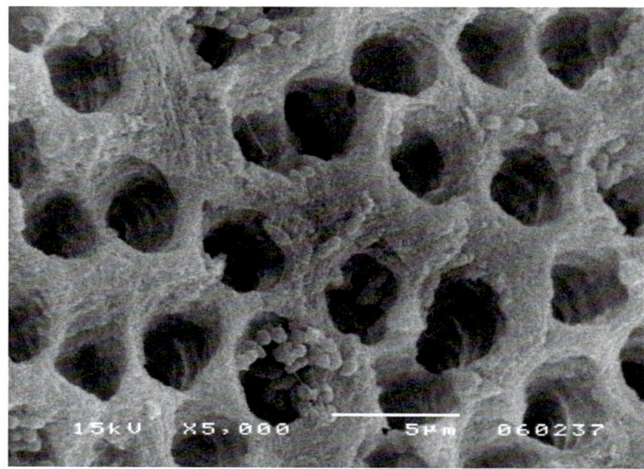

Fig. 8.5 SEM photomicrograph showing a superficial tubular infection that can be affected by the removal of the smear layer by a penultimate irrigation with EDTA and subsequent final irrigation with sodium hypochlorite

Table 8.4 Irrigation regimen for infected teeth: sequence, minimal contact time and minimal volume are proven to maximise the eradication of endodontic biofilms

	Volume	Concentration	Minimal contact time/ volume
Antimicrobial irrigant	NaOCl	1–2%	45′/10 mL
Chelating agent	EDTA	17%	1′(penultimate rinse)/0.5 mL
Adjuvant	Urea peroxide/EDTA gel	Variable	During shaping/*ad-lib*
Sequence	[NaOCL + EDTA + NaOCL] repeated n times + final rinse protocol (1' EDTA + final rinse with NaOCl)		
Activation	Passive ultrasonic irrigation (size 10 file to working length activated by touch with an ultrasonic tip)		

8.8 Avoid Iatrogenic Infection: *Primum Non Nocere*

A novel aspect of endodontic treatment is the possibility to cause nosocomial infections (*i.e.* cross-contamination from the clinical environment) [102]. The content of many endodontic consumables has been proven to be non-sterile even when packaged in sterile condition. Furthermore, non-sterile packaging is widely used in endodontics [103]. Among the consumable commonly used in the operative procedures, the gutta-percha is non-sterilised. The clinician should soak in Milton solution the gutta-percha cones prior to obturation for at least 60 seconds [104].

A major route of endodontic contamination can be ascribed to examination gloves. A recent paper had demonstrated the increase of the bacterial contamination of the gloves in the course of the endodontic procedure. Clinician should consider changing gloves at specific stages of the endodontic procedure: after access cavity, after master apical cone X-ray and/or prior to root canal obturation [34]. These steps together with the previously described operative protocols can reduce the chance of nosocomial infection of the root canal space.

8.9 To Dress or Not to Dress

Dressing has been often described as the safest means of achieving root canal sterility of the root canal space prior to obturation [105]. Systematic reviews revealed no difference in the outcome between one- and two-stage root canal treatment [106]. However, many controversies have haunted the topic. Type of dressing, time and repetition may have different effects, and a consensus has not been achieved on the gold standard in dressing [107].

The mostly agreed protocols require non-setting calcium hydroxide to fill the main canal lumen for at least 2 weeks. However, the high alkalinity upon which the disinfection mechanism relies is not sufficient to eradicate certain bacterial strains that are alkaliphile [69]. The data arising from the most recent CBCT studies reveal a different situation when considering the outcome of one-stage vs. two-stage root canal treatment [108]. The vast majority of study based on the traditional intraoral planar X-rays reported no difference between the two approaches [109]. However, the more sensitive CBCT-based analysis reveals a significantly better outcome for the two appointments endodontic treatment [108].

The ideal protocol to provide the maximum efficiency of dressing consists of non-setting calcium hydroxide inserted in each canal not beyond the working length and left in situ for at least 2 weeks with a satisfactory temporary restoration. Among the different types of material, coltosol and GIC provide a better seal compared with zinc phosphate and IRM [110]. Temporary restorations tend to lose coronal seal and allow bacterial microleakage after 2 weeks.

8.10 Advanced Disinfection Techniques

Despite the refinement in the protocols of shaping and irrigation, the relapse and persistence of endodontic infection pushed the researcher to analyse the potential factors limiting the effect of chemo-debridement. One of the main factors affecting the effectiveness of irrigation is the root canal anatomy complexity. The structure of the dentine microscopically limits the effect of irrigation within the dentinal tubules, and the dentinal composition as well can buffer the effect of irrigants. The fluid dynamic as well represents a major limitation in the contact time and shear stress of the irrigants against biofilm. The concept of stagnation plane beyond the tip of the needle limits the exchange of irrigants. Another issue recently described in literature is the presence of vapour lock or presence of a bubble of air at the apical third entrapped during the irrigation and shaping. The presence of bubble of air or dentinal debris plugs or other blockages closing the apex creates a closed system which limits the effect of irrigation [111, 112]. Patency filing and manual agitation of gutta-percha cone can disrupt the presence of bubbles of air.

In order to overcome the shortcomings of non-active irrigation, several alternatives and adjuvant system have been introduced. The passive ultrasonic irrigation (PUI) has been developed and tested extensively to improve the disruption of endodontic biofilm [113, 114]. The efficacy of PUI has been demonstrated [115]. The delivery of passive ultrasonic irrigation is very simple by flooding the canal with NaOCl, selecting a passive file reaching the full working length and touching with a periodontal probe to activate the irrigant for at least 20 s. More refined approaches can be used with endo-chuck or endosonore files as alternatives.

The use of negative pressure irrigation is theoretically advantageous; however, no evidence is present regarding an improved outcome [116]. The need to enlarge the apical portion of the canal to accommodate the cannula may not be possible in curved canals. The presence of debris is still visible in isthmuses and recesses of the root canal system.

More recently the use of sonic activation has been developed to overcome the potential limits of cavitation caused by PUI where bubbles of air could limit the contact time of irrigants [117]. Similarly to PUI the canal is flooded with the irrigant, and the tip of the appropriate size is activated for at least 20 s for each canal. The activation can be repeated for both EDTA and the NaOCl solutions.

8.11 Ozone

Ozone has been tested extensively in vitro to determine its effectiveness against biofilms and planktonic microbiota [118]. The current literature is lacking high-hierarchy studies [119, 120]. Ozone has limited action on *E. faecalis* [121].

8.12 Photodynamic Therapy

Photodynamic therapy is based on the incubation of the root canal space with a dye (photosensitiser) that once excited with light of the appropriated wave length will release free radical ions damaging the biofilm. One of the advantages of photodynamic therapy is the activity inside the dentinal tubules via optical scattering (Fig. 8.6a, b). Furthermore, certain bacterial species are targeted by the emitted light in absence of a photosensitiser due to the presence of endogenous protoporphyrin. Several studies showed potential application in vitro and in vivo, to date; however, photodynamic therapy can only be considered and adjuvant of the traditional irrigation methods [122–124]. Care needs to be paid in the clinical setting to limit the bleaching effect caused by sodium hypochlorite on the photosensitiser.

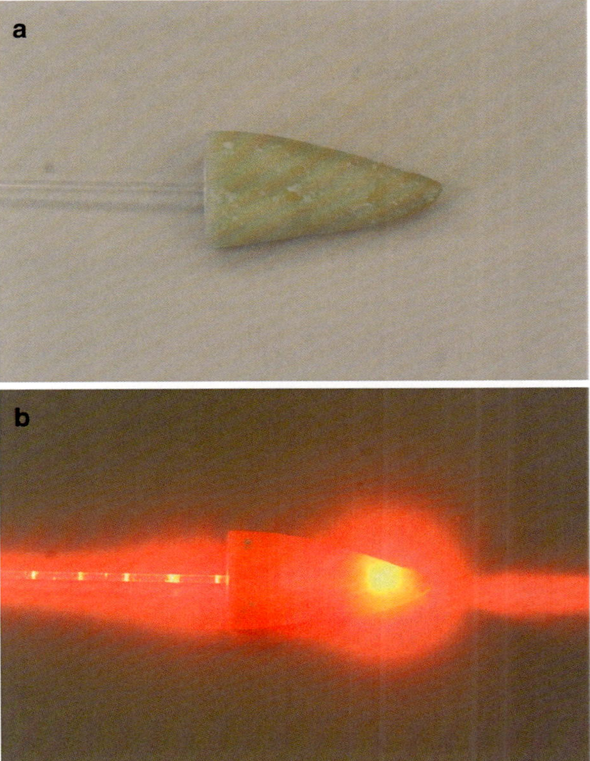

Fig. 8.6 (**a–b**) In vitro image of a PDT fibre inserted into the root canal system to the apex (**a**) and with the laser activated. To be noted the lateral scattering through the dentinal tubules and the foramen. The photodynamic effect is based on the previous incubation of the biofilm and the root canal system with a specific photosensitiser (e.g. *methylene blue*)

8.13 Future Development

The introduction of real-time detection of the presence of bacteria within the main lumen of the root canal treatment will allow a rapid determination of the most efficient protocol in removing the existing biofilm. The possibility to determine the endpoint of root canal treatment would create a direct feedback to the clinician, representing a surrogate endpoint. The use of functional dyes renders fluorescent the live pathogens present within the canal lumen. An experimental system has been developed to confirm the proof of principle. Technically with a rapid bacterial detection during root canal treatment, a paper point would be inserted in the root canal at the different stages of the treatment to collect the canal content; following a rapid dye incubation, the fluorescence emitted by the stained live bacteria will provide a feedback on the level of residual contamination of the canal [125].

References

1. Kakehashi S, Stanley HR, Fitzgerald RJ. The effects of surgical exposures of dental pulps in germ-free and conventional laboratory rats. Oral Surg Oral Med Oral Pathol. 1965;20:340–9.
2. Patel K, Schirru E, Niazi S, Mitchell P, Mannocci F. Multiple apical radiolucencies and external cervical resorption associated with varicella zoster virus: a case report. J Endod. 2016;42(6):978–83.
3. Slots J, Nowzari H, Sabeti M. Cytomegalovirus infection in symptomatic periapical pathosis. Int Endod J. 2004;37(8):519–24.
4. Siqueira JF Jr, Rocas IN. Clinical implications and microbiology of bacterial persistence after treatment procedures. J Endod. 2008;34(11):1291–301. e3
5. Stashenko P, Yu SM, Wang CY. Kinetics of immune cell and bone resorptive responses to endodontic infections. J Endod. 1992;18(9):422–6.
6. Siqueira JF Jr, Rocas IN. Diversity of endodontic microbiota revisited. J Dent Res. 2009;88(11):969–81.
7. Siqueira JF Jr, Rocas IN, Ricucci D, Hulsmann M. Causes and management of post-treatment apical periodontitis. Br Dent J. 2014;216(6):305–12.
8. Ricucci D, Siqueira JF Jr. Biofilms and apical periodontitis: study of prevalence and association with clinical and histopathologic findings. J Endod. 2010;36(8):1277–88.
9. Pasqualini D, Bergandi L, Palumbo L, Borraccino A, Dambra V, Alovisi M, et al. Association among oral health, apical periodontitis, CD14 polymorphisms, and coronary heart disease in middle-aged adults. J Endod. 2012;38(12):1570–7.
10. Siqueira JF Jr. Endodontic infections: concepts, paradigms, and perspectives. Oral Surg Oral Med Oral Pathol Oral Radiol Endod. 2002;94(3):281–93.
11. Debelian GJ, Olsen I, Tronstad L. Systemic diseases caused by oral microorganisms. Endod Dent Traumatol. 1994;10(2):57–65.
12. Tonetti MS, Van Dyke TE, Working group 1 of the joint EFPAAP workshop. Periodontitis and atherosclerotic cardiovascular disease: consensus report of the joint EFP/AAP workshop on periodontitis and systemic diseases. J Periodontol. 2013;84(4 Suppl):S24–9.
13. Teles R, Wang CY, Stashenko P. Increased susceptibility of RAG-2 SCID mice to dissemination of endodontic infections. Infect Immun. 1997;65(9):3781–7.
14. Khalighinejad N, Aminoshariae MR, Aminoshariae A, Kulild JC, Mickel A, Fouad AF. Association between systemic diseases and apical periodontitis. J Endod. 2016;42(10):1427–34.
15. Lopez-Lopez J, Jane-Salas E, Estrugo-Devesa A, Velasco-Ortega E, Martin-Gonzalez J, Segura-Egea JJ. Periapical and endodontic status of type 2 diabetic patients in Catalonia, Spain: a cross-sectional study. J Endod. 2011;37(5):598–601.
16. Wang CH, Chueh LH, Chen SC, Feng YC, Hsiao CK, Chiang CP. Impact of diabetes mellitus, hypertension, and coronary artery disease on tooth extraction after nonsurgical endodontic treatment. J Endod. 2011;37(1):1–5.
17. Fouad AF. Diabetes mellitus as a modulating factor of endodontic infections. J Dent Educ. 2003;67(4):459–67.
18. Hoppe CB, Oliveira JA, Grecca FS, Haas AN, Gomes MS. Association between chronic oral inflammatory burden and physical fitness in males: a cross-sectional observational study. Int Endod J. 2017;50(8):740–9.
19. Rocas IN, Siqueira JF Jr, Del Aguila CA, Provenzano JC, Guilherme BP, Goncalves LS. Polymorphism of the CD14 and TLR4 genes and post-treatment apical periodontitis. J Endod. 2014;40(2):168–72.
20. Oguntebi BR. Dentine tubule infection and endodontic therapy implications. Int Endod J. 1994;27(4):218–22.
21. Jacinto RC, Gomes BP, Ferraz CC, Zaia AA, Filho FJ. Microbiological analysis of infected root canals from symptomatic and asymptomatic teeth with periapical periodontitis and the antimicrobial susceptibility of some isolated anaerobic bacteria. Oral Microbiol Immunol. 2003;18(5):285–92.

22. Gomes BP, Pinheiro ET, Gade-Neto CR, Sousa EL, Ferraz CC, Zaia AA, et al. Microbiological examination of infected dental root canals. Oral Microbiol Immunol. 2004;19(2):71–6.
23. Sundqvist G, Figdor D, Persson S, Sjogren U. Microbiologic analysis of teeth with failed endodontic treatment and the outcome of conservative re-treatment. Oral Surg Oral Med Oral Pathol Oral Radiol Endod. 1998;85(1):86–93.
24. Distel JW, Hatton JF, Gillespie MJ. Biofilm formation in medicated root canals. J Endod. 2002;28(10):689–93.
25. Foschi F, Cavrini F, Montebugnoli L, Stashenko P, Sambri V, Prati C. Detection of bacteria in endodontic samples by polymerase chain reaction assays and association with defined clinical signs in Italian patients. Oral Microbiol Immunol. 2005;20(5):289–95.
26. Siqueira JF Jr, Rocas IN. Polymerase chain reaction-based analysis of microorganisms associated with failed endodontic treatment. Oral Surg Oral Med Oral Pathol Oral Radiol Endod. 2004;97(1):85–94.
27. Zehnder M, Guggenheim B. The mysterious appearance of enterococci in filled root canals. Int Endod J. 2009;42(4):277–87.
28. Tennert C, Fuhrmann M, Wittmer A, Karygianni L, Altenburger MJ, Pelz K, et al. New bacterial composition in primary and persistent/secondary endodontic infections with respect to clinical and radiographic findings. J Endod. 2014;40(5):670–7.
29. Chavez de Paz LE. Redefining the persistent infection in root canals: possible role of biofilm communities. J Endod. 2007;33(6):652–62.
30. Anderson AC, Hellwig E, Vespermann R, Wittmer A, Schmid M, Karygianni L, et al. Comprehensive analysis of secondary dental root canal infections: a combination of culture and culture-independent approaches reveals new insights. PLoS One. 2012;7(11):e49576.
31. Rocas IN, Siqueira JF Jr. Characterization of microbiota of root canal-treated teeth with post-treatment disease. J Clin Microbiol. 2012;50(5):1721–4.
32. Climo MW, Yokoe DS, Warren DK, Perl TM, Bolon M, Herwaldt LA, et al. Effect of daily chlorhexidine bathing on hospital-acquired infection. N Engl J Med. 2013;368(6):533–42.
33. Fukuda H, Lee J, Imanaka Y. Costs of hospital-acquired infection and transferability of the estimates: a systematic review. Infection. 2011;39(3):185–99.
34. Niazi SA, Vincer L, Mannocci F. Glove contamination during endodontic treatment is one of the sources of nosocomial endodontic Propionibacterium acnes infections. J Endod. 2016;42(8):1202–11.
35. Niazi SA, Clarke D, Do T, Gilbert SC, Mannocci F, Beighton D. Propionibacterium acnes and Staphylococcus epidermidis isolated from refractory endodontic lesions are opportunistic pathogens. J Clin Microbiol. 2010;48(11):3859–69.
36. Del Fabbro M, Samaranayake LP, Lolato A, Weinstein T, Taschieri S. Analysis of the secondary endodontic lesions focusing on the extraradicular microorganisms: an overview. J Investig Clin Dent. 2014;5(4):245–54.
37. Loesche WJ, Lopatin DE, Giordano J, Alcoforado G, Hujoel P. Comparison of the benzoyl-DL-arginine-naphthylamide (BANA) test, DNA probes, and immunological reagents for ability to detect anaerobic periodontal infections due to Porphyromonas gingivalis, Treponema denticola, and Bacteroides forsythus. J Clin Microbiol. 1992;30(2):427–33.
38. Yoneda M, Kita S, Suzuki N, Macedo SM, Iha K, Hirofuji T. Application of a chairside anaerobic culture test for endodontic treatment. Int J Dent. 2010;2010:942130.
39. Michailesco P, Boudeville P. Calibrated latex microspheres percolation: a possible route to model endodontic bacterial leakage. J Endod. 2003;29(7):456–62.
40. Jalalzadeh SM, Mamavi A, Abedi H, Mashouf RY, Modaresi A, Karapanou V. Bacterial microleakage and post space timing for two endodontic sealers: an in vitro study. J Mass Dent Soc. 2010;59(2):34–7.
41. Niazi SA, Al Kharusi HS, Patel S, Bruce K, Beighton D, Foschi F, et al. Isolation of Propionibacterium acnes among the microbiota of primary endodontic infections with and without intraoral communication. Clin Oral Investig. 2016;20(8):2149–60.

42. Aubin GG, Portillo ME, Trampuz A, Corvec S. Propionibacterium acnes, an emerging pathogen: from acne to implant-infections, from phylotype to resistance. Med Mal Infect. 2014;44(6):241–50.
43. Noguchi N, Noiri Y, Narimatsu M, Ebisu S. Identification and localization of extraradicular biofilm-forming bacteria associated with refractory endodontic pathogens. Appl Environ Microbiol. 2005;71(12):8738–43.
44. Signoretti FG, Endo MS, Gomes BP, Montagner F, Tosello FB, Jacinto RC. Persistent extraradicular infection in root-filled asymptomatic human tooth: scanning electron microscopic analysis and microbial investigation after apical microsurgery. J Endod. 2011;37(12):1696–700.
45. Ricucci D, Siqueira JF Jr. Apical actinomycosis as a continuum of intraradicular and extraradicular infection: case report and critical review on its involvement with treatment failure. J Endod. 2008;34(9):1124–9.
46. Stojicic S, Shen Y, Haapasalo M. Effect of the source of biofilm bacteria, level of biofilm maturation, and type of disinfecting agent on the susceptibility of biofilm bacteria to antibacterial agents. J Endod. 2013;39(4):473–7.
47. Niazi SA, Clark D, Do T, Gilbert SC, Foschi F, Mannocci F, et al. The effectiveness of enzymic irrigation in removing a nutrient-stressed endodontic multispecies biofilm. Int Endod J. 2014;47(8):756–68.
48. Ng YL, Mann V, Gulabivala K. A prospective study of the factors affecting outcomes of nonsurgical root canal treatment: part 2: tooth survival. Int Endod J. 2011;44(7):610–25.
49. Ng YL, Mann V, Gulabivala K. A prospective study of the factors affecting outcomes of nonsurgical root canal treatment: part 1: periapical health. Int Endod J. 2011;44(7):583–609.
50. McDonald A, Setchell D. Developing a tooth restorability index. Dent Update. 2005;32(6):343–4. 6-8
51. Bandlish RB, McDonald AV, Setchell DJ. Assessment of the amount of remaining coronal dentine in root-treated teeth. J Dent. 2006;34(9):699–708.
52. Al-Nuaimi N. The outcome of endodontically retreated teeth with varying degrees of coronal tooth structure loss: a prospective clinical study. London: King's College London; 2017.
53. Ramirez-Sebastia A, Bortolotto T, Roig M, Krejci I. Composite vs ceramic computer-aided design/computer-assisted manufacturing crowns in endodontically treated teeth: analysis of marginal adaptation. Oper Dent. 2013;38(6):663–73.
54. Pirani C, Chersoni S, Foschi F, Piana G, Loushine RJ, Tay FR, et al. Does hybridization of intraradicular dentin really improve fiber post retention in endodontically treated teeth? J Endod. 2005;31(12):891–4.
55. Fokkinga WA, Kreulen CM, Bronkhorst EM, Creugers NH. Composite resin core-crown reconstructions: an up to 17-year follow-up of a controlled clinical trial. Int J Prosthodont. 2008;21(2):109–15.
56. Nayyar A, Walton RE, Leonard LA. An amalgam coronal-radicular dowel and core technique for endodontically treated posterior teeth. J Prosthet Dent. 1980;43(5):511–5.
57. Fokkinga WA, Kreulen CM, Bronkhorst EM, Creugers NH. Up to 17-year controlled clinical study on post-and-cores and covering crowns. J Dent. 2007;35(10):778–86.
58. Safavi KE, Dowden WE, Langeland K. Influence of delayed coronal permanent restoration on endodontic prognosis. Endod Dent Traumatol. 1987;3(4):187–91.
59. Pratt I, Aminoshariae A, Montagnese TA, Williams KA, Khalighinejad N, Mickel A. Eight-year retrospective study of the critical time lapse between root canal completion and crown placement: its influence on the survival of endodontically treated teeth. J Endod. 2016;42(11):1598–603.
60. Reit C, Molander A, Dahlen G. The diagnostic accuracy of microbiologic root canal sampling and the influence of antimicrobial dressings. Endod Dent Traumatol. 1999;15(6):278–83.
61. Molander A, Warfvinge J, Reit C, Kvist T. Clinical and radiographic evaluation of one- and two-visit endodontic treatment of asymptomatic necrotic teeth with apical periodontitis: a randomized clinical trial. J Endod. 2007;33(10):1145–8.

62. Fabricius L, Dahlen G, Sundqvist G, Happonen RP, Moller AJ. Influence of residual bacteria on periapical tissue healing after chemomechanical treatment and root filling of experimentally infected monkey teeth. Eur J Oral Sci. 2006;114(4):278–85.
63. Sedgley CM, Lennan SL, Appelbe OK. Survival of Enterococcus faecalis in root canals ex vivo. Int Endod J. 2005;38(10):735–42.
64. Figdor D, Davies JK, Sundqvist G. Starvation survival, growth and recovery of Enterococcus faecalis in human serum. Oral Microbiol Immunol. 2003;18(4):234–9.
65. Portenier I, Waltimo T, Orstavik D, Haapasalo M. The susceptibility of starved, stationary phase, and growing cells of Enterococcus faecalis to endodontic medicaments. J Endod. 2005;31(5):380–6.
66. Sainsbury AL, Bird PS, Walsh LJ. DIAGNOdent laser fluorescence assessment of endodontic infection. J Endod. 2009;35(10):1404–7.
67. Tan BT, Messer HH. The quality of apical canal preparation using hand and rotary instruments with specific criteria for enlargement based on initial apical file size. J Endod. 2002;28(9):658–64.
68. Sjogren U, Figdor D, Persson S, Sundqvist G. Influence of infection at the time of root filling on the outcome of endodontic treatment of teeth with apical periodontitis. Int Endod J. 1997;30(5):297–306.
69. Lew HP, Quah SY, Lui JN, Bergenholtz G, Hoon Yu VS, Tan KS. Isolation of alkaline-tolerant bacteria from primary infected root canals. J Endod. 2015;41(4):451–6.
70. Vianna ME, Horz HP, Conrads G, Zaia AA, Souza-Filho FJ, Gomes BP. Effect of root canal procedures on endotoxins and endodontic pathogens. Oral Microbiol Immunol. 2007;22(6):411–8.
71. Goldfein J, Speirs C, Finkelman M, Amato R. Rubber dam use during post placement influences the success of root canal-treated teeth. J Endod. 2013;39(12):1481–4.
72. Ahmad IA. Rubber dam usage for endodontic treatment: a review. Int Endod J. 2009;42(11):963–72.
73. Ovaydi-Mandel A, Petrov SD, Drew HJ. Novel decision tree algorithms for the treatment planning of compromised teeth. Quintessence Int. 2013;44(1):75–84.
74. Maltz M, Jardim JJ, Mestrinho HD, Yamaguti PM, Podesta K, Moura MS, et al. Partial removal of carious dentine: a multicenter randomized controlled trial and 18-month follow-up results. Caries Res. 2013;47(2):103–9.
75. Matsushita-Tokugawa M, Miura J, Iwami Y, Sakagami T, Izumi Y, Mori N, et al. Detection of dentinal microcracks using infrared thermography. J Endod. 2013;39(1):88–91.
76. Abbott PV. Assessing restored teeth with pulp and periapical diseases for the presence of cracks, caries and marginal breakdown. Aust Dent J. 2004;49(1):33–9. quiz 45
77. Kahler W. The cracked tooth conundrum: terminology, classification, diagnosis, and management. Am J Dent. 2008;21(5):275–82.
78. Haueisen H, Gartner K, Kaiser L, Trohorsch D, Heidemann D. Vertical root fracture: prevalence, etiology, and diagnosis. Quintessence Int. 2013;44(7):467–74.
79. Patel S, Kanagasingam S, Mannocci F. Cone beam computed tomography (CBCT) in endodontics. Dent Update. 2010;37(6):373–9.
80. Qualtrough AJ, Mannocci F. Endodontics and the older patient. Dent Update. 2011;38(8):559–62. 64-6
81. Nair PN. On the causes of persistent apical periodontitis: a review. Int Endod J. 2006;39(4):249–81.
82. Witherspoon DE, Small JC, Regan JD. Missed canal systems are the most likely basis for endodontic retreatment of molars. Tex Dent J. 2013;130(2):127–39.
83. Saunders WP, Saunders EM. Effect of noncutting tipped instruments on the quality of root canal preparation using a modified double-flared technique. J Endod. 1992;18(1):32–6.
84. Foschi F, Nucci C, Montebugnoli L, Marchionni S, Breschi L, Malagnino VA, et al. SEM evaluation of canal wall dentine following use of Mtwo and ProTaper NiTi rotary instruments. Int Endod J. 2004;37(12):832–9.

85. Shuping GB, Orstavik D, Sigurdsson A, Trope M. Reduction of intracanal bacteria using nickel-titanium rotary instrumentation and various medications. J Endod. 2000;26(12):751–5.
86. Boutsioukis C, Gogos C, Verhaagen B, Versluis M, Kastrinakis E, Van der Sluis LW. The effect of apical preparation size on irrigant flow in root canals evaluated using an unsteady computational fluid dynamics model. Int Endod J. 2010;43(10):874–81.
87. Peters OA, Peters CI, Schonenberger K, Barbakow F. ProTaper rotary root canal preparation: effects of canal anatomy on final shape analysed by micro CT. Int Endod J. 2003;36(2):86–92.
88. Love RM, Jenkinson HF. Invasion of dentinal tubules by oral bacteria. Crit Rev Oral Biol Med. 2002;13(2):171–83.
89. Peters OA. Current challenges and concepts in the preparation of root canal systems: a review. J Endod. 2004;30(8):559–67.
90. Parashos P, Linsuwanont P, Messer HH. A cleaning protocol for rotary nickel-titanium endodontic instruments. Aust Dent J. 2004;49(1):20–7.
91. Rossi-Fedele G, Guastalli AR, Dogramaci EJ, Steier L, De Figueiredo JA. Influence of pH changes on chlorine-containing endodontic irrigating solutions. Int Endod J. 2011;44(9):792–9.
92. Giardino L, Savoldi E, Ambu E, Rimondini R, Palezona A, Debbia EA. Antimicrobial effect of MTAD, Tetraclean, Cloreximid, and sodium hypochlorite on three common endodontic pathogens. Indian J Dent Res. 2009;20(3):391.
93. Boutsioukis C, Lambrianidis T, Verhaagen B, Versluis M, Kastrinakis E, Wesselink PR, et al. The effect of needle-insertion depth on the irrigant flow in the root canal: evaluation using an unsteady computational fluid dynamics model. J Endod. 2010;36(10):1664–8.
94. Retamozo B, Shabahang S, Johnson N, Aprecio RM, Torabinejad M. Minimum contact time and concentration of sodium hypochlorite required to eliminate Enterococcus faecalis. J Endod. 2010;36(3):520–3.
95. Siqueira JF Jr, Rocas IN, Favieri A, Lima KC. Chemomechanical reduction of the bacterial population in the root canal after instrumentation and irrigation with 1%, 2.5%, and 5.25% sodium hypochlorite. J Endod. 2000;26(6):331–4.
96. Baumgartner JC, Cuenin PR. Efficacy of several concentrations of sodium hypochlorite for root canal irrigation. J Endod. 1992;18(12):605–12.
97. Basrani BR, Manek S, Mathers D, Fillery E, Sodhi RN. Determination of 4-chloroaniline and its derivatives formed in the interaction of sodium hypochlorite and chlorhexidine by using gas chromatography. J Endod. 2010;36(2):312–4.
98. Violich DR, Chandler NP. The smear layer in endodontics - a review. Int Endod J. 2010;43(1):2–15.
99. Prado M, Santos Junior HM, Rezende CM, Pinto AC, Faria RB, Simao RA, et al. Interactions between irrigants commonly used in endodontic practice: a chemical analysis. J Endod. 2013;39(4):505–10.
100. Sobhani OE, Gulabivala K, Knowles JC, Ng YL. The effect of irrigation time, root morphology and dentine thickness on tooth surface strain when using 5% sodium hypochlorite and 17% EDTA. Int Endod J. 2010;43(3):190–9.
101. Buck R, Eleazer PD, Staat RH. In vitro disinfection of dentinal tubules by various endodontics irrigants. J Endod. 1999;25(12):786–8.
102. Vidana R, Sillerstrom E, Ahlquist M, Lund B. Potential for nosocomial transmission of Enterococcus faecalis from surfaces in dental operatories. Int Endod J. 2015;48(6):518–27.
103. Roth TP, Whitney SI, Walker SG, Friedman S. Microbial contamination of endodontic files received from the manufacturer. J Endod. 2006;32(7):649–51.
104. Gomes BP, Vianna ME, Matsumoto CU, Rossi Vde P, Zaia AA, Ferraz CC, et al. Disinfection of gutta-percha cones with chlorhexidine and sodium hypochlorite. Oral Surg Oral Med Oral Pathol Oral Radiol Endod. 2005;100(4):512–7.
105. Siqueira JF Jr, de Uzeda M. Disinfection by calcium hydroxide pastes of dentinal tubules infected with two obligate and one facultative anaerobic bacteria. J Endod. 1996;22(12):674–6.
106. Sathorn C, Parashos P, Messer HH. Effectiveness of single- versus multiple-visit endodontic treatment of teeth with apical periodontitis: a systematic review and meta-analysis. Int Endod J. 2005;38(6):347–55.

107. Teles AM, Manso MC, Loureiro S, Silva R, Madeira IG, Pina C, et al. Effectiveness of two intracanal dressings in adult Portuguese patients: a qPCR and anaerobic culture assessment. Int Endod J. 2014;47(1):32–40.
108. Davies A, Patel S, Foschi F, Andiappan M, Mitchell PJ, Mannocci F. The detection of periapical pathoses using digital periapical radiography and cone beam computed tomography in endodontically retreated teeth - part 2: a 1 year post-treatment follow-up. Int Endod J. 2016;49(7):623–35.
109. Penesis VA, Fitzgerald PI, Fayad MI, Wenckus CS, BeGole EA, Johnson BR. Outcome of one-visit and two-visit endodontic treatment of necrotic teeth with apical periodontitis: a randomized controlled trial with one-year evaluation. J Endod. 2008;34(3):251–7.
110. Madarati A, Rekab MS, Watts DC, Qualtrough A. Time-dependence of coronal seal of temporary materials used in endodontics. Aust Endod J. 2008;34(3):89–93.
111. Psimma Z, Boutsioukis C, Vasiliadis L, Kastrinakis E. A new method for real-time quantification of irrigant extrusion during root canal irrigation ex vivo. Int Endod J. 2013;46(7):619–31.
112. Tay FR, Gu LS, Schoeffel GJ, Wimmer C, Susin L, Zhang K, et al. Effect of vapor lock on root canal debridement by using a side-vented needle for positive-pressure irrigant delivery. J Endod. 2010;36(4):745–50.
113. Niazi SA, Al-Ali WM, Patel S, Foschi F, Mannocci F. Synergistic effect of 2% chlorhexidine combined with proteolytic enzymes on biofilm disruption and killing. Int Endod J. 2015;48(12):1157–67.
114. van der Sluis LW, Versluis M, Wu MK, Wesselink PR. Passive ultrasonic irrigation of the root canal: a review of the literature. Int Endod J. 2007;40(6):415–26.
115. Bhuva B, Patel S, Wilson R, Niazi S, Beighton D, Mannocci F. The effectiveness of passive ultrasonic irrigation on intraradicular Enterococcus faecalis biofilms in extracted single-rooted human teeth. Int Endod J. 2010;43(3):241–50.
116. Mancini M, Cerroni L, Iorio L, Armellin E, Conte G, Cianconi L. Smear layer removal and canal cleanliness using different irrigation systems (EndoActivator, EndoVac, and passive ultrasonic irrigation): field emission scanning electron microscopic evaluation in an in vitro study. J Endod. 2013;39(11):1456–60.
117. Paragliola R, Franco V, Fabiani C, Mazzoni A, Nato F, Tay FR, et al. Final rinse optimization: influence of different agitation protocols. J Endod. 2010;36(2):282–5.
118. Huth KC, Quirling M, Maier S, Kamereck K, Alkhayer M, Paschos E, et al. Effectiveness of ozone against endodontopathogenic microorganisms in a root canal biofilm model. Int Endod J. 2009;42(1):3–13.
119. Case PD, Bird PS, Kahler WA, George R, Walsh LJ. Treatment of root canal biofilms of Enterococcus faecalis with ozone gas and passive ultrasound activation. J Endod. 2012;38(4):523–6.
120. Plotino G, Cortese T, Grande NM, Leonardi DP, Di Giorgio G, Testarelli L, et al. New technologies to improve root canal disinfection. Braz Dent J. 2016;27(1):3–8.
121. Estrela C, Estrela CR, Decurcio DA, Hollanda AC, Silva JA. Antimicrobial efficacy of ozonated water, gaseous ozone, sodium hypochlorite and chlorhexidine in infected human root canals. Int Endod J. 2007;40(2):85–93.
122. Foschi F, Fontana CR, Ruggiero K, Riahi R, Vera A, Doukas AG, et al. Photodynamic inactivation of Enterococcus faecalis in dental root canals in vitro. Lasers Surg Med. 2007;39(10):782–7.
123. Soukos NS, Chen PS, Morris JT, Ruggiero K, Abernethy AD, Som S, et al. Photodynamic therapy for endodontic disinfection. J Endod. 2006;32(10):979–84.
124. Chiniforush N, Pourhajibagher M, Shahabi S, Kosarieh E, Bahador A. Can antimicrobial photodynamic therapy (aPDT) enhance the endodontic treatment? J Lasers Med Sci. 2016;7(2):76–85.
125. Herzog DB, Hosny NA, Niazi SA, Koller G, Cook RJ, Foschi F, et al. Rapid bacterial detection during endodontic treatment. J Dent Res. 2017;96(6):626–32.

Complications of Endodontic Surgery

9

Igor Tsesis, Tamar Blazer, Shlomo Elbahary, and Eyal Rosen

9.1 Introduction

The main goal of a surgical endodontic treatment is to prevent the invasion of bacteria and their by-products from the root canal system into the periradicular tissues [1, 2]. Surgical endodontic treatment may be indicated for teeth with apical periodontitis, when a nonsurgical retreatment is impractical [3–6].

In modern surgical endodontic treatment, magnification devices are used to enable a precise surgical procedure. The root end is cut with minimal bevel, retrograde canal preparation is performed with the aid of an ultrasonic tip to a depth of 3–4 mm, and root-end filling is placed [7]. The advantages of this technique include better identification of root apices, and it requires smaller osteotomies and shallower resection angles that enable to preserve the cortical bone and the root length [1, 8]. In addition, under magnification and illumination, it is possible to detect on the resected root surface isthmusi, cracks, and lateral canals [1]. The modern technique is considered an efficient and predictable treatment with a long-term success rate of over 90% [2, 4–6].

Like any treatment modality, surgical endodontics is exposed to risk of complications, defined as "any undesirable, unintended and direct result of surgery affecting the patient, which would not have occurred had the surgery gone as well as could reasonably be hoped" [9]. The practitioner should try to minimize complications by the application of an appropriate surgical technique and to efficiently

I. Tsesis (✉) • S. Elbahary • E. Rosen
Department of Endodontology, Maurice and Gabriela Goldschleger School of Dental Medicine, Tel Aviv University, Tel Aviv, Israel
e-mail: dr.tsesis@gmail.com; dr.eyalrosen@gmail.com

T. Blazer
Department of Endodontics and Dental Traumatology, Graduate School of Dentistry, Rambam Health Care Campus, Haifa, Israel
e-mail: tamar.blazer@gmail.com

P. Jain (ed.), *Common Complications in Endodontics*,
https://doi.org/10.1007/978-3-319-60997-3_9

identify and manage complications in case they occur in order to prevent long-term damage [6].

This chapter is aimed to provide endodontic practitioners with knowledge and practical tools to incorporate an evidence-based approach for prevention and management of surgical complications, in their daily practice.

9.1.1 Soft Tissue Complications in Endodontic Surgery

Endodontic surgery involves soft tissue wounding during the flap elevation [10] to enable proper surgical access to the root apex [1, 11]. In the esthetic zone, adequate flap design is crucial in order to achieve satisfactory esthetic results [6, 12].

Flap procedure possesses risks of complications, such as delayed healing and periodontal defect formation [11] that sometimes may adversely affect the long-term survival of the tooth and/or cause esthetic and functional problems [10, 12–14]. These flap-related complications may be associated with patient-specific factors or with the surgical technique [1, 6, 10, 12–17].

Following the surgery, the wound heals either by "repair" (when the injured tissues are replaced with a scar tissue) or by "regeneration" (when the original injured tissues are reestablished) [18, 19]. From a clinical point of view, scar formation may be a significant esthetic problem, especially in the esthetic zone [6, 20].

Gingival recession may be caused by incorrect repositioning of the flap, compromised blood circulation of the flap, and flap contraction (Fig. 9.1) [10, 13, 14, 16, 17, 21–23]. Thus, it is important to preserve the root-associated tissues and to reposition a tension-free flap [6]. *Flap necrosis* may occur because of insufficient blood supply. Therefore, the vertical releasing incisions should be parallel or converging to the coronal part of the flap; the base of the flap should be wider than the free margin; and it is crucial to avoid crashing of the tissue with the surgical instruments [1, 6, 13]. *Flap tearing* may occur as a result of poor flap design with an insufficient incision that causes flap tension. The flap should be reflected as one unit, with sufficient length of releasing incisions [1, 6, 13].

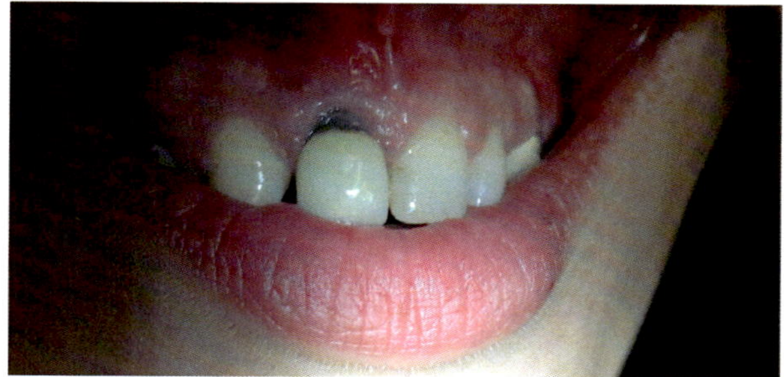

Fig. 9.1 Gingival recession following intrasulcular incision in the area of maxillary central incisor (PFM crown)

Separation of the wound margins may occur within the first week after surgery. This complication may result from tissue failure rather or improper suturing techniques. The wound margins may be closed again or left to heal depending upon the margins extent and the surgeon's judgment of the clinical scenario [6].

The presence of a *periodontal disease* may adversely affect the outcome of the endodontic surgery [24, 25] and is associated with higher risk of complications [6, 26, 27]. When performing endodontic surgery in teeth with periodontal lesions, the endodontic success rate may be less than 80%, compared to more than 90% for cases without periodontal lesions [24].

Gingival morphology has a significant impact on the risk of soft tissue-related complications following endodontic surgery. There are two types of anatomical "gingival biotypes" [28]: "thin gingival biotype" is characterized by a highly scalloped marginal gingiva with slender teeth, delicate and translucent appearance, and with a narrow attached gingival [13, 17, 29]. "Thick gingival biotype" is characterized with a bulky scalloped marginal gingiva in short and wide teeth, broad attached gingiva, fibrotic and resilient tissue, flat soft tissue, and large amount of attached gingival [6, 13, 17, 29]. Patients with thin gingival biotypes may be at a higher risk for recession development following the surgery [6, 14, 17, 29]. On the other hand, patients with thick gingival biotype may be more prone to infra-bony defect formation and deeper probing pocket depth following the endodontic surgery [10, 12–14, 17, 28, 29].

Adequate incision design is crucial and several principles should be applied: horizontal and severely angled vertical incisions or incisions over radicular eminences should not be performed [27, 30, 31]; the incisions should facilitate flap repositioning over a solid bone [27, 31]; the incisions should avoid muscle attachments [27, 31]; the vertical incision extension should facilitate the positioning of the retractor during surgery on a solid bone without tension [1, 27, 31]; and the extent of the horizontal incision should enable adequate surgical access with minimal stretching of the soft tissue [1, 6, 27, 31].

The flap should be designed as "full thickness" to include the entire mucoperiosteal tissues. Full-thickness flaps maintain the supra-periosteal blood vessels and result in less tissue trauma and ensuing bleeding [1, 6, 27, 31]. It is recommended to minimize as possible the time of the operation and perform a short-duration surgery in order to prevent flap ischemia and necrosis [6].

Sutures are supposed to help the repositioning of the flap and secure the flap edges until the wound has healed enough to withstand the functional stresses [32, 33]. However, improper use of sutures may lead to inflammation, delayed healing [31], and tissue strangulation (Fig. 9.2) [6, 26]. The suturing technique should allow wound closure and flap stabilization for at least 3 days. The sutures should be passive and avoid stretching, tearing, or compromising the blood circulation of the tissue [6, 26, 32, 33].

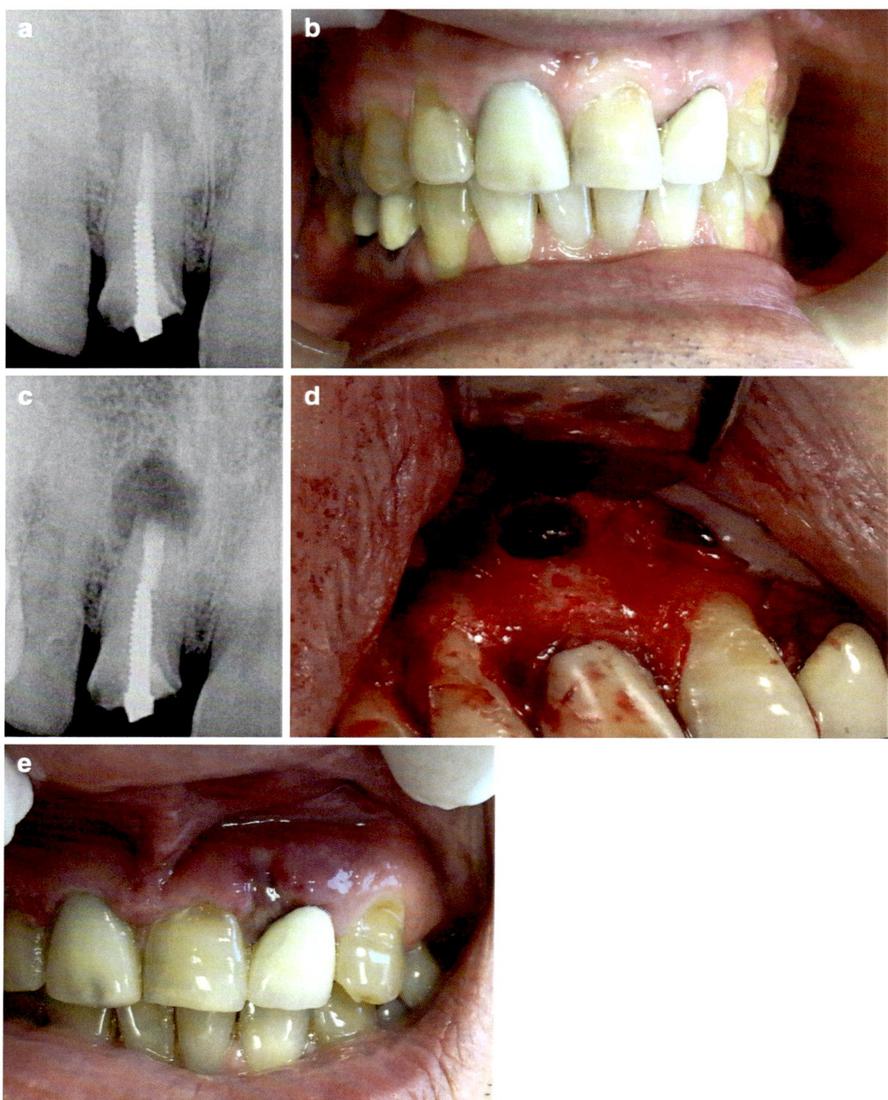

Fig. 9.2 (**a**) Maxillary *right* lateral incisor with periapical lesion—preoperative radiograph. (**b**) Maxillary *right* lateral incisor—preoperative clinical photograph. (**c**) Immediate postoperative radiograph following root-end preparation and filling. (**d**) Intraoperative photograph following flap elevation and osteotomy. (**e**) One month following surgical procedure—acute inflammation of gingiva

9.1.2 Periapical Osteotomy and Curettage

The main goal of the osteotomy in endodontic surgery is to provide an adequate access for the surgical management of the apical part of the root [1, 2, 4–6, 18, 34]. However, when the size of the osseous defect is extensive, osseous regeneration of the wound may not occur, and the defect might heal by fibrous connective tissue [6, 18, 35, 36]. Enlarged osteotomy directed toward the coronal margin may potentially lead to perio-endo communication, endanger the adjacent anatomical structures, and cause a damage to neighboring teeth [1, 6, 24, 37]. With the modern microsurgical techniques, the size of the required osteotomy decreased, to about 4–5 mm in diameter, a diameter large enough to allow the surgical manipulations and at the same time reducing the potential risk [1, 6].

Excessive heat generated during osteotomy preparation may generate heat [38, 39], interrupting the blood flow, and may cause decreased osteoclastic and osteoblastic activity, dehydration, and desiccation, with resulting osteocytic degeneration and osteonecrosis [6, 38, 39]. The factors that may influence the amount of heat generation are the drill design, the drilling technique, and the bone characteristics [6, 40]. Only light brushing motions using a high-speed bur with the copious amount of irrigation should be applied for endodontic surgery [6].

Periapical curettage is aimed to remove pathological tissue and enable access to the surgical site. The curettage may potentially jeopardize adjacent anatomical structures such as the maxillary sinus, the nasal cavity, and neurovascular bundles [6]. The inflammatory endodontic lesions (either cyst or granuloma) are the responses of the periradicular tissues to irritants from the infected root canal, and it is usually not necessary to completely curette all the involved periradicular tissues during the surgery [6, 41].

9.1.3 Complications During Root-End Management

Root-end management involves a root-end resection and retrograde preparation and filling of the apical part of the root canal [42].

Root-end resection was traditionally recommended in order to remove the contaminated apical part of the root canal and to provide access for retrograde cavity preparation and obturation [1, 43]. It was suggested that at least 3 mm of the root end should be removed [44]. However, in some cases, excessive root-end resection may dangerously reduce the crown-to-root ratio (CRR) [44, 45]. Recent studies suggest that root-resected teeth are not prosthodontically compromised unless there is also periodontal bone loss. Therefore, preserving the suggested ideal 1:2 CRR must not compromise the main goal of the surgery [46, 47].

Missed root canals may compromise the success of the whole surgical procedure. Inadequate root resection or limited visualization of the root anatomy is the main cause of missed root canals [48].

Ultrasonic tips are used to prepare a retrograde cavity to a depth of 3–4 mm [16, 49]. However, during the use of ultrasonic endodontic tips, a fracture of the tip can occur, and dentinal cracks may develop [50]. Therefore, light touch with moderate power setting and copious irrigations should be employed while operating the ultrasonic tips [42].

9.2 Bleeding in Endodontic Surgery

A damage to blood vessels during the surgical procedure may lead to hemorrhage [51–55]. While a severe hemorrhage is rare in endodontic surgery, when happens it may cause serious systemic complications [53, 56]. In patient with bleeding disorders, excessive bleeding may occur even if only small blood vessels were damaged during the surgical procedure [6, 53, 56].

In cases when the bleeding is not penetrating the oral mucosa or the skin, a localized collection of the blood in the oral mucosa or facial tissues may cause a discoloration resulting in the formation of hematoma. Hematomas can last for up to 2 weeks and usually require no treatment [6]. Rarely, an excessive hematoma developed in the floor of the mouth may even lead to potentially life-threatening scenarios [57].

Mild hemorrhage is relatively common during endodontic surgery, and although it is usually not life threatening, it may cause complications and may even compromise the prognosis of the treatment [52]. Adequate bleeding control is therefore essential since it improves visualization of the surgical site, minimizes the operating time, and enables the dry field for proper placement of retrograde filling materials [6, 52, 55]. Minor bleeding is still common and should be controlled by a variety of means such as digital compression, gauze tamponade, cauterization, suturing of the bleeding vessel (ligation), and by adjunct topical hemostatic agents [1, 6, 52, 54, 55, 58–61].

The goals of local anesthesia during endodontic surgery are to achieve profound anesthesia that is necessary for the patient comfort and cooperation, together with proper hemostasis, achieved by administrating a local anesthesia agent with vasoconstrictor [1, 51, 54, 55, 60]. Usually, 1:100,000 epinephrine concentration should be sufficient to achieve proper hemostasis [6, 27].

Occasionally, a secondary bleeding phase is observed after an infiltration of local anesthetic with vasoconstrictor. This phenomenon, termed "the rebound phenomenon" [62], may last for hours, and it is usually impossible to reestablish hemostasis by additional injections [63]. Thus, the more complicated and hemostasis-dependent procedures (such as the root-end management) should be done first [6, 31, 63].

9.3 Nerve Injury During Endodontic Surgery

Most routine surgical procedures may lead to nerve injury [1, 6, 64, 65]. In addition, nerve injuries may be caused indirectly by postsurgical pressure increase applied on the nerve bundle by the development of an intra-alveolar hematoma, or edema inside the mandibular canal, or by a prolonged pressure increase from neuritis [66]. However, direct trauma to the nerve bundle during surgery is the most frequent cause of nerve injury and may occur through nerve compression, stretching, cutting, overheating, and accidental puncture [6, 67–71]. Most cases of inferior alveolar nerve (IAN) injuries have been reported in second mandibular molars [1, 6, 64, 72].

The use of cone-beam CT (CBCT) may facilitate the evaluation of the true extent of the periapical (PA) lesions and the relationship of the PA lesions and root apices to anatomical landmarks such as adjacent neurosensory structures, thus enabling a more predictable surgical approach [73–79]. Following surgical procedure, the practitioner needs to detect any possible signs of altered sensation [69, 71, 72, 80]. Early symptoms that may suggest possible nerve injury are acute pain during or after the surgical procedure or neurosensory alterations, such as paresthesia [6, 81].

The long-term prognosis of altered sensation following endodontic surgery is not fully elucidated, but it may be related to the type and extent of injury and to the intervention protocol and timing [64, 71, 72, 82–84]. It seems that most patients, especially those with a relatively low extent of injury, whom were treated immediately and properly, tend to improve with time [84]. When nerve injury is suspected, a timely mannered clinical approach aimed to prevent permanent damage and to enable a better clinical and medicolegal response is of outmost importance [6, 64].

9.3.1 Maxillary Sinus Complications

The roots of maxillary premolars and molars may lie in proximity to the maxillary sinus floor [85]. In many cases, it is the periapical granuloma or cyst extending into the sinus cavity, causing sinusitis of dental origin. This was shown for the first time in a study by Bauer [86] and later was termed “endo-antral syndrome” (EAS) by Selden [87]. The reported frequency of sinusitis of dental origin varies considerably, between 4.6 and 47% [88] of all sinusitis cases. These represent risk factors for perforation of the Schneiderian membrane during periapical surgery.

Frequencies of Schneiderian membrane perforations vary from 9.6 to 50% [89]. Sinus membrane perforations could be detrimental, causing inhibition of ciliary activity, thereby reducing the resistance to infection [90]. Clinical signs and symptoms include nasal bleeding, sinus obstruction, and acute or chronic sinus infections [90]. However, Ericson et al. [91] and then Watzek et al. (1997) [108] found no significant difference in the healing rate between patients with and without intraoperative sinus exposure. Moreover, later on, it was also demonstrated that as long as foreign materials and root apex are not allowed to enter the sinus cavity during root-end preparation, a Schneiderian membrane perforation is not detrimental to the clinical outcome [92].

9.3.2 Postoperative Pain, Swelling, and Infection

Postoperative pain and swelling are common complications of surgical procedures [93], and their intensity depends on the degree of tissue damage and inflammatory response. Inflammation may occur due to the surgical wound alone or as a result of the tissue injury combined with surgical site infection [6, 94].

Swelling may begin minutes to hours after the surgical procedure (Fig. 9.3) and is the consequence of hemorrhage and edema (an accumulation of fluid in a tissue) that can continue for several days [94]. Following the surgery, bleeding usually stops within minutes because of clotting, and the swelling is usually caused by edema [6].

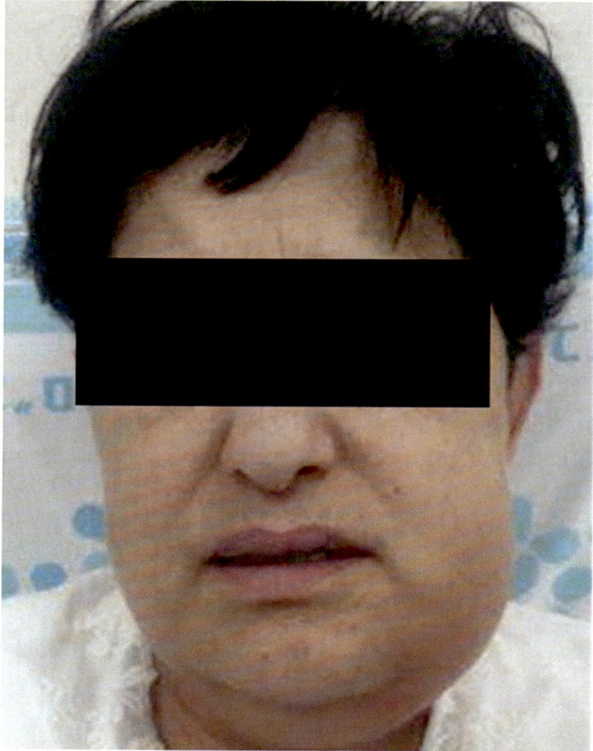

Fig. 9.3 Postoperative swelling following endodontic surgery in the first *left* mandibular molar tooth

Pain is an unpleasant sensory and emotional experience associated with actual or potential damage or described in terms of such damage [95]. The maximum severity of pain usually occurs during the first 24 h [96], and the maximum swelling occurs between the first and second postoperative days. However, between 45 and 66% of patients present either with moderate swelling or with no swelling at all [6, 96].

Several possible factors affecting the risk and intensity of postsurgical symptoms were reported, including the type of surgical technique (traditional vs. modern surgical technique [2, 96–98]), poor oral hygiene, [99], smoking [99], preoperative medication [100], type of local anesthesia [101], type of root-end filling material [102], and the patient's age or gender [99]. However, because it is more efficient to prevent than to treat pain, the concept of "preemptive analgesia" was suggested (i.e., to prevent postoperative pain by preventing the establishment of central sensitization) [103, 104]. It includes the administration of a drug that blocks painful inputs from entering the central nervous system before the surgical procedure, in order to attenuate the development of changes that manifest as increased pain during or following the surgery [6, 104, 105].

Tsesis et al. [100] premedicated all patients treated surgically by the modern endodontic surgical technique, with a single 8 mg dose of oral dexamethasone preoperatively and two single 4 mg doses 1 and 2 days postoperatively. One day postoperatively, 76% of the patients were completely pain-free, less than 4% had moderate pain, and 65% did not report any swelling [100].

No consensus exists regarding the use of antibiotics in endodontic surgery [93, 106]. The prevention of surgical site infection is best managed by maintenance of oral hygiene measures and the use of antiseptic mouth washes immediately preoperatively and postoperatively [6]. Antibiotics should be considered mainly for immunocompromised patients or when signs of systemic involvement develop following the surgery. A surgical reentry might be also indicated for surgical drainage and to explore and debride the apical tissues [6, 107].

References

1. Kim S, Kratchman S. Modern endodontic surgery concepts and practice: a review. J Endod. 2006;32(7):601–23.
2. Tsesis I, Rosen E, Schwartz-Arad D, Fuss Z. Retrospective evaluation of surgical endodontic treatment: traditional versus modern technique. J Endod. 2006;32(5):412–6.
3. Johnson BR, Witherspoon D. Periradicular surgery. In: Cohen S, Hargreaves KM, editors. Pathways of the pulp. 9th ed. St. Louis, MO: Mosby, Elsevier; 2006. p. 724–85.
4. Tsesis I, Rosen E, Taschieri S, Telishevsky Strauss Y, Ceresoli V, Del Fabbro M. Outcomes of surgical endodontic treatment performed by a modern technique: an updated meta-analysis of the literature. J Endod. 2013;39(3):332–9.
5. Tsesis I, Faivishevsky V, Kfir A, Rosen E. Outcome of surgical endodontic treatment performed by a modern technique: a meta-analysis of literature. J Endod. 2009;35(11):1505–11.
6. Complications in Endodontic Surgery. Prevention, identification and management. Berlin: Springer; 2014.

7. Rubinstein RAKS. Short-term observation of the results of endodontic surgery with the use of surgical operation microscope and super-EBA as root end filling material. J Endod. 1999;25:43–8.
8. Strbac GD, Schnappauf A, Giannis K, Moritz A, Ulm C. Guided modern endodontic surgery: a novel approach for guided osteotomy and root resection. J Endod. 2017;43(3):496–501.
9. Angelos P. Complications, errors, and surgical ethics. World J Surg. 2009;33(4):609–11.
10. von Arx T, Salvi GE, Janner S, Jensen SS. Scarring of gingiva and alveolar mucosa following apical surgery: visual assessment after one year. Oral Surg. 2008;1:178–89.
11. Taschieri S, Del Fabbro M, Francetti L, Perondi I, Corbella S. Does the papilla preservation flap technique induce soft tissue modifications over time in endodontic surgery procedures? J Endod. 2016;42(8):1191–5.
12. Ahmad I. Anterior dental aesthetics: gingival perspective. Br Dent J. 2005;199(4):195–202.
13. Trombelli L, Farina R. Flap designs for periodontal healing. Endod Top. 2012;25:4–15.
14. von Arx T, Salvi GE, Janner S, Jensen SS. Gingival recession following apical surgery in the esthetic zone: a clinical study with 70 cases. Eur J Esthet Dent. 2009;4(1):28–45.
15. Ainamo J, Loe H. Anatomical characteristics of gingiva. A clinical and microscopic study of the free and attached gingiva. J Periodontol. 1966;37(1):5–13.
16. Ferguson MW, Whitby DJ, Shah M, Armstrong J, Siebert JW, Longaker MT. Scar formation: the spectral nature of fetal and adult wound repair. Plast Reconstr Surg. 1996;97(4):854–60.
17. Fischer KR, Grill E, Jockel-Schneider Y, Bechtold M, Schlagenhauf U, Fickl S. On the relationship between gingival biotypes and supracrestal gingival height, crown form and papilla height. Clin Oral Implants Res. 2014;25(8):894–8.
18. Tsesis I, Rosen E, Tamse A, Taschieri S, Del Fabbro M. Effect of guided tissue regeneration on the outcome of surgical endodontic treatment: a systematic review and meta-analysis. J Endod. 2011;37(8):1039–45.
19. Chi CS, Andrade DB, Kim SG, Solomon CS. Guided tissue regeneration in endodontic surgery by using a bioactive resorbable membrane. J Endod. 2015;41(4):559–62.
20. Peck S, Peck L, Kataja M. The gingival smile line. Angle Orthod. 1992;62(2):91–100. discussion 1-2
21. Enoch S, Moseley R, Stephens P, Thomas DW. The oral mucosa: a model of wound healing with reduced scarring. Oral Surg. 2008;1(1):11–21.
22. Palumbo A. The anatomy and physiology of the healthy periodontium. In: Panagakos F, editor. Gingival diseases -their aetiology, prevention and treatment: InTech; 2011.
23. Velvart P, Ebner-Zimmermann U, Ebner JP. Comparison of papilla healing following sulcular full-thickness flap and papilla base flap in endodontic surgery. Int Endod J. 2003;36(10):653–9.
24. Kim E, Song JS, Jung IY, Lee SJ, Kim S. Prospective clinical study evaluating endodontic microsurgery outcomes for cases with lesions of endodontic origin compared with cases with lesions of combined periodontal-endodontic origin. J Endod. 2008;34(5):546–51.
25. Lui JN, Khin MM, Krishnaswamy G, Chen NN. Prognostic factors relating to the outcome of endodontic microsurgery. J Endod. 2014;40(8):1071–6.
26. Miloro M, Ghali GE, Larsen P. Peterson's. Principles of oral and maxillofacial surgery. 3rd ed. Shelton, CT: Shelton People's Medical Publishing House; 2012.
27. Lindhe J, Lang NP, Karring T. Clinical periodontology and implant dentistry. 5th ed. Oxford, UK: Blackwell Publishing Ltd.; 2008.
28. Kahn S, Almeida RA, Dias AT, Rodrigues WJ, Barceleiro MO, Taba M Jr. Clinical considerations on the root coverage of gingival recessions in thin or thick biotype. Int J Periodontics Restorative Dent. 2016;36(3):409–15.
29. De Rouck T, Eghbali R, Collys K, De Bruyn H, Cosyn J. The gingival biotype revisited: transparency of the periodontal probe through the gingival margin as a method to discriminate thin from thick gingiva. J Clin Periodontol. 2009;36(5):428–33.
30. Cutright DE, Hunsuck EE. Microcirculation of the perioral regions in the Macaca Rhesus. II. Oral Surg Oral Med Oral Pathol. 1970;29(6):926–34.
31. Morrow SG, Rubinstein RA. Endodontic surgery. In: Ingle JI, editor. Endodontics. 5th ed. Hamilton: BC Decker Inc.; 2002.

32. Selvig KA, Biagiotti GR, Leknes KN, Wikesjo UM. Oral tissue reactions to suture materials. Int J Periodontics Restorative Dent. 1998;18(5):474–87.
33. Silverstein LH, Kurtzman GM, Shatz PC. Suturing for optimal soft-tissue management. J Oral Implantol. 2009;35(2):82–90.
34. Lin L, Chen MY, Ricucci D, Rosenberg PA. Guided tissue regeneration in periapical surgery. J Endod. 2010;36(4):618–25.
35. Andreasen JO, Rud J. Modes of healing histologically after endodontic surgery in 70 cases. Int J Oral Surg. 1972;1(3):148–60.
36. Grzesik WJ, Narayanan AS. Cementum and periodontal wound healing and regeneration. Crit Rev Oral Biol Med. 2002;13(6):474–84.
37. Kratchman SI. Endodontic microsurgery. Compendium. 2007;28(6):324–31.
38. Heinemann F, Hasan I, Kunert-Keil C, Gotz W, Gedrange T, Spassov A, et al. Experimental and histological investigations of the bone using two different oscillating osteotomy techniques compared with conventional rotary osteotomy. Ann Anat. 2012;194(2):165–70.
39. Lavelle C, Wedgwood D. Effect of internal irrigation on frictional heat generated from bone drilling. J Oral Surg. 1980;38(7):499–503.
40. Augustin G, Zigman T, Davila S, Udilljak T, Staroveski T, Brezak D, et al. Cortical bone drilling and thermal osteonecrosis. Clin Biomech (Bristol, Avon). 2012;27(4):313–25.
41. Lin LM, Gaengler P, Langeland K. Periradicular curettage. Int Endod J. 1996;29(4):220–7.
42. Corbella S, Del-Fabbro M, Rosen E, Taschieri S. Complications in root-end management. In: Tsesis I, editor. Complications in endodontic surgery: prevention, identification and management. Berlin: Springer; 2014. p. 89–100.
43. Lin S, Platner O, Metzger Z, Tsesis I. Residual bacteria in root apices removed by a diagonal root-end resection: a histopathological evaluation. Int Endod J. 2008;41(6):469–75.
44. Roy R, Chandler NP, Lin J. Peripheral dentin thickness after root-end cavity preparation. Oral Surg Oral Med Oral Pathol Oral Radiol Endod. 2008;105(2):263–6.
45. Grossmann Y, Sadan A. The prosthodontic concept of crown-to-root ratio: a review of the literature. J Prosthet Dent. 2005;93(6):559–62.
46. Cho SY, Kim E. Does apical root resection in endodontic microsurgery jeopardize the prosthodontic prognosis? Restor Dent Endod. 2013;38(2):59–64.
47. Jang Y, Hong HT, Chun HJ, Roh BD. Influence of apical root resection on the biomechanical response of a single-rooted tooth-part 2: apical root resection combined with periodontal bone loss. J Endod. 2015;41(3):412–6.
48. Vertucci FJ. Root canal anatomy of the human permanent teeth. Oral Surg Oral Med Oral Pathol. 1984;58(5):589–99.
49. Del Fabbro M, Tsesis I, Rosano G, Bortolin M, Taschieri S. Scanning electron microscopic analysis of the integrity of the root-end surface after root-end management using a piezoelectric device: a cadaveric study. J Endod. 2010;36(10):1693–7.
50. Peters CI, Peters OA, Barbakow F. An in vitro study comparing root-end cavities prepared by diamond-coated and stainless steel ultrasonic retrotips. Int Endod J. 2001;34(2):142–8.
51. Israels S, Schwetz N, Boyar R, McNicol A. Bleeding disorders: characterization, dental considerations and management. J Can Dent Assoc. 2006;72(9):827.
52. Penarrocha-Diago M, Maestre-Ferrin L, Penarrocha-Oltra D, von Arx T. Influence of hemostatic agents upon the outcome of periapical surgery: dressings with anesthetic and vasoconstrictor or aluminum chloride. Med Oral Patol Oral Cir Bucal. 2013;18(2):e272–8.
53. Reich W, Kriwalsky MS, Wolf HH, Schubert J. Bleeding complications after oral surgery in outpatients with compromised haemostasis: incidence and management. Oral Maxillofac Surg. 2009;13(2):73–7.
54. Samudrala S. Topical hemostatic agents in surgery: a surgeon's perspective. AORN J. 2008;88(3):S2–11.
55. Witherspoon DE, Gutmann JL. Haemostasis in periradicular surgery. Int Endod J. 1996;29(3):135–49.
56. Moghadam HG, Caminiti MF. Life-threatening hemorrhage after extraction of third molars:case report and management protocol. J Can Dent Assoc. 2002;68(11):670–4.

57. Goldstein BH. Acute dissecting hematoma: a complication of oral and maxillofacial surgery. J Oral Surg. 1981;39(1):40–3.
58. Gupta G, Prestigiacomo CJ. From sealing wax to bone wax: predecessors to Horsley's development. Neurosurg Focus. 2007;23(1):E16.
59. Livaditis GJ. Comparison of monopolar and bipolar electrosurgical modes for restorative dentistry: a review of the literature. J Prosthet Dent. 2001;86(4):390–9.
60. Sileshi B, Achneck HE, Lawson JH. Management of surgical hemostasis: topical agents. Vascular. 2008;16(Suppl 1):S22–8.
61. Soballe PW, Nimbkar NV, Hayward I, Nielsen TB, Drucker WR. Electric cautery lowers the contamination threshold for infection of laparotomies. Am J Surg. 1998;175(4):263–6.
62. Lindorf HH. Investigation of the vascular effect of newer local anesthetics and vasoconstrictors. Oral Surg Oral Med Oral Pathol. 1979;48(4):292–7.
63. Gutmann JL, Harrison JW. Surgical endodontics. Boston: Blackwell Scientific Publications; 1991.
64. Rosen E, Goldberger T, Taschieri S, Del Fabbro M, Corbella S, Tsesis I. The prognosis of altered sensation after extrusion of root canal filling materials: a systematic review of the literature. J Endod. 2016;42(6):873–9.
65. Moiseiwitsch JR. Avoiding the mental foramen during periapical surgery. J Endod. 1995;21(6):340–2.
66. Park SH, Wang HL. Implant reversible complications: classification and treatments. Implant Dent. 2005;14(3):211–20.
67. Annibali S, Ripari M, La Monaca G, Tonoli F, Cristalli MP. Local accidents in dental implant surgery: prevention and treatment. Int J Periodontics Restorative Dent. 2009;29(3):325–31.
68. Gallas-Torreira MM, Reboiras-Lopez MD, Garcia-Garcia A, Gandara-Rey J. Mandibular nerve paresthesia caused by endodontic treatment. Med Oral. 2003;8(4):299–303.
69. Givol N, Rosen E, Bjorndal L, Taschieri S, Ofec R, Tsesis I. Medico-legal aspects of altered sensation following endodontic treatment: a retrospective case series. Oral Surg Oral Med Oral Pathol Oral Radiol Endod. 2011;112(1):126–31.
70. Grotz KA, Al-Nawas B, de Aguiar EG, Schulz A, Wagner W. Treatment of injuries to the inferior alveolar nerve after endodontic procedures. Clin Oral Investig. 1998;2(2):73–6.
71. Juodzbalys G, Wang H, Sabalys G. Injury of the inferior alveolar nerve during implant placement: a literature review. J Oral Maxillofac Res. 2011;2(1):e1.
72. Pogrel MA. Damage to the inferior alveolar nerve as the result of root canal therapy. J Am Dent Assoc. 2007;138(1):65–9.
73. AAE, AAOMR. AAE and AAOMR joint position statement - use of cone-beam-computed tomography in endodontics. 2010.
74. Bornstein MM, Lauber R, Sendi P, von Arx T. Comparison of periapical radiography and limited cone-beam computed tomography in mandibular molars for analysis of anatomical landmarks before apical surgery. J Endod. 2011;37(2):151–7.
75. de Paula-Silva FW, Wu MK, Leonardo MR, da Silva LA, Wesselink PR. Accuracy of periapical radiography and cone-beam computed tomography scans in diagnosing apical periodontitis using histopathological findings as a gold standard. J Endod. 2009;35(7):1009–12.
76. Kamburoglu K, Kilic C, Ozen T, Yuksel SP. Measurements of mandibular canal region obtained by cone-beam computed tomography: a cadaveric study. Oral Surg Oral Med Oral Pathol Oral Radiol Endod. 2009;107(2):e34–42.
77. Patel S. New dimensions in endodontic imaging: part 2. Cone beam computed tomography. Int Endod J. 2009;42(6):463–75.
78. Pinsky HM, Dyda S, Pinsky RW, Misch KA, Sarment DP. Accuracy of three-dimensional measurements using cone-beam CT. Dentomaxillofac Radiol. 2006;35(6):410–6.
79. Simonton JD, Azevedo B, Schindler WG, Hargreaves KM. Age- and gender-related differences in the position of the inferior alveolar nerve by using cone beam computed tomography. J Endod. 2009;35(7):944–9.
80. Givol N, Rosen E, Taicher S, Tsesis I. Risk management in endodontics. J Endod. 2010;36(6):982–4.
81. Froes FG, Miranda AM, Abad Eda C, Riche FN, Pires FR. Non-surgical management of paraesthesia and pain associated with endodontic sealer extrusion into the mandibular canal. Aust Endod J. 2009;35(3):183–6.

82. Leung YY, Fung PP, Cheung LK. Treatment modalities of neurosensory deficit after lower third molar surgery: a systematic review. J Oral Maxillofac Surg. 2012;70(4):768–78.
83. Seddon HJ. A classification of nerve injuries. Br Med J. 1942;2(4260):237–9.
84. Pogrel MA, Jergensen R, Burgon E, Hulme D. Long-term outcome of trigeminal nerve injuries related to dental treatment. J Oral Maxillofac Surg. 2011;69(9):2284–8.
85. Tian XM, Qian L, Xin XZ, Wei B, Gong Y. An analysis of the proximity of maxillary posterior teeth to the maxillary sinus using cone-beam computed tomography. J Endod. 2016;42(3):371–7.
86. Bauer WH. Maxillary sinusitis of dental origin. Am J Orthod Oral Surg. 1943;29(3): B133–B51.
87. Selden HS. The interrelationship between the maxillary sinus and endodontics. Oral Surg Oral Med Oral Pathol. 1974;38(4):623–9.
88. Melen I, Lindahl L, Andreasson L, Rundcrantz H. Chronic maxillary sinusitis. Definition, diagnosis and relation to dental infections and nasal polyposis. Acta Otolaryngol. 1986;101(3–4):320–7.
89. Persson G. Periapical surgery of molars. Int J Oral Surg. 1982;11(2):96–100.
90. Pignataro L, Mantovani M, Torretta S, Felisati G, Sambataro G. ENT assessment in the integrated management of candidate for (maxillary) sinus lift. Acta Otorhinolaryngol Ital. 2008;28(3):110–9.
91. Ericson S, Finne K, Persson G. Results of apicoectomy of maxillary canines, premolars and molars with special reference to oroantral communication as a prognostic factor. Int J Oral Surg. 1974;3(6):386–93.
92. Hauman CH, Chandler NP, Tong DC. Endodontic implications of the maxillary sinus: a review. Int Endod J. 2002;35(2):127–41.
93. Mansoor J. Pre- and postoperative management techniques. Part 3: before and after - endodontic surgery. Br Dent J. 2015;218(6):333–5.
94. AAE. Glossary of endodontic terms. 8th ed.; 2012.
95. Merskey H, Bogduk N. International Association for the Study of Pain. IASP Task Force on Taxonomy. Classification of chronic pain. 2nd ed. Seattle: IASP Press; 1994.
96. Garcia B, Larrazabal C, Penarrocha M. Pain and swelling in periapical surgery. A literature update. Med Oral Patol Oral Cir Bucal. 2008;13(11):E726–9.
97. Kvist T, Reit C. Postoperative discomfort associated with surgical and nonsurgical endodontic retreatment. Endod Dent Traumatol. 2000;16(2):71–4.
98. Tsesis I, Shoshani Y, Givol N, Yahalom R, Fuss Z, Taicher S. Comparison of quality of life after surgical endodontic treatment using two techniques: a prospective study. Oral Surg Oral Med Oral Pathol Oral Radiol Endod. 2005;99(3):367–71.
99. Garcia B, Penarrocha M, Marti E, Gay-Escodad C, von Arx T. Pain and swelling after periapical surgery related to oral hygiene and smoking. Oral Surg Oral Med Oral Pathol Oral Radiol Endod. 2007;104(2):271–6.
100. Tsesis I, Fuss Z, Lin S, Tilinger G, Peled M. Analysis of postoperative symptoms following surgical endodontic treatment. Quintessence Int. 2003;34(10):756–60.
101. Meechan JG, Blair GS. The effect of two different local anaesthetic solutions on pain experience following apicectomy. Br Dent J. 1993;175(11–12):410–3.
102. Chong BS, Pitt Ford TR. Postoperative pain after root-end resection and filling. Oral Surg Oral Med Oral Pathol Oral Radiol Endod. 2005;100(6):762–6.
103. Khan AA, Dionne RA. COX-2 inhibitors for endodontic pain. Endod Top. 2002;3:31–40.
104. Dahl JB, Moiniche S. Pre-emptive analgesia. Br Med Bull. 2004;71:13–27.
105. Dionne R. Preemptive vs preventive analgesia: which approach improves clinical outcomes? Compend Contin Educ Dent. 2000;21(1):48. 51-4, 6
106. Lindeboom JA, Frenken JW, Valkenburg P, van den Akker HP. The role of preoperative prophylactic antibiotic administration in periapical endodontic surgery: a randomized, prospective double-blind placebo-controlled study. Int Endod J. 2005;38(12):877–81.
107. Yingling NM, Byrne BE, Hartwell GR. Antibiotic use by members of the American Association of Endodontists in the year 2000: report of a national survey. J Endod. 2002;28(5):396–404.
108. Watzek G1, Bernhart T, Ulm C. Complications of sinus perforations and their management in endodontics. Dent Clin North Am. 1997;41(3):563–83.

Endodontic-Periodontal Relationship 10

Mehmet Omer Gorduysus

10.1 Introduction

The tooth, dental pulp, and the tooth supporting tissues (periodontium) are viewed as one biologic unit which is called dentoalveolar unit. The periodontal ligament, gingiva, cementum, and alveolar bone are the components of periodontium. A healthy periodontium is essential for the functions of a tooth and also for the health of the pulpal tissue. The interrelationship of these structures influences each other during health, function, and disease. This relationship between periodontal and endodontic diseases was first discovered by Simring and Goldberg in 1964 [1]. The periodontium and pulp have embryonic, anatomic, and functional interrelationship. Ectomesenchymal cells proliferate to form the dental papilla and follicle, which are the precursors of the periodontium and the pulp respectively. This embryonic development gives rise to anatomical connections, which remain throughout life [2].

The periodontal-endodontic lesions are characterized by the involvement of the pulp and periodontal disease in the same tooth. This is a unique biological relation and makes the diagnosis complicated and difficult because a single lesion may present signs of both endodontic and periodontal involvement. Generally, the majority of pulpal and periodontal lesions are the result of bacterial infection. This suggests that one disease may be the result or cause of the other or even originated from two different and independent processes which are associated with their advancement [3]. Diagnosis is further complicated by the fact that these diseases are viewed as independent entities. Diagnosis, differential diagnosis, etiopathogenesis of the problems, treatment approaches, decision-making, and prognosis of those clinical situations are really challenging problems in endodontics and periodontology.

M.O. Gorduysus, D.D.S., Ph.D.
Professor, Department of Preventive and Restorative Dentistry,
University of Sharjah, College of Dental Medicine, Sharjah, UAE
e-mail: ogorduysus@yahoo.com

P. Jain (ed.), *Common Complications in Endodontics*,
https://doi.org/10.1007/978-3-319-60997-3_10

The purpose of this chapter, while emphasizing upon pulpal-periodontal tissues interactions and endodontic-periodontal interrelationships, is to also talk about clinical considerations, treatment protocol and approach, and their possible solutions from an endodontic aspect.

10.2 Pathways of Communication

Pulpal and periodontal tissues are closely related, and the disease transmission between these two lesions has been demonstrated by many studies, demonstrating microbiological similarities between infected root canals and advanced periodontitis [4–7]. Other than these microbial findings, similarities in the composition of cellular infiltrates also suggest the existence of communication between the pulp and the periodontal tissues [8]. These findings infer that cross-contamination between the pulp and periodontal tissues is possible. Pulpal and periodontal problems are responsible for more than 50% of tooth mortality [9]. Periodontal disease is a slowly progressing disease that may have an atrophic effect on the dental pulp.

Three main pathways in the development of periodontal-endodontic lesions are [10]:

1. Dentinal tubules
2. Lateral and accessory canals
3. Apical foramen

Endodontic and periodontal sites have similar embryological and developmental process and that make the bilateral interactions more easier besides the other common pathways. Any problem in any compartment of that biological unit (dentoalveolar unit) may affect the other one (as primary or secondary reason like a domino effect). The relations between endodontic and periodontal tissues were mentioned and defined by Simring and Goldberg at first in the literature [3], and later it was used as a concept and term to describe the inflammatory elements and procedures between the two tissues. An erupting tooth is surrounded by squamous epithelium and a connective tissue. The pulpal tissue and supporting tissues around the tooth in both periapical and gingival sides are connective tissues. Therefore the effects of the noxious stimuli and microorganisms are similar on these tissues because of the characteristic similarities of the pulpal, periodontal, and periapical tissues. These tissues are very similar embryologically, developmentally, and structurally. Also from the point of healing capacity and potential of healing are very similar because in fact periodontal, periapical, and pulpal tissues are the continuation of each other. As a connective tissue, their reaction to inflammation, their collagen metabolism, and their immunological and physiological responses are more or less the same. In both (endodontic and periodontal tissues), the reactions can be acute or chronic, but in endodontium generally the reactions are acute, and in periodontium the reactions are generally chronically observed.

The possible pathways for ingress of bacteria and their products into these tissues can broadly be divided into: anatomical/physiological and nonphysiological/pathologic pathways [11].

10.3 Anatomical/Physiological Pathways

Anatomical structures such as apical foramen and lateral and accessory canals are the main routes of the interactions between the pulp and periodontium. They create very special and intimate connections between the periodontal and pulpal tissues (Fig. 10.1).

In case of endodontic lesions, the pathway of inflammation is through the apical foramen, furcation canals, and lateral accessory canals to the periodontium resulting in a 1 ° endodontic lesion, sometimes progressing toward 2 ° periodontal involvement. In case of periodontal lesions, the progression of periodontitis is by way of lateral canal and apex to induce a 2 ° endodontic lesion. True combined and concomitant endodontic-periodontal lesions are a mixture of the two, and it is difficult to differentiate the primary reason and the source.

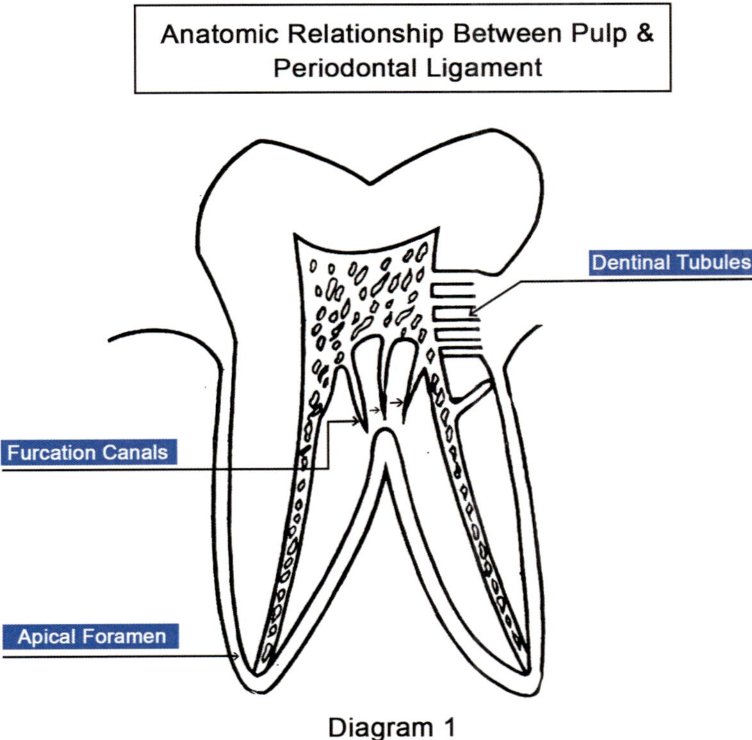

Fig. 10.1 Anatomic relationship between pulp and periodontium

10.3.1 Apical Foramen

The pulp and periodontal tissues are derived from mesenchymal tissues of the tooth germ. The blood supply maintains a connection between these tissues via the apical foramen and lateral canals throughout the development of the tooth. The apical foramen is the main and most direct route of communication between the periodontium and the pulp. Although periodontal disease can have a damaging effect on the pulp tissue, total disintegration of the pulp is only possible if bacterial plaque involves the apical foramen, thus, compromising the vascular supply. Following the total necrosis of the pulp, various bacterial products like enzymes, metabolites, antigens, etc. reach the periodontium through the apical foramen, initiating an inflammatory response.

Pulp exposures, periodontitis, and caries lesions are of significant importance in the development of periodontal-endodontic lesions. If these lesions are not well treated and the canals are not disinfected and sealed completely, it may account for the progression of the lesion or even for the endodontic reinfection [12–14].

10.3.2 Lateral Canals

In addition to the apical foramen, there are a number of branches connecting the main root canal with the periodontal ligament. These root canal ramifications were first described nearly 100 years ago and are known as "accessory canals." As the root develops, ectomesenchymal channels get incorporated, either due to the dentin formation around existing blood vessels or breaks in the continuity of the Hertwig's root sheath, to become lateral or accessory canals [15]. The term accessory canal is nowadays used to describe any ramification that connects the root canal system to the periodontal ligament [11].

Lateral canals contain connective tissue and vessels which connect the circulating system of the pulp with that of the periodontal ligament. The radiographic indications of the presence of lateral canals are localized thickening of periodontal ligament on the lateral root surface or a frank lateral lesion. The majority of the accessory canals are found in the apical part of the root and lateral canals in the molar furcation region. The percentage of these lateral canals and their frequency on the root surface are as follows: apical third 17%, coronal third 1.6%, and body of the root 8.8% [16]. According to Bender et al., the periodontal endodontic problems were much more frequent in the molars than in the anterior teeth because of the greater number of accessory canals present in the molars.

10.3.3 Dentinal Tubules

In addition to the abovementioned pathways, the dentinal tubules are also important as other main ways to create interaction between the pulpal and periodontal tissues [10] (Fig. 10.2a, b). Periodontal disease, scaling, root planning, surgical procedures,

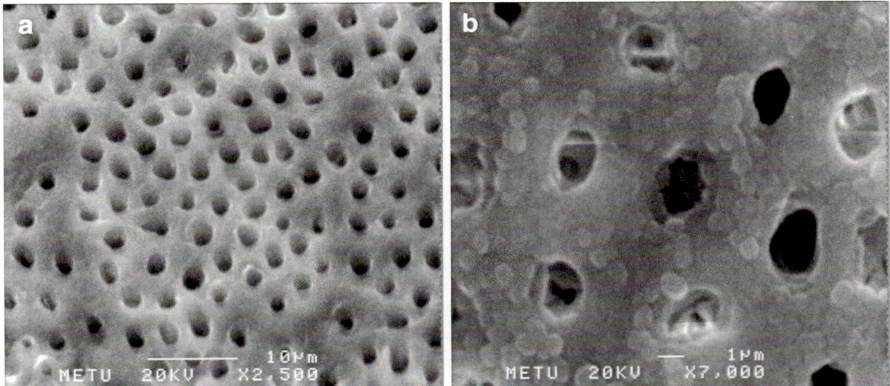

Fig. 10.2 (**a**, **b**) Dentinal tubules under SEM (Scanning Electron Microscope). (These pictures were taken from the study of Prof Mehmet Omer Gorduysus, pictures were taken in Middle East Technical University, Ankara-Turkey). On the *left* side, the clean dentinal tubules are seen. Tubules as hollow tubes are very unique pathways between periodontium and pulpal tissues. The cementum does not cover the dentin in the cervical area all the time, and the exposed tubules allow microorganisms and noxious stimuli into the canals. On the right side (**b**), the smear layer and microorganisms around the dentinal tubules are visible

developmental grooves, and gap joint at the cementoenamel junction may lead to exposed dentin [17]. As a very classical and established example, passage of microorganisms between the pulp and periodontal tissues is possible through these tubules, when the dentinal tubules are exposed in areas of denuded cementum [18].

According to Adriaens et al. [5], the bacteria coming from the periodontal pockets may contaminate the pulp through the dentinal tubules that would be exposed during root planning and scaling, serving as a microorganism reservoir resulting in the recolonization of the treated root surface. In contradiction to this, some studies [18, 19] have stated that because even with the removal of the cementum during the periodontal therapy in the vital teeth, the pulp tissue is protected against the harmful agents through forming reparative dentin. Moreover, the dentinal fluids move toward the exterior surface, thereby reducing the diffusion of the harmful products of the bacteria on the exposed dentin.

10.4 Nonphysiological/Pathologic Pathways

Another form of the communication is due to the iatrogenic perforations which occur while using either rotary instruments or due to the improper handling of the endodontic instruments [20]. When root perforation occurs, communications between the root canal system and periradicular tissues often reduce the prognosis of treatment. At the site of perforation, an inflammatory reaction in periodontal ligament occurs and leads to the formation of a lesion which can progress as a conventional primary endodontic lesion (Fig. 10.3).

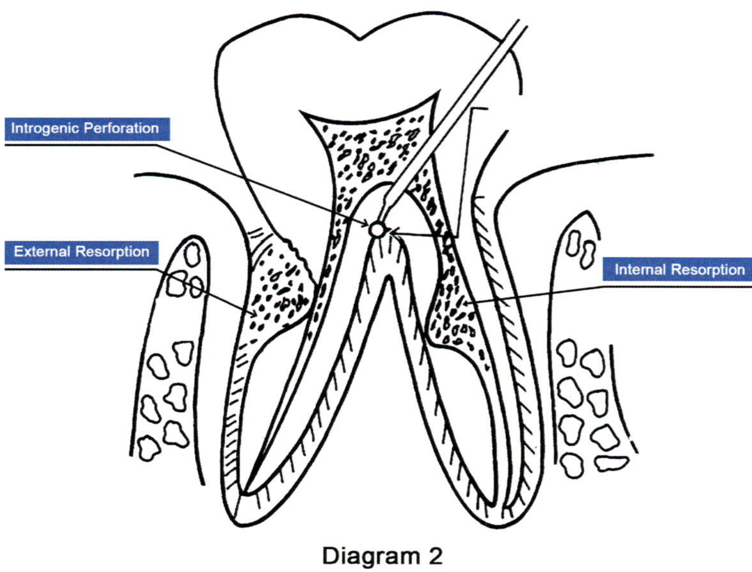

Fig. 10.3 Pathologic pathways between pulp and periodontium

Another way of communication between periodontal and pulpal tissues is vertical root fractures caused by trauma which can occur in both vital and non-vital teeth. The incidence of root fractures is more in the roots that are filled with lateral condensation technique and the teeth restored with intracanal posts [11]. They serve as a bridge for pulp contamination. If the periodontium had a previous inflammation, it may lead to dissemination of the inflammation which can result in pulp necrosis [21].

Developmental defects (Figs. 10.4 and 10.5a–c), abnormalities, and malformations, i.e., fusion, gemination, dens in dente, dens invaginatus, dens eviginatus, immediate bifurcation ridge (furcation is very cervically located); enamel, dentinal, and cemental abnormalities; or developmental problems, i.e., cemental agenesis, hypoplasia, amelogenesis imperfecta, and dentinogenesis imperfecta also can be itemized among the pathological pathway-causing situations. Physiological and pathological resorptions (transient, pressure, replantation resorption, internal resorption, etc.) also fall under this category (Figs. 10.6 and 10.7).

Wide-open apex and related infections, coronal leakage and unsuccessful coronal restorations, extrusion kind or rapid orthodontic movements, deep restorations, secondary caries, bone loss of the tooth supporting area, periodontal pockets,

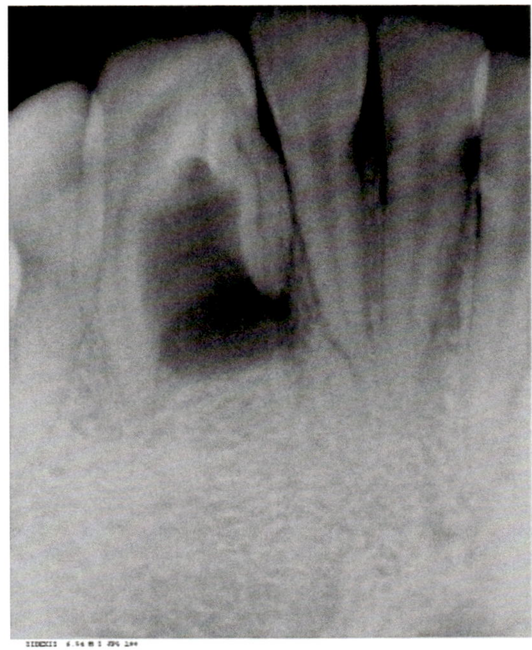

Fig. 10.4 Mandibular *right* lateral tooth represents developmental abnormality and related that in the X-ray periapical radiolucency. This is an example for endo-perio lesion-related developmental defects and malformations (from the archive of Prof. Mehmet Omer Gorduysus, author of the chapter)

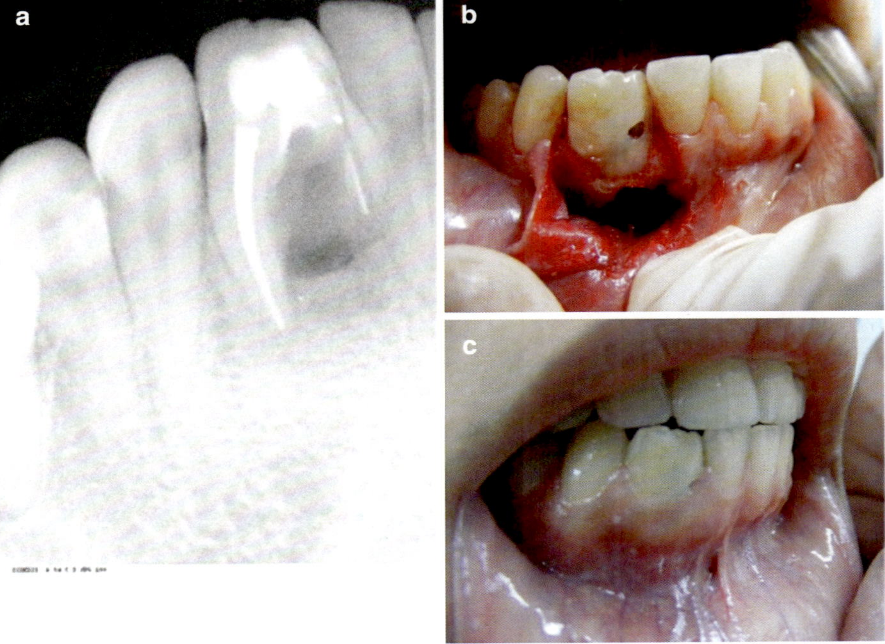

Fig. 10.5 (**a–c**) Following the root canal therapy, surgery, and restoration (from the archive of Prof Mehmet Omer Gorduysus, author of the chapter)

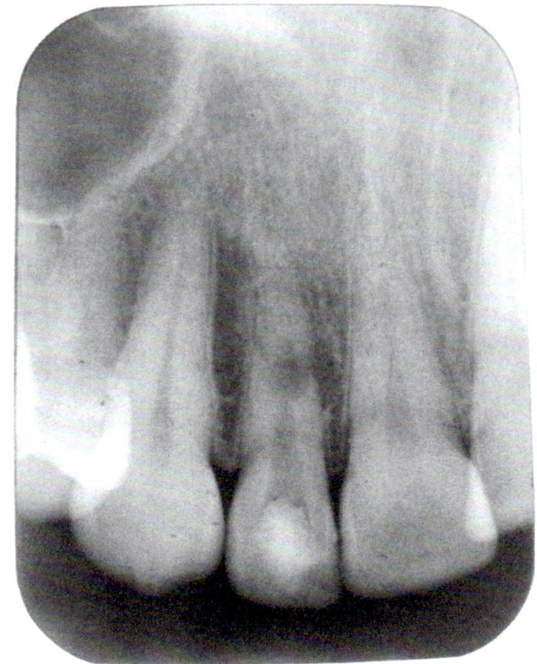

Fig. 10.6 In the *middle* third of the root (tooth 22), an internal resorption was observed radiographically which is communicated to periodontium. Patient had endodontic and periodontal clinical symptoms. The root canal was calcified at the apical third of the tooth. (From the archive of Prof Mehmet Omer Gorduysus, author of the chapter)

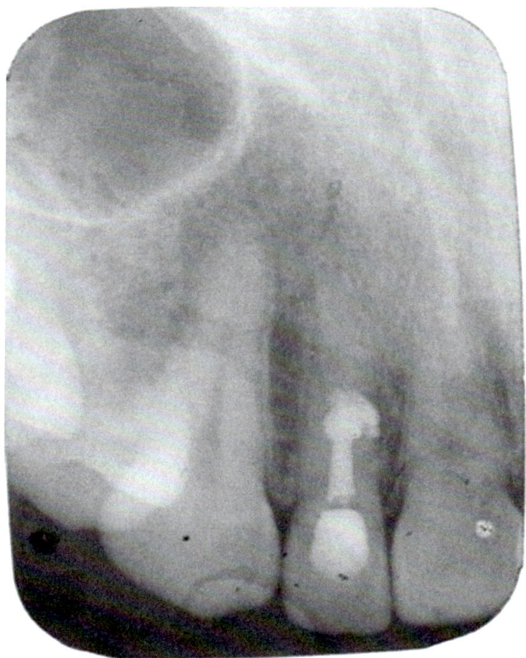

Fig. 10.7 The resorption area was obturated with injectable gutta-percha (Obtura II) and followed up. (From the archive of Prof Mehmet Omer Gorduysus, author of the chapter)

unsuccessful endodontic surgical applications, weak retrograde fillings, flora changes during the dental replantation and transplantation, and sinus tracts (fistula) are all possible pathological pathways. Besides these, extruded gutta-percha or posts beyond the apex also create a chronic irritation as foreign material. Amalgam particles, separated particles of absorbent paper cones and other materials, and calculus are extrinsic irritating factors and may cause pathological pathways between endodontium and periodontium.

10.5 Etiopathogenesis

10.5.1 Effect of Periodontal Lesions on the Pulp

High percentage of pulpal inflammation and degeneration has been reported in periodontally involved teeth than in teeth with no periodontal disease [22]. Research shows that periodontal disease has no effect on the pulp till it involves the apex or the periodontal breakdown has exposed an accessory canal to the oral environment [3, 23].

Microbial agents are the main etiologic factors involved in these lesions. The formation of bacterial plaque on denuded root surfaces, following periodontal disease, has the potential to induce pathologic changes in the pulp through lateral or accessory canals. Hence, a deleterious effect of periodontal disease on the pulp can occur and produce pulpitis and is often referred as retrograde pulpitis [1].

The effect of periodontal lesions on the pulp can result in atrophic and other degenerative changes like reduction in the number of pulp cells, dystrophic mineralization, fibrosis, reparative dentin formation, inflammation, and resorption. The explanation for atrophic changes is the disruption of blood flow through the lateral canals, which leads to localized areas of coagulation necrosis in the pulp. These areas are subsequently walled off from the rest of the healthy pulp tissue by collagen and dystrophic mineralization. With slowly advancing periodontal disease, cementum deposition may obliterate lateral canals before pulpal irritation occurs. Hence, this is the reason why not all periodontally involved teeth demonstrate pulpal atrophy and canal narrowing.

The causative agents of periodontal disease are found in the sulcus and are continually challenged by host defenses. An immunologic or inflammatory response is elicited in response to this microbiologic challenge. The speed of the pathogenesis increases generally as the immunity and resistance of the patients becomes lower. Noxious stimuli such as chemicals, rubber dam, broaches, local trauma, brushing style, etc., all may increase the "pathogenesis," and thus the endo-perio interfacing situations may accelerate. Either physiological or pathological pathways come into function and synergize with the help of predisposing factors. This results in the formation of granulomatous tissue in the periodontium. When periodontal disease extends from the gingival sulcus toward the apex, the inflammatory products attack the periodontal ligament and the surrounding alveolar bone. A clear-cut relationship between progressive periodontal disease and pulpal involvement, however, does not exist. The most common periodontal lesion produced by the pulp disease is the localized apical granuloma. It is produced by the diffusion of bacterial products through the root apex, with the formation of vascular granulation tissue. Subsequently, resorption of the alveolar bone and occasionally of the root itself may occur [24].

As these inflammatory changes increase in intensity, there is clinical evidence of bone loss, pain, infection, and abscess which increases the tooth mobility and leads to sinus tract and fistula formation. These situations may be categorized as acute or chronic or subacute exacerbations or flare-ups and sometimes may be a part of the clinical observations. Besides the individual factors, the pathogenicity of the microorganisms and the virulence are also important.

Resorption of the sides of the roots is frequently found adjacent to the granulation tissue overlying the roots. When the periodontal lesions are deep, resorption may also be found within the root canals and at the apical foramen. Since this resorptive process extends into the dentin peripherally toward the pulp, and the activating factors are produced from the periodontal lesion, this known as peripheral inflammatory root resorption (PIRR) was proposed [25].

10.5.1.1 Effects of Periodontal Treatment Procedures on the Dental Pulp

Commonly, the teeth become hypersensitive after periodontal procedures like scaling and root planning, gingivectomy or deep curettage, and lengthening of clinical crowns. This may be due to the influence of the periodontal diseases on the status of the pulp. When the periodontal disease extends apically, the cementum gets necrosed or removed, and the dentin or a lateral canal may get exposed. Dentinal tubules get exposed as a result and act as a channel of communication thus irritating the pulp. Root planning and scaling may result in the rupture of the vessels and destruction of the neurovascular bundle in the lateral canals, provoking a reduction of the blood supply and consequently leading to pulp alterations. If less than 2 mm of dentin remains after procedures like scaling and root planning (especially in mandibular anteriors), pulpal changes would occur in the teeth. Thus frequent periodontal procedures of long duration may cause pulpal pain.

The increase in intensity of pain may be explained by one or both of the following two reasons. Firstly, the smear layer formed on the root surface by the scaling procedures will be dissolved within a few days. This, in turn, will decrease the peripheral resistance to fluid flow across dentin. Thereby, pain sensations are more readily evoked. Secondly, open dentinal tubules serve as pathways for diffusive transport of bacterial elements in the oral cavity to the pulp, which is likely to cause a localized inflammatory pulpal response [4].

Drugs/chemical agents used for the cauterization of inflamed gingival tissues can also cause damage to the dental pulp via the exposed dentinal tubules.

Root conditioning using citric acid, though beneficial in the treatment of periodontal disease, unfortunately also removes the smear layer, an important pulp protector. Cotton and Siegel reported that citric acid, when applied to freshly cut dentin, has a toxic effect on the human dental pulp [26]. However, several other studies have concluded that pulpal changes after the application of citric acid does not show any significant changes in the pulp [27, 28].

10.6 Pulpal Diseases and the Periodontium

10.6.1 Effects of Endodontic Infection on the Periodontium

It has been demonstrated that intra pulpal infection tends to promote epithelial down growth along a denuded dentin surface. An endodontic infection if untreated is a local modifying risk factor for periodontitis by way of the apex and lateral or accessory canals.

Necrosis of the pulp can result in rapid and widespread destruction of periodontium, the production of radiolucency at the apex of the tooth, in the furcation or at various points along the root. It has been demonstrated that periodontal treatment of teeth with pulpal necrosis and periapical radiolucency resulted in impaired periodontal healing [26]. Retrograde periodontitis caused by pulpal disease is a common cause of severe, localized destruction of periodontal tissues and manifests as periodontal pocket formation, purulent inflammatory exudates, angular bone loss, swelling and bleeding of the gingival tissues, and increased tooth mobility. Therefore, it is essential that pulpal infections be treated first, before undertaking periodontal procedures.

10.7 Classification

The most commonly used classification was given by Simon et al. [29] (Fig. 10.8). According to this classification, endo-perio lesions can be classified into:

1. Primary endodontic lesion
2. Primary periodontal lesion
3. Primary endodontic lesion with secondary periodontal involvement
4. Primary periodontal lesion with secondary endodontic involvement
5. True combined lesion

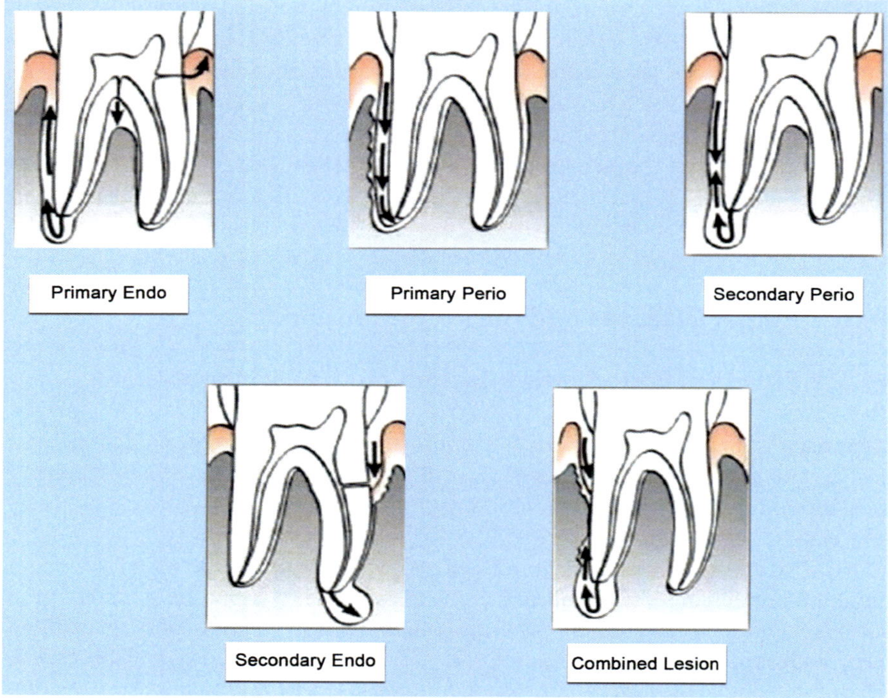

Fig. 10.8 Diagrammatic representation of endo-perio lesions based on the classification by Simon JH, Glick DH, Frank JL [29]

10.8 Primary Endodontic Lesions

An acute exacerbation of a chronic apical lesion on a tooth with a necrotic pulp may drain coronally through the periodontal ligament into the gingival sulcus [10]. Dental pulp with inflammatory changes is the essential and main reason. Most common causes are traumatic injuries, caries, and restorative procedures.

The necrotic pulp may drain through the apical foramen, lateral canal, or through the accessory canals at the furcal area. This condition may clinically mimic the presence of a periodontal abscess. In reality, however, it would be a sinus tract originating from the pulp that opens into the periodontal ligament. The pocket that forms is narrow and has little or no local factors. Radiographs with gutta-percha cone tracing the sinus tract will point toward the origin of the lesion. Root canal treatment is the treatment of choice. Prognosis is excellent with complete and rapid resolution of the lesion in most cases.

10.9 Primary Periodontal Lesions

Periodontium is the essential and main cause of the process. These lesions are primarily related to the accumulation of plaque and calculus. Pockets may be deep and wide [10]. In this process, chronic periodontitis progresses apically along the root surface. In most cases, pulpal tests indicate a clinically normal pulpal reaction. The prognosis depends on the efficacy of periodontal treatment [10].

10.9.1 Combined Lesions

10.9.1.1 Primary Endodontic Lesions with Secondary Periodontal Involvement

Untreated endodontic lesion results in destruction of periapical alveolar bone and in multirooted teeth bone in the interradicular area. Later drainage into gingival sulcus, plaque and calculus follow path of tract leading to periodontal involvement.

10.9.1.2 Periodontal Lesions with Secondary Endodontic İnvolvement

The apical progression of a periodontal pocket continues till the apical tissues are involved. The pulp may become necrotic as a result of infection entering via lateral canals or the apical foramen. Prognosis is better in molar teeth than in single-rooted teeth [30]. Although the pulp is exposed to bacteria via patent dentinal tubules, it is quite capable of repair and healing. Production of reparative dentin and reduced canal diameter may result, but pulp tissue remains relatively unaffected. Unless periodontal disease has progressed to involve the tooth apex, the effect of periodontal disease on the pulp is negligible.

As mentioned earlier, the treatment of periodontal disease can also lead to secondary endodontic involvement. It is possible for a blood vessel within a lateral canal to be severed by a curette and for the microorganisms to be pushed into the area during treatment, resulting in pulp inflammation and necrosis [10].

10.9.1.3 True Combined Lesions

True combined endodontic periodontal disease occurs less frequently than other endodontic-periodontal problems. It is formed when an endodontic lesion progressing coronally joins an infected periodontal pocket progressing apically [29]. These lesions occur independently of each other and are indistinguishable. The two lesions can either merge or exist separately. Merged lesions form by ongoing marginal attachment loss or by exacerbations of apical periodontitis.

The degree of attachment loss in this type of lesion is invariably large, and the prognosis is questionable. This is particularly true in single-rooted teeth. In molar teeth, root resection can be an alternative treatment. The radiographic appearance of combined endodontic periodontal disease may be similar to that of a vertically fractured tooth.

Clinically, necrotic pulp or failing endodontic treatment with presence of local factors (plaque and calculus), deep pockets, and periodontitis are present in varying degrees [31, 32]. Immediate sealing of root perforations, root canal therapy, advanced endodontic surgery, periodontal therapy with procedures such as hemisection, root resection may be required treatment options [6]. In most cases, periapical healing may be anticipated following successful endodontic treatment. The periodontal tissues, however, may not respond well to treatment and will depend on the severity of the combined disease. Prognosis depends on the amount of destruction caused by periodontal disease [31, 33] (Table 10.1).

Table 10.1 Features of endo-perio lesions

Lesion	Pain	Periodontal pocketing	Pulp vitality	Radiographic features
Primary endodontic	Moderate to severe pain	None unless sinus tract is present	Non-vital	Possible periapical radiolucency
Primary periodontic	None to moderate pain	Moderate	Vital	Decreased crestal bone height
Primary endodontic with secondary periodontal involvement	Moderate to severe pain	Evident/possibility of a sinus	Non-vital	Radiolucency extends from the apex to the sulcus with decreased crestal bone height
Primary periodontic with secondary endodontic involvement	None unless acute endo	Severe	Vital	Bone loss approaching the apex
Combined lesions	Moderate to severe	Severe connecting with the periapex	Non-vital	Bone loss extending till the apex

10.9.2 Concomitant Pulpal and Periodontal Lesions

This additional group of lesions was proposed by Belk and Gutmann [34]. In this scenario, both diseases coexist (endodontic and periodontal) with different etiologies. Thus the lesions will consist of an endodontic lesion and a noncommunicating periodontal lesion. Both the diseases should be treated individually in such a case.

10.9.3 Iatrogenic Lesion

A new endodontic-periodontal interrelationship classification, based on the primary disease with its secondary effect, suggests iatrogenic lesions as another group. This group consists mainly of endodontic lesions which caused by following various treatment procedures (as discussed earlier) [35].

10.10 Diagnosis

Diagnosis of primary endodontic disease and primary periodontal disease usually present no clinical difficulty. In primary periodontal disease, the pulp is vital and responsive to testing. In primary endodontic disease, the pulp is infected and non-vital. However, primary endodontic disease with secondary periodontal involvement, primary periodontal disease with secondary endodontic involvement, or true combined diseases are clinically and radiographically very similar. Accurate diagnosis can be achieved by careful history taking, examination, and objective and subjective findings [2, 10, 11, 13, 36–50] (Table 10.2).

Table 10.2 Features to differentiate between lesions of endodontic and periodontic origin

If of endodontic origin	If of periodontic origin
Non-vital pulp	Vital pulp (except in advanced lesions)
Sharp throbbing pain	Dull, chronic pain
Swelling	Swelling confined to the attached mucosa
Tracing the sinus tract points to apical area or in the region of a lateral canal	Sinus tract tracing leads to mid root
Mobility in acute stages only	Generalized mobility
Sinus tract is narrow and maybe tortuous	Sinus tract is wide in the cervical area and can be easily probed. This is due to the extensive loss of periodontal structures
Bone loss (crestal and furcal)	Generalized crestal bone loss (either horizontal or vertical)

The following steps in diagnosis, aids in deciding an appropriate treatment plan [10]:

10.10.1 Visual Examination

Examination of soft tissues, alveolar mucosa, and attached gingiva is carried out to check for any signs of inflammation, ulcerations, or sinus tracts. Frequently, the presence of a sinus tract is associated with a necrotic pulp. The teeth are examined for any caries, defective restorations, erosions, abrasions, cracks, fractures, and discolorations like "pink spot" which is indicative of internal resorption.

10.10.2 Radiographs

Radiographic examination helps in detection of carious lesions, defective restorations, root fractures, periradicular radiolucency, thickened periodontal ligament, and alveolar bone loss. Correct interpretation of apical and periodontal lesions is important in diagnosing the etiology of the lesion. Radiographic changes can be detected only after inflammation or bacterial by-products originating from the dental pulp cause sufficient enough demineralization of the cortical bone. It is difficult to identify bone loss caused due to endodontic disease in the initial stages as periradicular bone resorption from endodontic origin is confined to only cancellous bone. However, periodontal disease causing alveolar bone loss and the presence of calculus can be effectively detected by radiographs.

10.10.3 Palpation and Percussion

Palpation may be performed by applying firm digital pressure to the mucosa covering the roots and apices. With the index finger, the mucosa is pressed against the underlying cortical bone. This will detect the presence of periradicular abnormalities or "hot" zones that produce painful response to digital pressure [51].

Percussion indicates the presence of a periradicular inflammation. An abnormal positive response indicates inflammation of the periodontal ligament that may be either from pulpal or periodontal origin. This test should be performed gently, especially in highly sensitive teeth.

10.10.4 Mobility

The integrity and consistency of the attachment apparatus, level of inflammation in periodontal ligament, degree of mobility, pocket depth, amount of gingival bleeding, and amount of bone loss give an idea about the periodontal status.

Tooth mobility is directly proportional to the extent of inflammation in the periodontal ligament [10]. Hypermobility is quite common in cases of primary endodontic involvement and should not be confused with true mobility caused by periodontal destruction. In cases of primary endodontic pathology, the mobility resolves within a week of initiating endodontic therapy.

10.10.5 Pulp Testing

Teeth with vital pulps will react to cold test with sharp brief pain response that usually does not last more than few seconds. An intense and prolonged pain response often indicates irreversible pulpitis and lack of response may indicate pulp necrosis.

10.10.6 Periodontal Pocket Probing

The presence of a deep solitary pocket in the absence of periodontal disease may indicate the presence of a lesion of endodontic origin or a vertical root fracture. Periodontal probing is important for diagnosis and helps in differentiating between endodontic and periodontal disease.

In periodontal disease, bone loss always begins at the crestal bone level and progresses apically. The typical lesion is conical in contour. The probing may start from a sulcus depth within normal limits, then gradually step down a slope to the apical extent of the lesion, and then step up again on the other side to a sulcus depth within normal limits. Such a conical-shaped probing indicates periodontal pathosis.

Endodontic or periodontal disease may sometimes develop a fistulous sinus track (Fig. 10.9). These may open anywhere on the oral mucosa or facial skin. Intraorally, the opening is usually visible on the attached buccal gingiva or in the vestibule. Sinus tracking is done by inserting a semirigid radiopaque material into the sinus track until resistance is met. A radiograph is then taken, which reveals the path and the origin of the inflammatory process [10].

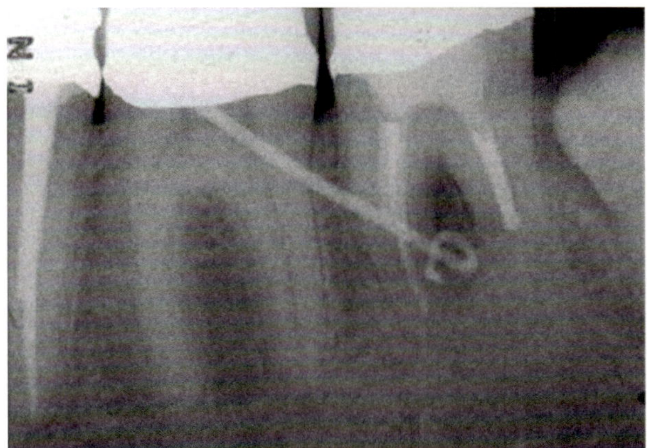

Fig. 10.9 A size 30 gutta-percha has been inserted from the orifice of the sinus tract and reaches the furca area between mesial and distal roots of tooth number 37. In the clinic this technique is very useful to understand the real source of the infection and which tooth is the cause of the problem. (From the archive of Prof Mehmet Omer Gorduysus, author of the chapter)

10.10.7 Acute or "Blowout" Lesions

When a patient presents with a localized swelling involving the gingival sulcus, it may be difficult to determine whether the swelling is due to a periodontal involvement or of endodontic origin [30, 52]. There is usually normal sulcus depth all the way around the tooth until the area of the swelling is probed. At the edge of the swelling, the probe drops significantly to a level near the apex of the tooth, and the probing depth remains the full width of the swelling. At the opposite edge of the swelling, probing is once again within normal limits. The width of the detached gingiva can be as broad as the entire buccal or lingual surface of the tooth. This swelling can be characterized as having "blown out" [9] the entire attachment on that side. In such a case, only endodontic treatment will suffice and complete periodontal reattachment occurs within 1 week in most cases.

10.11 Treatment Protocol

From the diagnostic point of view, it is important to realize that as long as the pulp remains vital, although inflamed or scarred, it is unlikely to produce irritants that are sufficient to cause pronounced marginal breakdown of the periodontium.

The prognosis of the tooth should always be considered carefully before the commencement of any treatment procedure. If the prognosis is weak and/or hopeless, the clinical application is very challenging especially from the endodontic aspect, restorability of the tooth is questionable, and if the patient is not suitable for a lengthy, costly, and invasive treatment, extraction is an alternative at the beginning. This should be analyzed carefully and in detail. If extraction is not an alternative, treatment plan should be considered for endo and perio separately or together depending on the classification of the case.

10.11.1 Clinical Considerations

A periodontal defect should always be suspected to harbor bacteria and should therefore be treated endodontically. If the remaining dentition is periodontally healthy and a vertical root fracture has been ruled out, healing of the attachment apparatus can be expected after endodontic treatment without any periodontal treatment. In general, when primary disease of one tissue, i.e., pulp or periodontium, is present and secondary disease is just starting, always treat the primary disease first [10, 30, 53, 54].

But in cases, when the secondary disease is also established and chronic, both primary and secondary diseases must be treated. By and large, endodontic therapy precedes periodontal therapy. Periodontal therapy may or may not be required, depending on disease status. The complete healing of destroyed periodontal support usually occurs following endodontic treatment. On the other hand, the complete resolution of extensive destruction following the treatment of chronic periodontitis is less predictable. It is important to realize that it is clinically not possible to determine the extent to which one or the other of the two disorders (endodontic or periodontal) has affected the supporting tissues.

Therefore, the treatment should first focus on the pulpal infection. The second phase includes a period of observation, whereby the extent of periodontal healing resulting from the endodontic treatment is evaluated. Reduced probing depth can usually be expected within a couple of weeks while bone regeneration may require several months before it can be radiographically detected. Thus, periodontal therapy, including deep scaling with and without periodontal surgery, should be postponed until the result of the endodontic treatment can be properly evaluated.

In a *primary endodontic lesion*, when the pulp is non-vital and infected, conventional endodontic therapy alone will resolve the lesion. Surgical endodontic therapy is not necessary, even in the presence of large periradicular radiolucencies and periodontal abscesses. If primary endodontic lesions persist, despite extensive endodontic treatment, the lesion may have secondary periodontal involvement, or it may be a true combined lesion.

In case of *secondary periodontal involvement*, the tooth now requires both endodontic and periodontal treatments. If the endodontic treatment is adequate, the prognosis depends on the severity of the plaque-induced periodontitis and the efficacy of periodontal treatment. With endodontic treatment alone, only part of the lesion will heal. If tooth has vertical crack, the prognosis will not be bright. If the tooth is multirooted and if the problem is only related to one of the roots (but not the palatal root), the root amputation or hemisection can be taken into consideration. First initiate root canal treatment, and canals may be filled with calcium hydroxide paste, which has bactericidal, anti- inflammatory, and proteolytic property, inhibiting resorption and favoring repair. Treatment results should be evaluated after 2–3 months, and only then should periodontal treatment be considered. This allows sufficient time for initial tissue healing and better assessment of the periodontal condition. Prognosis of primary endodontic disease with secondary periodontal involvement depends on periodontal treatment and patient response [24].

Primary endodontic lesions with secondary periodontal involvement may also occur as a result of root perforation during root canal treatment, or where pins or posts have been misplaced during coronal restoration. In such a situation, this perforation repair must be sealed properly, and misplaced pin or post should be removed. If the root perforation is situated close to the alveolar crest, it may be required to raise a flap and repair the defect with an appropriate filling material. MTA is one of the most recommended materials to repair the perforation.

Frequently an accumulation of plaque and calculus is observed clinically, and the pockets are wider. Plaque and calculus should be eliminated periodontally. Prognosis depends on the stage of the periodontal disease the periodontal treatment. Periodontal site can be painful because of the accumulation of plaque and tartars in the periodontal pocket, and as a result of them related the loss of the attachment, a mobility can be observed. If the treatment is in the early stages of the disease, prognosis is good. Sometimes extra-grafting techniques are necessary to be able to solve the problem if there is a large amount of recession around the root surface due to deep periodontal pocket for covering the root surface.

Primary periodontal lesions should be treated first by proper hygiene phase therapy. An advanced periodontal lesion can be detected clinically. Chronic periodontitis progresses apically along the root surface. Poor restorations which may make oral hygiene maintenance problematic for the patient should be removed. Periodontal surgery is performed only after the completion of hygiene phase therapy, if required. Frequently an accumulation of plaque and calculus can be observed clinically, and the pockets are wider. Plaque and calculus should be eliminated periodontally. Prognosis depends on the stage of the periodontal disease. Mobility may be observed due to the loss of the attachment. If the disease is in the early stages, prognosis is good.

Periodontal therapy sometimes may consist of procedures (new attachment techniques, gingivectomy, apically displaced flap, hemisection, or root resection) that attempt to promote regeneration. In such cases, root canal therapy is not indicated unless pulp vitality test results show change. Reevaluation must be performed periodically after treatment to check for any change in the pulpal status. But, the prognosis is entirely dependent on the periodontal therapy, in such cases.

Periodontal lesions with secondary endodontic involvement may present as reversible pulpal hypersensitivity, which can be treated purely by periodontal therapy. Periodontal treatment removes noxious stimuli, and secondary mineralization of dentinal tubules allows the resolution of hypersensitivity. But if pulpal inflammation is irreversible, root canal treatment is carried out, followed by periodontal treatment.

Pulp is affected indirectly because of deep periodontal pocket. Physiological (natural pathways) or iatrogenic reasons may be the cause of this process. Tooth may become mobile. Root canal therapy and periodontal therapy should be applied together. Prognosis depends on the severity of the periodontal problem. Generally when this occurs, the tooth is non-vital. The prognosis of periodontal lesions is poorer than endodontic lesions and is dependent on the apical extensions of the lesion. As the lesion advances, the prognosis approaches that of a true combined lesion [55].

True combined lesions are treated initially as for primary endodontic lesions with secondary periodontal involvement. Generally the true combined lesions are the most difficult endo-perio problems to be treated, and the treatment is challenging. Periodontal pockets are very deep, and in some cases, the probe can even reach to the apex or to the apical third of the root. The first question to ask yourself should be "can this periodontal problem be treated and how would be the prognosis." Both periodontal and endodontic therapy should be performed, but prognosis generally depends on the severity and extent of the periodontal disease and the efficacy of the periodontal therapy.

It is essential to understand that in endo-perio lesions, the endodontic treatment is the more predictable of the two. However the success of endodontic therapy is dependent on the completion of periodontal therapy. The complete treatment of both aspects of endo-perio lesions is essential for successful long-term results.

In molar teeth, root resection can be considered as a treatment alternative if not all roots are severely involved. Prior to surgery, palliative periodontal therapy should be completed and root canal treatment carried out on the roots to be saved. The prognosis of an affected tooth can be improved by increasing bony support, which can be achieved by bone grafting and guided tissue regeneration. These advanced treatment options are based on responses to conventional periodontal and endodontic treatment over an extended time period. Generally the true combined lesions are the most difficult endo-perio problems for to be treated. Figures 10.10, 10.11, 10.12, and 10.13 show some clinical example of true combined lesion.

Concomitant pulpal and periodontal lesions can cause true combined lesions at the end. Again, it is not easy to differentiate between the causative factors. Reasons can be either periodontal or endodontic. Treatment approach should be considered

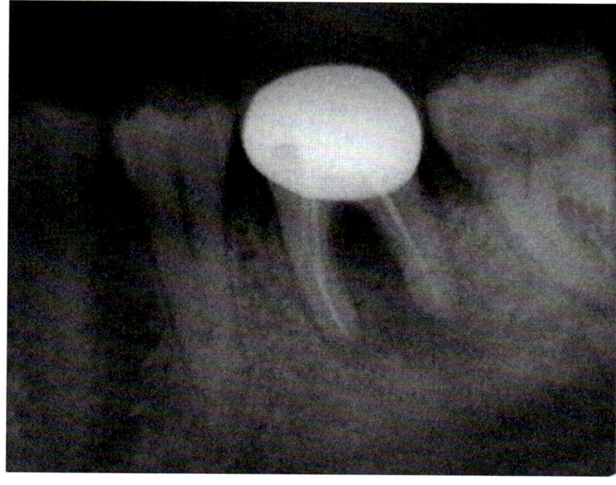

Fig. 10.10 Preoperative radiograph in a *left* mandibular first molar, an old crown which the marginal adaptation was lost, a substandard, weak, and unsuccessful (failured) endodontic root canal obturation, periapical involvement, and a big furcal lesion were observed. Examinations revealed and was decided as a true combined lesion. Crown was removed, endodontic retreatment and periodontal curettage at the furcal site were applied

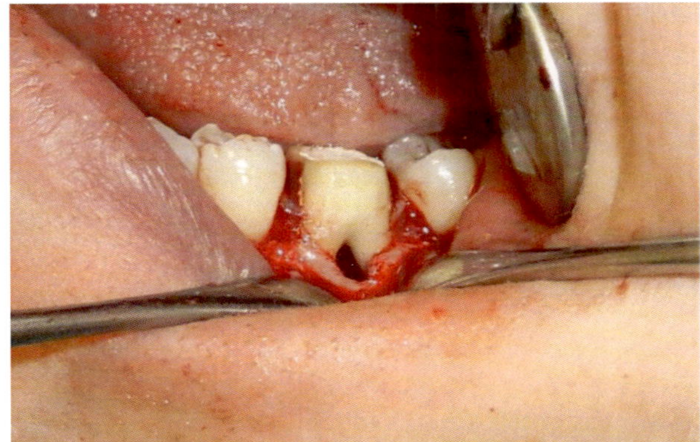

Fig. 10.11 During the periodontal curettage to the furca, granulation and inflammatory tissues were eliminated

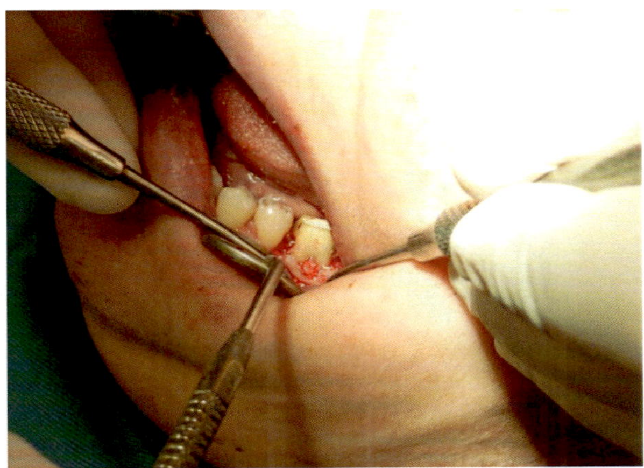

Fig. 10.12 Graft material application to the surgical site to regenerate the tissues

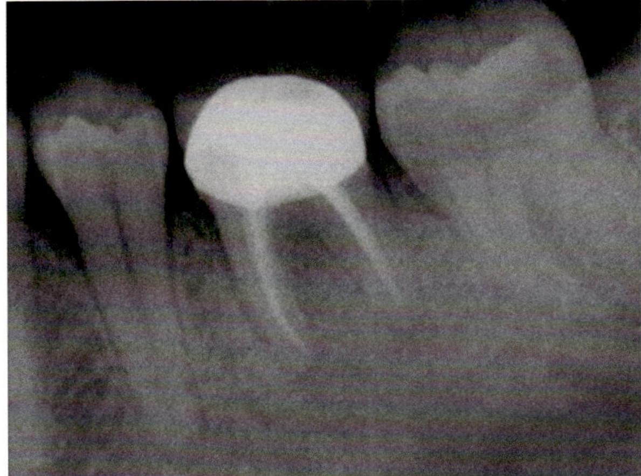

Fig. 10.13 Postoperative radiograph of the case (1 year). Endodontic retreatment was completed, and periodontal surgery was successful. In the bifurcation of the tooth, healing was seen radiographically and clinically. This true combined lesion case was healed successfully. (From the archive of Prof Mehmet Omer Gorduysus, author of the chapter)

Table 10.3 A comparative chart for the prognosis and severity of the endo-perio cases

Primary endodontic lesion	++++
Primary periodontal lesions	+++
Primary endodontic lesions with secondary periodontal involvement	+++
Periodontal lesions with secondary endodontic involvement	++
True combined lesions	+
Concomitant pulpal and periodontal lesions	+
Iatrogenic lesions	++

as combined lesions, and the etiological factors must be eliminated. In *iatrogenic lesions*, the etiology should be eliminated.

As it can be seen from Gorduysus' "endo-perio problems prognosis chart" (Table 10.3), showing a scoring index for the prognosis, the most successful prognosis comes with the primary endodontic lesions. Most risky or guarded prognosis is true combined lesions and concomitant pulpal and periodontal lesions. For a better success beyond this chart, the skills and ability of the operator and patient immunity and defense factors, along with many local and general factors may also affect the success of the cases.

10.11.2 Sequencing Treatment for Endo-Perio Lesions

Research and literature indicate that combined periodontal and endodontic therapy is essential for the successful healing of a periodontal-endodontic lesion. Either endodontic or periodontic treatment alone would not lead to a satisfactory prognosis, if both disease entities are present and that both must be considered together [56, 57]. Treatment protocol recommendations are shown in Appendix 10.1.

However, the problem arises over which lesion came first and which caused the clinical problem. It is generally agreed that pulpal disease can/may initiate a periodontal disease, but the opposite theory is controversial. Simring and Goldberg [1] postulated that endodontic therapy is indicated in the treatment of periodontal disease that does not respond to periodontal therapy.

It has been suggested that periodontal disease has no effect on the pulp, at least until it involves the apex [3]. On the other hand, several studies suggested that the effect of periodontal disease on the pulp is degenerative in nature and has a direct inflammatory effect [23, 58]. Therefore, treatment of combined lesions should aim at eliminating both the problems. In acute cases, it is of paramount importance to diagnose the source of the pain and/or swelling and delineate it to be endodontic or periodontal. This problem should be treated first as a priority.

Conclusion

Endo-perio cases always must be considered from both sides as two different entities. Generally in endo-perio lesions, the endodontic treatment is the more predictable of the two. However the success of endodontic therapy is dependent on the completion of periodontal therapy. The complete treatment of both aspects of endo-perio lesions is essential for successful long-term results. The limitations of the prognosis always should be explained clearly to the patients.

Appendix 10.1: Treatment Protocol Recommendations

Endo perio lesions
Primary endo
Primary perio
Combined lesion
Endodontic therapy
Periodontal therapy
Primary endo and secondary perio
Primary perio and secondary endo
First do endo therapy followed by simple hygienetherapy
Iatrogenic causes
Palliativeperio therapy and endo treatment
Evaluate after 3 months
PA resolution
PA lesion persists
Mobility
No Mobility
Splinting
Surgical/Non Surgical/regenrative procedure depending on the depth of the pocket
If hopeless prognosis-extract
Root resection, hemisection, bicuspidization, or any other surgical procedure

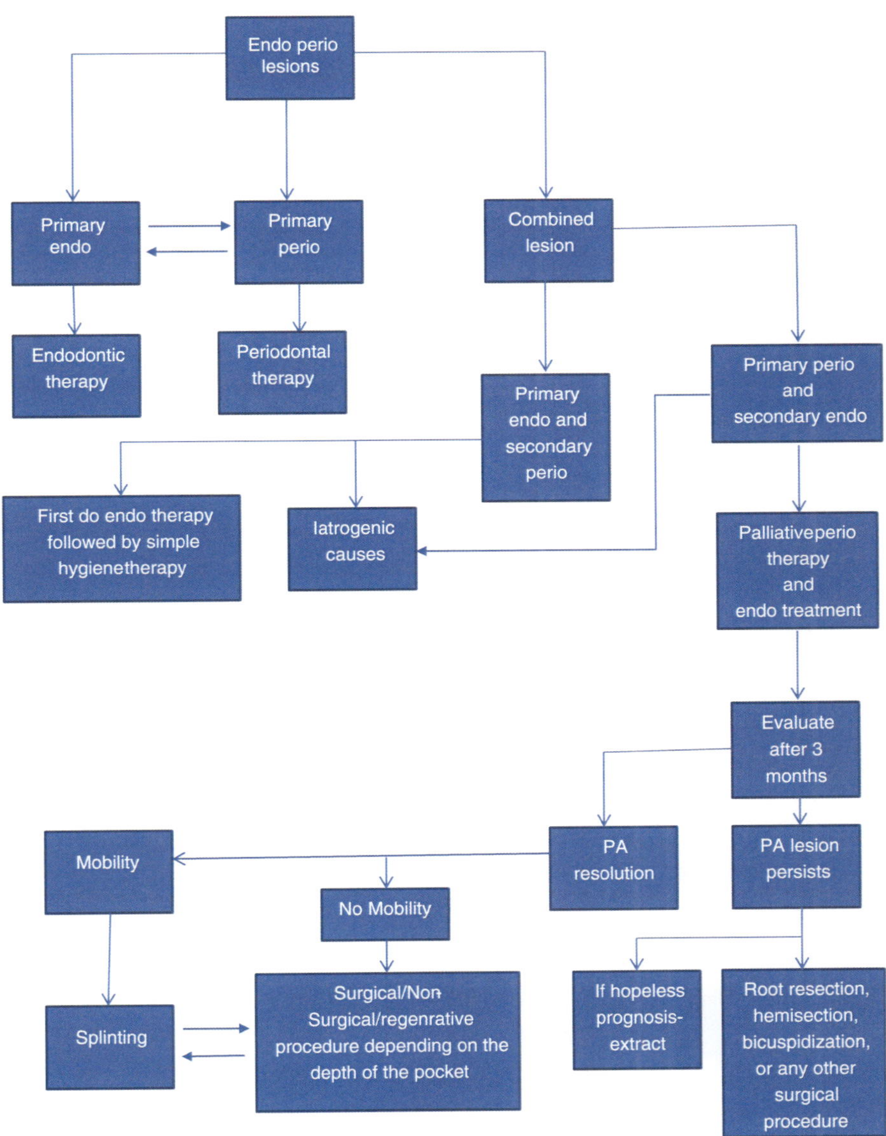

References

1. Simring M, Goldberg M. The pulpal pocket approach: retrograde periodontitis. J Periodontol. 1964;35:22–48.
2. Mandel E, Machton P, Torabinejad M. Clinical diagnosis and treatment of endodontic and periodontal lesions. Quintessence Int. 1993;24:135–9.
3. Czarnecki RT, Schilder H. A histological evaluation of the human pulp in teeth with varying degrees of periodontal disease. J Endod. 1979;5(8):242–53.
4. Adriaens PA, de Boever JA, Loesche WJ. Bacterial invasion in root cementum and radicular dentin of periodontally diseased teeth in humans: a reservoir of periodontopathic bacteria. J Periodontol. 1988;59(4):222–30.
5. Adriaens PA, Edwards CA, de Boever JA, Loesche WJ. Ultrastructural observations on bacterial invasion in cementum and radicular dentin of periodontally diseased human teeth. J Periodontol. 1988;59(8):493–503.
6. Haapasalo M, Ranta H, Ranta K, Shah H. Blackpigmented Bacteroides spp. in human apical periodontitis. Infect Immun. 1986;53(1):149–53.
7. Trope M, Tronstad L, Rosenberg ES, Listgarten M. Darkfield microscopy as a diagnostic aid in differentiating exudates from endodontic and periodontal abscesses. J Endod. 1988;14(1):35–8.
8. Jansson L, Ehnevid H, Blomlöf L, Weintraub A, Lindskog S. Endodontic pathogens in periodontal disease augmentation. J Clin Periodontol. 1995;22(8):598–602.
9. Bender IB. Factors influencing radiographic appearance of bony lesions. J Endod. 1982;8:161–70.
10. Rotstein I, Simon JH. Diagnosis, prognosis and decision making in the treatment of combined periodontal-endodontic lesions. Periodontol 2000. 2004;34:265–303.
11. Zehnder M, Gold SI, Hasselgren G. Pathologic interaction in pulpal and periodontal tissues. J Clin Periodontol. 2002;29:663–71.
12. Madison S, Wilcox LR. An evaluation of coronal microleakage in endodontically treated teeth. Part III: in vivo study. J Endod. 1988;14(9):455–8.
13. Ray HA, Trope M. Periapical status of endodontically treated teeth in relation to the technical quality of the root filling and the coronal restoration. Int Endod J. 1995;28(1):12–8.
14. Saunders WP, Saunders EM. Assessment of leakage in the restored pulp chamber of endodontically treated multirooted teeth. Int Endod J. 1990;23(1):28–33.
15. Solomon C, Chalafin H, Kellert M. The endodontic periodontal lesion, a rational approach to treatment. J Am Dent Assoc. 1995;126:473–9.
16. DeDeus QD. Frequency location and direction of the lateral, secondary and accessory canals. J Endod. 1975;1:361–6.
17. Simon JHS, Dorgan H, Ceresa LM, Silver GK. The radicular groove: its potential clinical significance. J Endod. 2000;26:295–8.
18. Seltzer S, Bender IB, Nazimov H, Sinai I. Pulpitis induced interradicular periodontal changes in experimental animals. J Periodontol. 1967;38:124–9.
19. Seltzer S, Bender IB, Ziontz M. The interrelationship of pulp and periodontal disease. Oral Surg Med Oral Pathol. 1963;16(12):1474–90.
20. Jew RCK, Weine FS, Keene JJ Jr, Smulson MH. A histologic evaluation of periodontal tissues adjacent to root perforations filled with Cavit. Oral Surg Oral Med Oral Pathol. 1982;54(1):124–35.
21. Andreasen JO, Andreasen FM, Skeie A, Hjørting-Hansen E, Schwartz O. Effect of treatment delay upon pulp and periodontal healing of traumatic dental injuries: a review article. Dent Traumatol. 2002;18(3):116–28.
22. Bender IB, Seltzer S. The effect of periodontal disease on the dental pulp. Oral Surg Oral Med Oral Pathol. 1972;33:458–74.
23. Langeland K, et al. Periodontal disease, bacteria, and pulpal histopathology. Oral Surg Oral Med Oral Pathol. 1974;37:257–70.
24. Mhairi RW. The pathogenesis and treatment of endo-perio lesions. CPD Dent. 2001;2:9–95.

25. Lindhe J. Clinical periodontology and implant dentistry. 4th ed. Oxford: Blackwell Munksgaard; 2003. p. 339–45.
26. Cotton WR, Siegel RL. Human pulpal response to citric acid cavity cleanser. J Am Dent Assoc. 1978;96:639–44.
27. Yeung S, Clarke N. Pulpal effect of citric acid applied topically to root surfaces. Oral Surg Oral Med Oral Pathol. 1983;56:317–20.
28. Kitchings SK, del Rio CE, Aufdemorte DE, Meffert RM, Lane JJ. The pulpal response to topically applied citric acid. Oral Surg Oral Med Oral Pathol. 1984;58:199–206.
29. Simon JH, Glick DH, Frank AL. The relationship of endodontic-periodontic lesions. J Clin Periodontol. 1972;43:202.
30. Walton RE, Torabinejad M. Principles and practice of endodontics. 3rd ed. Philadelphia: W B Saunders Company; 2002. p. 467–84.
31. Kerns DG, Glickman GN. Endodontic and periodontal interrelationships. In: Cohen S, Hargreaves KM, editors. Pathways of the pulp. 9th ed. St.Louis: Mosby Inc.; 2006. p. 650–67.
32. Didilescu A, et al. Current concepts on the relationship between Pulpal and Periodontal diseases. TMJ. 2008;58:1–2.
33. Rotstein I, Simon JHS. Diagnosis, Prognosis and decision-making in the treatment of combined Periodontal-endodontic lesions. Periodontology 2000. 2004;34:165–203.
34. Belk CE, Gutmann JL. Perspectives, controversies, and directives on pulpal-periodontal relationship. J Can Dent Assoc. 1990;56:1013–7.
35. Pretinder S. Endo-Perio Dilemma: a brief review. Dent Res J. 2011;8(1):39–47.
36. Bhaskar SN. Periapical lesion types, incidence and clinical features. Oral Surg Oral Med Oral Pathol. 1996;21:657–71.
37. Orstavik D, Pit Ford TR. Essential endodontology prevention and treatment of apical periodontitis. Malden, MA: Blackwell Science; 1998. p. 45–6.
38. Görduysus O. Pulpa-Periodonsiyum Etkileşimleri, Endodontik-Periodontik İlişkiler, Klinik Düşünceler ve Tedavi Yaklaşımları (Book chapter in Turkish). Book Chapter: Pulpal-periodontal interactions, clinical considerations and treatment approaches. In: Çağlayan G, editor. Periodontoloji. 1st ed. Ankara-Turkey: Hacettepe Yayınları, , Hacettepe Publications; 2010. p. 401–21.
39. Jenkins WM, Allan CJ. Guide to. periodontics. 3rd ed. California: Wright Publishing Company; 1994. p. 146–52.
40. Harrington GW, Natkin E. External resorption associated with bleaching of pulpless teeth. J Endod. 1979;5(11):344–8.
41. Cvek M, Lindvall AM. External root resorption following bleaching of pulpless teeth with oxygen peroxide. Endod Dent Traumatol. 1985;1(2):56–60.
42. Dahlen G. Microbiology and treatment of dental abscesses and periodontal-endodontic lesions. Periodontology 2000. 2002;28:206–33.
43. Paul BF, Hutter JW. The Enodontic-periodontal continuum revisited: new insights into etiology, diagnosis and treatment. J Am Dent Assoc. 1997;128:1541–8.
44. Bergenholtz G, Lindhe J. Effect of experimentally induced marginal periodontitis and periodontal scaling on the dental pulp. J Clin Periodontol. 1978;5:59–73.
45. Jansson L, Ehnevid H, Lindskog S, Blomlöf L. The influence of endodontic infection on progression of marginal bone loss in periodontitis. J Clin Periodontol. 1995;22:729–34.
46. Miyashita H, Bergenholtz G, Gröndahl K. Impact of endodontic conditions on marginal bone loss. J Periodontol. 1998;69:158–64.
47. Wilcox LR, Diaz-Arnold A. Coronal leakage of permanent lingual access restorations in endodontically treated anterior teeth. J Endod. 1989;12:584–7.
48. Heling I, Gorfil C, Slutzky H, Kopolovich K, Zalkind M, Slutzky-Goldberg I. Endodontic failure caused by inadequate restorative procedure: review and treatment recommendations. J Prosthet Dent. 2002;87:674–8.
49. Torabinejad M, Lemon RL. Procedural accidents. In: Walton RE, Torabinejad M, editors. Principles and practice of endodontics. 2nd ed. Philadelphia: W.B. Saunders; 1996. p. 306–23.
50. Mathews DC, Tabash M. Detection of localized tooth-related factors that predispose to periodontal infections. Periodontology 2000. 2004;34:136–50.

51. Sigurdsson A. Pulpal diagnosis. Endod Top. 2003;5:12–25.
52. Harrington GW. The perio-endo question: differential diagnosis. Dent Clin N Am. 1979;23:673–90.
53. Harrington GW, Steiner DR, Ammons WF. The periodontal-endodontic controversy. Periodontol 2000. 2000;30:123–30.
54. Meng HX. Periodontic-endodontic lesions. Ann Periodontal. 1999;4:84–9.
55. Newman M, Takei H, Klokkevold P, Carranza F. Clinical periodontology. 10th ed. St. Louis: Saunders; 2006. p. 88–90.
56. Schilder H. Endodontic-periodontal therapy. In: Grossman L, editor. Endodontic practice. 6th ed. Philadelphia: Lea and Febiger; 1965.
57. Simon P, Jacobs D. The so-called combined periodontal-pulpal problem. Dent Clin N Am. 1969;13:45–52.
58. Mandi FA. Histological study of the pulp changes caused by periodontal disease. J Br Endod Soc. 1972;6:80–2.

Endodontics in Geriatric Patient

11

Mehmet Omer Gorduysus

11.1 Introduction

Tooth retention has increased significantly in the older adults, and dentists are now challenged by the need to preserve their teeth. Endodontic procedures in the elderly have been considered challenging from a technical perspective in view of the likelihood of the root canal system being "sclerosed."

Geriatrics is the branch of science that focuses on health promotion, prevention, and treatment of disease and disability in later life. The term geriatrics comes from a Greek word *geron* which means old man and *iatros* meaning healer. It is different from gerontology, which is the study of the aging process itself. Geriatric dentistry (*gerodontology*) is the delivery of dental care to older adults involving diagnosis, prevention, and treatment of problems associated with normal aging and age-related diseases as part of an interdisciplinary team with other health professionals [1, 2]. It focuses upon patients with chronic physiological, physical, and/or psychological changes or morbid conditions/diseases.

Geriatric endodontics (*geroendodontics*) is a branch of endodontics and gerodontology to provide elder people good-quality endodontic therapy to ensure them a better quality of oral health and overall to improve their life quality by saving teeth through endodontic treatment. It is mainly about the effect of aging on diagnosis of pulpal and periapical disease and successful root canal therapy.

The dental management of the elderly population is different from that of the rest of the population as special considerations for age-related concerns are required. Therefore, a multidisciplinary approach/team with special knowledge and skills is required to provide oral health care to the elderly. Endodontic considerations in the

M.O. Gorduysus, D.D.S., Ph.D.
Professor, Department of Preventive and Restorative Dentistry, College of Dental Medicine, University of Sharjah, Sharjah, UAE
e-mail: ogorduysus@yahoo.com, mgorduysus@sharjah.ac.ae

P. Jain (ed.), *Common Complications in Endodontics*,
https://doi.org/10.1007/978-3-319-60997-3_11

elderly patients are quite similar to those in the younger patients. At the same time, it can be quite challenging from a technical perspective due to the modifications in the teeth morphology, namely, the pulp space system being obliterated. The combination of an increase in pathosis and dental needs coupled with greater expectations has resulted in more endodontic procedures for older adults.

The purpose of this chapter is to outline the role of endodontics in helping older adults achieve the goal of retaining healthy teeth and satisfactory oral function into old age.

Geriatric endodontics is gaining a more significant role as can be seen from the demographic data on aging population of the world (source: UN):

- 1900—10–17 million people over 65 years (less than 1% of the world population of that time).
- 1992—362 million over 65 years (6.2% of the world population).
- 2030—(estimated) 2–2.5 billion people over 65 years (20% of the world population).
- 2035—26% of the world population will be over 65 years old.

An endodontist working with geriatric patients must be able to:

1. Identify the oral conditions common to older individuals, particularly which goes with pathology which increases in frequency with age.
2. Obtain a through medical and medication history from aged patients.
3. Obtain a psychosocial history which describes factors influencing the older patients' dental needs and ability to obtain care.
4. Coordinate dental care with other health-care disciplines, i.e., medicine, pharmacy, social work, nursing, etc.
5. Understand and be able to perform clinical procedures with geriatric patients that consider their special needs with good clinical skills and competency.

Preserving the continuum of dental arch and protecting the integrity of gnatostomotogic system, enhancing the retention of a removable prosthesis especially when loss of the tooth will result in a free-end saddle, keeping strong retainers for the fixed prosthesis, maintaining occlusal contact in a reduced dentition, keeping last standing molars to help preserve the vertical dimension and bone, maintaining periodontal health, and helping them lead a pain-free life are very crucial for teeth and gnatostomatic system-related points in old.

11.2 Categorizing

Categorizing the geriatric patients as groups from the easiest to most complex will be helpful to our clinical strategies [1]. Chronological age refers to age as measured by calendar time since birth, while functional age or physiological age is based on performance capacities. Scientists have divided the study of the older population into several categories based on chronological age:

- New-old (55–64 years)
- Young-old (65–74 years) [3]
- Middle-old/older old (75–84 years) [4]
- Old-old/oldest old (85-plus years) [5]

Ettinger and Beck [6] developed a functional definition of the elderly based upon an older person's physical ability to seek dental services. Functional ability is the standard that differentiates an individual's capability to maintain activity.

- The functionally independent older adult (70%).
- The frail older adult (14%)—these are persons with chronic conditions that create major limitations in mobility. Another way to classify the frail elderly is to count the seniors who have one or more physical or mental disabilities. This includes the medically compromised and homebound living in the community, as well as those institutionalized in nursing homes.
- The functionally dependent older adult (5%).

11.3 The Challenge

Teeth are subjected to various physiological wear and tear, as well as pathological disease conditions in one's lifetime. Old age is associated with several risk factors, specific to the oral cavity as well. Managing this compromised dentition with a multitude of risk factors is indeed a multifaceted challenge.

The general risk factors include various medical problems, medication-induced side effects, and psychological problems. The risk factors related specifically to oral cavity are gingival recession, presence of restorations, removable partial dentures, and age-related odontometric changes.

11.4 Medical Problems and Considerations for Geriatric Patients

At the outset, old age must not be confused with ill health. In older adults, as with younger adults, successful outcome of endodontic procedures depends on elimination of pathogenic bacteria from the pulp space and prevention of reinfection. But, nonetheless, some general considerations should be kept in mind which are pertinent to the elderly. The patient should be able to sit comfortably in the dental chair and tolerate a lengthy course of treatment. This may not be possible in patients with, for example, chronic back conditions or transient cerebral ischemia.

There are few medical contraindications to root canal treatment. Situations, which may contraindicate endodontic intervention, include patients requiring radiotherapy to the head and neck region and patients with poor compliance, for example, patients with Parkinson's disease, tremors, or dementia.

Most of the patients over 60 years of age are medically compromised and are on medication. Most commonly seen medical conditions are hypertension, chronic respiratory diseases, cardiovascular diseases, diabetes, osteoporosis, joint and rheumatoid problems, Parkinson's disease, and Alzheimer's. All dental practitioners should be familiar with the course and the complications associated with these disease conditions and the prophylactic guidelines provided for various medical conditions [7]. Patients with cardiovascular diseases are more susceptible to physical or emotional stress during dental treatment. Therefore, treatment plan should include low-stress protocols and shorter appointments. Local anesthesia with vasoconstrictors should not be administered to patients with unstable angina and uncontrolled hypertension or people with recent myocardial infarction and coronary bypass graft. Prophylactic antibiotic may be necessary for patients with history of high-risk cardiac conditions while undertaking endodontic therapy [8]. Similarly, dental treatment appointments for diabetic patients should be scheduled with consideration given to patients' normal meal and insulin schedule. Patients with diabetes often have cardiovascular diseases and are more susceptible to infection if the disease is not properly controlled.

In the presence of acute infections, hypoglycemic control needs to be altered in consultation with a physician. Dentists also need to keep in mind various drug interactions and adverse drug reactions as many elderly patients may be undergoing multiple drug therapy. Careful evaluation of patient's medical and drug history, in consultation with the patient's physician, is essential for proper optimization of patient care [9]. Systemic conditions and their considerations during endodontic therapy are covered in detail in the next chapter.

11.5 Psychological

Many elderly patients suffer from depression due to loneliness or feeling of neglect. Senile dementia is a common phenomenon seen among the elderly that can cause memory loss, confusion, difficulty in making decisions, and comprehension and alter ability to learn new tasks associated with the treatment modality [10, 11]. Hearing and vision impairment can further worsen the situation. All these may lead to problems in cooperating during treatment. Such patients are psychologically more fragile and oversensitive. Some of them may feel tired quickly, are impatient, ask many questions, may become nervous and unstable easily, and have strong far memory but not actual memory (appointments, etc. easily can be forgotten). Psychological problems in the elderly differ in each country depending on the social infrastructure.

11.6 Age-Related Changes

Tooth tissue and supporting structures undergo a number of changes as a person ages. These maybe a result of incremental effects of wear, disease, and habits. Old pulps are frequently described as being "sclerosed" or "calcified." Pulp space diminishes throughout life by the deposition of regular secondary dentine [12]. This occurs most commonly in pulp horns and on the floor and roof of the pulp chamber in molars, which may be converted from a large rectangular cavern in the young, to a flat disc in the elderly.

Pulp space is further reduced by reactionary and reparative dentine (formerly classified together as tertiary or irritation dentine). These changes are again mostly confined to the coronal reaches of the canal system where external irritants have greatest impact. Increased pulp fibrosis may present challenges for canal negotiation, with the potential to compact fibrous pulp tissue and cause obstructions which may be as difficult to overcome as hard tissue ledge or blockage. Coronally, these are usually encountered as pulp stones.

There is considerable reduction in density of odontoblasts due to these changes. Reparative capacity of the pulp following injury (tooth preparation, micro leakage, etc.) gets reduced [12]. Compensatory changes occur as a result of aging or disease. The greater thickness of dentine and the reduced volume of pulp in the elderly may compensate to some extent for the compromised response of the pulp, thus allowing the preparation to be deeper. Attrition, a compensatory change, acts as a stabilizing factor between loss of bony support and excessive leverage from occlusal forces imposed on the teeth. In addition, a reduction in the overjet of the teeth may be seen manifesting as an edge-to-edge contact of anterior teeth due to the proximal wear of posterior teeth [12, 13].

Main differences in teeth of geriatric patients from an endodontic viewpoint are (geriatric patients vs. young age) the pulpal changes. The pulpal tissue volume is reduced leading to increased pulpal calcification and sclerosed/calcified canals, making access difficult.

Delaying reactions to pulp testings by aging and increase of complicating factors such as administering interligamentery injections (more damaging) and other injection techniques, rubber dam isolation techniques may need modifications because of badly broken-down coronal structures in old patients, and this may cause restorative problems, locating the canal orifice in calcified teeth becomes more difficult (in olders we see very often), repair of periapical tissues following endo-treatment seems late in geriatric patients, and dose of anesthetics and medicaments might need to be reduced [14–18].

Briefly reviewing the effects of aging on pulpal functions will be very useful and helpful to understand the biological basis of the pulpal treatments and clinical approaches, decisions/challenges, and management of the problems in geriatric patients [19–33]. The pulp is a dynamic connective tissue and pulp response changes with age. The reasons can be attributed and linked with two considerations (biological reasons):

1. Structural and dimensional (histologic) changes.
2. Tissue changes that occur in response to irritation from injury

11.6.1 Structural Changes

By aging (or conditions that may lead to aging of the pulp, i.e., irritations, occlusal trauma and premature contacts, caries, periodontal involvements), the volume of pulp tissue reduces. Changes in cellular, extracellular, and supportive elements of the pulp are seen, and pulpal cells decrease in number and appear less active (odontoblasts and fibroblasts). There is also a decrease in supportive elements (blood vessels, nerves) and ground substance while the thickness of collagen fibers increases. Fewer cells are available to replace injured odontoblasts, and overall ability to recover from injury becomes more limited.

While secondary dentine formation and dentine thickness increase, the volume of pulp space reduces. Pulp stones (denticles) are more common, generally in the coronal pulp, whereas diffuse (linear) calcifications are more predominant in the radicular pulp along with dystrophic calcifications, perivascular calcifications, and perineural calcifications. Peritubular and sclerotic dentine formation increases while tubule diameters become less. There is reduced dentine permeability in geriatric patients. All these changes are directly related to the change in size and shape of pulp space, thus making the clinical applications more challenging and difficult.

There are dramatic dimensional changes as well, besides the structural changes. Specifically in the molars, the pulp floor and the roof can be seen approaching each other, and the shape can/may develop into a disclike (flattened) pulp chamber. In the anteriors, occluded pulp chamber and tight canals (very recessed) are seen. The height of the pulp chamber, canal diameter and reduction in the canal curvature (due to calcifications), and the thickness of the roof of the pulp chamber roof are other considerations causing limitations during endodontic therapy in geriatric patients.

The effects of aging on the size of the apical foramen also affect the endodontic treatment in older individuals. There is an increase in the cementum deposition. The size of the apical foramen becomes smaller and may shift further from anatomic apex. The difference between anatomic and radiographic apex increases in the radiographs based on these changes, and reaching to the full working length may become very difficult. Modifications of treatment procedures may be required in geriatric group based on these biological realities and changes.

11.6.2 Tissue Responses

Cumulative insults reduce the vascularity and cell content of the pulp, with an increase in fibrosis. This, adding to the relatively thicker overlying dentine, means that old pulps may be less sensitive to thermal changes and less easy to stimulate for the purpose of diagnosis. Most pulp breakdown in the elderly is in fact without the classic symptoms of reversible and irreversible pulpitis [15].

Possible false-negative response to electric and thermal tests in older patients can be based on the biological changes mentioned above. It does not imply that the tooth is necrotic. There is no conclusive evidence that systemic or medical conditions directly affect (decrease) pulp resistance to injury but may decrease the healing capacity (theoretically atherosclerosis may affect vessels, but pulpal atherosclerosis has not been demonstrated). At the same time, indirect effects of systemic diseases to pulpal resistance to injury are a proven research (i.e., diabetes, rheumatoid arthritis, multiple sclerosis, other autoimmune diseases and immune deficiency problems).

Endodontics has been successively performed on patients ranging from age 2 to 100 years and over. It can be easily said that since the first day, the teeth appear in the oral cavity till the last day of human life; root canal therapy can be applied successfully. Endodontics is less traumatic than extraction and implants in geriatric age group patients. Elder patients (also babies) are not fragile to touch; they just need more care and competency to work with.

11.7 Medical History

A thorough medical history is more important in these patients because they are likely to suffer from chronic diseases and take more medications. Sensitivity to medications, drug intolerance, and potential interactions with drugs prescribed for dental treatment are to be anticipated. Some older patients may need assistance in filling out the forms. Consultation with family, guardian, and/or physician is necessary. Possible symptoms of undiagnosed illness may be present.

Some common problems encountered are:

1. Increased incidence of root sensitivity that is hard to control
2. Increased incidence of caries especially subgingival root caries which is difficult to restore in the interproximal regions resulting in restoration failure and continued decay
3. Tooth wear in the form of attrition, abrasion, and erosion
4. Increased susceptibility to cracks, cuspal fracture, craze lines due to loss of resiliency and decreased organic component of teeth
5. Temporomandibular joint dysfunction and decreased vertical dimension owing to compensating bite because of loss of teeth
6. Less tilting and supraeruption because of decreased eruptive forces of teeth
7. Increased incidence of periodontal problems and a need for combined endodontic-periodontic treatment

11.8 Chief Complaint

These patients have fewer complaints and dental pain usually is indicative of either pulpal or periodontal pain. Patients must be allowed to explain in their own words. The dental practitioner must be alert for any visual/auditory handicaps, patient's dental knowledge, and his/her ability to communicate, at all given times. A disease process usually arises as an acute problem in children, but assumes a more chronic or less dramatic form in elderly. Pain associated with vital pulps (that which is caused by heat, cold, sweets, or referred pain) seems to be reduced by age, and the severity of symptoms is diminished.

11.9 Dental History

The history may be as obvious as a recent pulp exposure and restorations or as subtle as a routine crown preparation years ago (a degenerative process may start following the overzealous dental efforts or over preparations).

11.10 Subjective Symptoms

Pulpal symptoms are usually chronic in elder patients. If pain cannot be localized, one must rule out other sources of orofacial pain. Some subjective symptoms may be exaggerated or pretended (use your clinical experience to differentiate).

11.11 Objective Signs

Oral mucosal check is very important because of the risk of oral cancer which is increasing with age (leukoplakia, etc.). Commissures are more fragile, and conditions such as angular cheilitis, angular stomatitis, fissures, hyperpigmentation, bleeding skin, etc. are possible due to dryness of the skin around the mouth. Secondary dentine formation occurs throughout lifetime and may eventually result in almost complete pulp obliteration. In maxillary anterior teeth, the dentine is formed on the lingual wall of the pulp chamber; in molar teeth the greatest deposition occurs on the floor of the pulp chamber (Fig. 11.1a, b). In such cases, pulp may appear receded. There is an increased incidence of root sensitivity which is difficult to control, increased incidence of subgingival root caries in the interproximal areas which is difficult to restore, and increased susceptibility to cracks, cuspal fractures, and craze lines due to loss of resiliency and organic component of the teeth and asymptomatic pulpal exposure in multirooted teeth.

As age increases, canal size decreases. Reparative dentine resulting from restorative procedures, trauma, and tooth wear in the form of attrition, abrasion, erosion, and recurrent caries also contributes to diminution of canal and chamber size. There is also decreased vertical dimension and temporomandibular joint dysfunction due to compensation bite related to loss of teeth. This may lead to limited mouth opening and increased muscular fatigue thus posing a challenge during instrumentation.

Periodontal disease may be the principal problem for such senior dentate patients, and there is always an increased incidence of combined endodontic-periodontic treatment (Fig. 11.2a, b). Besides all these deep periodontal pockets, chronic food accumulations, halitosis, and root and dentinal sensitivity are seen.

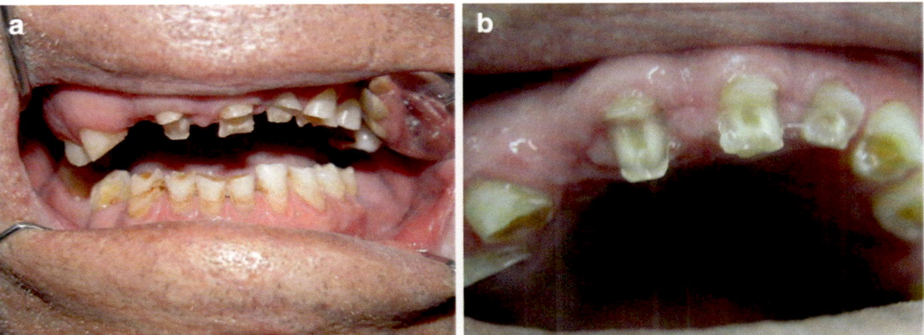

Fig. 11.1 (**a, b**) Male patient, 70 years old, no systemic problem, strong attrition, secondary dentine formation and calcifications in pulp chamber, and vertical dimensional loss. This sort of clinical situations may restrict access cavity preparations even it seems easy at the first moment. Because of heavy calcifications in the pulp chamber and in the root canal, pulpal recessions of root canal recapitulation might be challenging

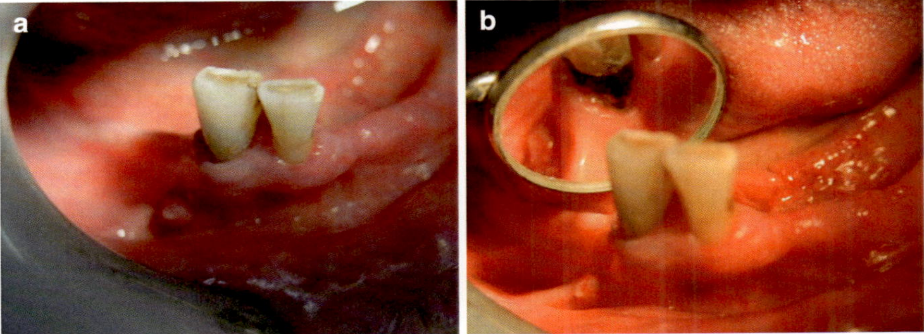

Fig. 11.2 (**a, b**) A 73-year-old female patient, no systemic disorder. A sinus tract in the related site and also tooth wearing is examined. Mandibular crest was edentulous except these two teeth. Also in the lingual side, a circular root caries was detected. Sinus tract was linked with that deep chronic caries. Patient was not reporting any sign and symptoms

11.12 Pulp Testing

The reduced neural and vascular component of aged pulps, the overall reduced pulp volume, and the change in character of the ground substance create an environment that responds with difficulty to both stimuli and irritants. Therefore thermal electrical pulp tests are mostly deceptive in elderly patients and not very much reliable. The response to stimuli may be weaker than in the more highly innervated younger one. Extensive restorations, pulp recession, and excessive calcifications are limitations in both performing and interpreting results of electrical and thermal pulp testing.

Such tests must be avoided in patients with pacemakers. A test cavity and selective anesthesia test is not valuable in elderly patients. Discoloration of single tooth may indicate pulp death, or it may be a sign of aging in elderly patients (generally this is normal).

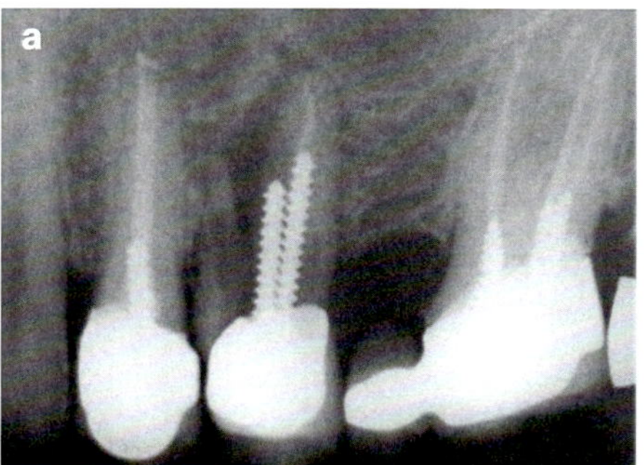

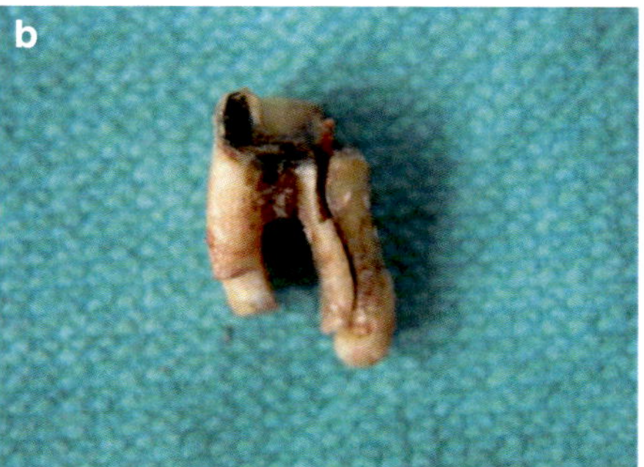

Fig. 11.3 (**a, b**) A 70-year-old female patient applied to clinic with pain with her tooth number 14. In the radiograph, a post-related fracture was detected. Tooth was extracted. The radiograph and the picture of the tooth after extraction is seen

11.13 Radiographs

Radiographic images generally show pulp calcifications, pulp recession, pulp stones, increased cementum formation at apex (hypercementosis), small and narrow canals, decreased osteosclerosis and condensing osteitis, deep proximal caries, root caries, and deep and extensive restorations. Midroot disappearance of a detectable canal may indicate bifurcation rather than calcification. The incidence of some odontogenic and nonodontogenic cysts and tumors characteristically increases with age besides the risk of osteosclerosis and condensing osteitis in the radiographs. Resorptions associated with chronic apical periodontitis significantly alter the shape of apex and the anatomy of the foramen through inflammatory osteoclastic activity. Sometimes root fractures are also seen (Fig. 11.3a, b).

11.14 Treatment Considerations

11.14.1 General

Short appointments and if possible single visit are better for the elderly patients. Practitioners' ability to perform the treatment is important (competency and experience). Endodontic surgery is not the first option, and re-treatment alternatives must be given priority.

Good communication should be established and maintained with all the patients. Relatives or patient's trusted friends should be included in consultations if their judgment is valued by the patient or needed for consent. Procedures should be explained in detail. Obtaining signed consent to the outlined treatment is encouraged and may be useful if the patient is forgetful. The patient's limited life expectancy should not appreciably alter treatment plans and surely is no excuse for extractions or poor root canal treatment. It is important that each geriatric patient be kept well informed of risks and alternatives at all stages. Treatment for the medically compromised patients must be done after consulting with the physician.

11.15 Patient Comfort

The ideal time of day for scheduling appointments must take into consideration patients' daily personal, eating, and resting habits as well as any medication schedule. Morning appointments are preferable for most older patients. Chair positioning and comfort may be of greater importance for the elderly than younger. If necessary patient should be offered assistance in the operatory. When it comes to the number of sittings, functionally independent patients who can tolerate stress can be treated in a single sitting. For patients who cannot tolerate prolonged mouth opening, shorter multiple appointments would be required. As much work as possible should be performed at each visit, and a restroom break should be offered at intervals as the patient's needs indicate. Jaw fatigue should be prevented by using bite blocks.

11.16 Anesthesia

The need for anesthesia depends on pulp vitality status and cervical positioning of rubber dam clamp. During anesthesia in geriatric patients, the anatomic landmarks are more prominent; hence, anesthetic should be deposited more slowly. Teeth with necrotic pulp should be treated without anesthesia (optional) or minimal anesthesia. Where possible, it is best to allow the patient's response to instrumentation through apical foramen to determine/confirm the working length or need for adjustment and reduce risk of over instrumentation and inoculation of canal contents into the periapical tissue. Electronic apex locator is best for the elderly patients.

The reduced width of PDL makes needle placement for supplementary intraligamentary injections more difficult. Avoid intraosseous anesthesia as much as possible. But if required, smaller amounts of solution (3% mepivacaine instead of 2% lidocaine) should be used during intraosseous anesthesia. Intra-pulpal anesthesia is difficult to achieve due to the reduced volume of the pulp chamber, thus making the diffusion into the canals much more difficult.

11.17 Orthostatic Hypotension

At the completion of the appointment, the patient should not be brought to a different position abruptly. Orthostatic hypotension is a frequent occurrence in the older adult with quick positional changes. Allowing the patient to sit for a minute or two before escorting the patient to the reception area helps them regain their balance.

11.18 Endodontic Considerations in the Elderly

As already mentioned, there are many technical challenges encountered during the root canal treatment of the elderly starting from diagnosis to various stages in the therapy. Increased bulk of dentine and increased pulpal fibrosis may diminish the response to traditional vitality testing. Hence, it will be wrong to assume that the pulp is non-vital and carry out the treatment without other supporting evidences [34]. Certain systemic conditions may preclude the use of epinephrine, reducing the duration of anesthesia warranting reinjections [35].

11.18.1 During Access and Orientation

Access and canal negotiation probably present the greatest challenge in geriatric endodontics [16]. The physiological changes in the pulp space should be analyzed in the preoperative radiograph in order to prevent any complications [36]. If antibiotic is necessary, prescribe minimum doses. Rubber dam must be used (tilted teeth may be excluded during the access preparation until you locate the pulp chamber because of the misorientation problems). Reduction in salivary flow and gag reflex reduces the need for saliva ejector. Isolation should be carried out for single tooth preferably.

The effects of access preparation on existing restoration and the possible need for the actual removal of the restoration should be discussed with the patient before the procedure as well as the removal of the artificial crown prior to access preparation. If patient has multiple restorations, removal of them and coronal disassembling are necessary.

In anterior teeth, the pulp retreats progressively in a cervical direction, becoming narrower. In roots, deposition is always concentric toward the center of the mass of dentine. Deposition is often pronounced more in the coronal parts of the canal, with deeper areas of root canals remaining widely patent even in old age [13]. These points are important to remember during the search for root canals. The clinician should always look in the middle of masses of dentine and must not assume that because a canal is narrow coronally it will not open into a manageable system at a deeper level.

Safe-ended, slow-speed burs have to be used in order to not damage the pulp chamber floor. Use of magnification (operating microscope gives the best result or magnifying glasses, 2.5X–3.5X) is an advantage during the identification of canal orifices. Another aid in the treatment of geriatric patients is the use of transillumination. The pulp stones can be visualized often with additional light and magnification [37, 38]. Ultrasonic troughing tips are especially useful in cutting through the calcifications that cover the canal orifices. Proper planning is required for over-erupted, tilted teeth with reduced clinical crown height [39].

Entry to a calcified canal system should be carefully planned, and care should be taken to identify features of the pulp space from an accurate preoperative radiograph, with attention to the expected depth of patent pulp space and long axis orientation. In most cases, a high-speed medium tapered diamond bur will be sufficient to outline the cavity and gain initial penetration. Define a classic cavity outline, with a narrower and more cervically placed starting point in the case of calcified anterior teeth.

Orientation should be constantly checked and rechecked and the cavity inspected periodically for extent and alignment. Special care should be taken to inspect the cavity at a depth at which it is anticipated the pulp will be entered. If the initial access bur has not entered the canal, it is time to reconsider alignment. In such a situation, it is possible that the clinician may be at the correct level, but needs to bypass it on any side. Exposure of radiographs is important to confirm the progress and realignment. Under no circumstances should the clinician progress beyond the expected entry depth without careful consideration, else the bur could enter the periodontal ligament.

Once the clinician has reached the extent of a medium tapered diamond bur in good orientation, but without entry, it is advisable to change to less aggressive, slow-speed burs to continue the procedure. Ideal are instruments with narrow necks to allow the active head to be observed at all times. Working with magnification, there are often visual clues to give an idea about penetration, owing to the altered color, texture, and translucency of the mineralized deposits in the former pulp space, in comparison to the surrounding primary dentine. Some researchers suggest the use of fine ultrasonic cutting tips to gently advance apically. These instruments may, however, cause drying and burning of dentine, which can distract the natural features of the tooth, alter color and translucency, and lead to misdirected preparation.

At intervals, probing should be attempted firmly with a DG16 canal probe to help locate a small puncture spot into the pulp space. If no such luck, carefully attempt to align burring and probing and continue until a stick is found or until a decision is made that entry will not be secured.

In the case of multirooted teeth, the chamber should be fully unroofed. Safe-ended, high-speed burs (Endo Z or Diamendo, Maillefer) are ideal and avoid injury to the chamber floor. Pulp stones should be removed. Most often heavy probing with a DG16 is sufficient to fragment/remove stones. Ultrasonic scalers are also useful tools for fragmentation and elimination. Again, care should be exercised to avoid damage to the pulp chamber floor.

Figure 11.4a, b are showing a successfully treated tooth by following the recommendation here. Avoid using barbed broaches because of their high risk of fracture;

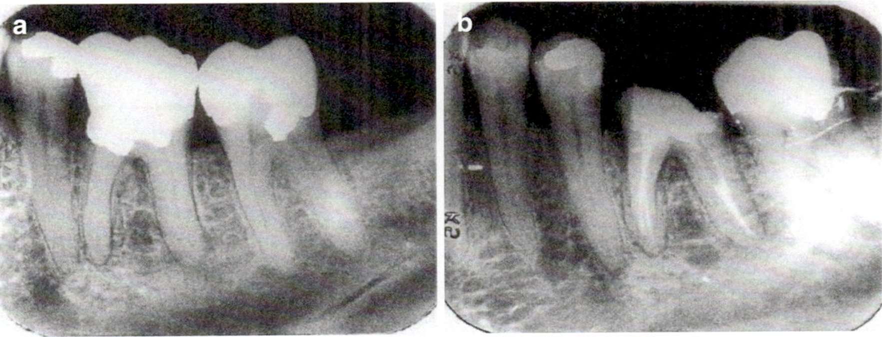

Fig. 11.4 (**a, b**) A 68-year-old female patient. Before and after her treatment. Coronal disassembling was done, and all defective and previous restorations were removed. Tight and narrow canals were prepared properly and obturated. A post-space was also prepared for a further restoration in the distal canal

coronal tooth structure may have to be sacrificed for better access (at times even complete removal of crown) and widening of axial walls for visibility. Perforations are more likely to occur as the pulp chamber is calcified and disclike. Immediate sealing with an appropriate root repair material (MTA recommended) improves the prognosis significantly.

If you feel fatigued as the operator and are unable to locate the canals, reschedule the patient. In such a case, second appointment will be more productive.

11.18.2 During Preparation

Unlike in young patients where the cemento-dentinal junction is situated usually around 0.5–1 mm from the outer surface of the root, in geriatric cases, this distance becomes greater because of continued cementum formation at the apex [40]. Since the canals are much narrower, it takes more time, effort, and care to prepare the root canal and reduce the risk of binding and separation [41].

Difficulty in locating apical constriction as:

- It is 0.5–2.5 mm from radiographic apex.
- Clinicians' tactile sense is reduced.
- Reduced periapical sensitivity in older patients.
- Use of electronic apex locator limited in heavily restored teeth.

Calcification of older canals is much more concentric and linear, and this allows easier penetration once canals are found. Flaring of canal is advised early in the procedure for better irrigation and to reduce binding of instruments. NiTi rotary instrumentation provides a more efficient method of shaping the calcified and curved root canals. Longer canals are more commonly seen because of increased cementum deposition. Prefer to use instruments with no rake angle and use of the crown down preparation technique is preferred.

Lubricants are always helpful to ease the glide path during entry. Small files, typically 21 mm size 10, or dedicated entry files (Pathfinder files C+ files) with increased rigidity are gently advanced into the canal in a watch-winding motion, rotating the instrument lightly between the forefinger tip and thumb. If progress and rotation of the instrument between the finger and thumb become tight, resist the temptation to drive on. The instrument should be withdrawn at this stage (picking motion) to free/disengage it from the canal walls, and irrigant/lubricant should be used. Progress continues in this manner as the instrument progresses apically.

As mentioned earlier, it should be kept in mind that canals are often narrower coronally than they are apically.

Progress is not always smooth despite careful instrumentation and copious irrigation/lubrication. If the negotiating instrument/file does not advance well apically, the clinician should determine tactile feel of the instrument in the canal. If the instrument is advanced with a watch-winding motion and engages within the canal and demonstrates a tugging or sticky sensation on removal, this is tight resistance. This suggests that the instrument is engaging a fine/narrow canal orifice, and with patience and persistence, it will progress toward the deeper parts of the canal.

If, on the contrary, the instrument sails loosely through the canal and hits an obstruction with no tactile sticky sensation, this is loose resistance. This is often an "apical calcification," a rare event deep in a canal system. The explanation is that the canal is curving, and the operator should apply a smooth curve to the apical 2–3 mm of the file before reinserting and negotiating around the walls to find a sticking spot. Despite best efforts, canals are not always negotiated to definitive length, and decision-making should balance the risks of attempting to cut further, perhaps in an iatrogenic path, or to accept the outcome. This decision will be influenced by the pathological state and the restorative plan for the tooth, and decisions should always be made with proper patient information and consent. If one canal of a multirooted tooth is difficult to enter, work should continue in the other canals through a pulp chamber flooded with sodium hypochlorite, and a further attempt should be made to negotiate later in the appointment.

Problems are common while progressing from the initial size 10 instrument to the size 15 file, which is 50% wider. In such cases, use of half-sized files may help gain path for the enlarging tools to follow such as Golden Mediums (Maillefer/Dentsply), which include instruments in sizes 12.5, 17.5, and 22.5.

11.18.3 During Obturation

Obturation techniques that do not require large midroot taper and overzealous forces to canal walls during condensation are preferred. A lateral condensation technique with a bio-ceramic sealer and coated cones is ideal and less time-consuming. Warm gutta-percha techniques are recommended (System B, Touch 'n Heat, Obtura). Root fractures may occur when much taper is given to the canals, and post failures are likely to occur with parallel posts. Permanent coronal restorations should be scheduled as soon as possible, and intermediate restorative materials should be selected and properly placed to maintain a seal coronally (IRM, glass ionomer, etc.). Six-month recall period to evaluate repair radiographically may not be adequate to evaluate success and failure in the presence of periapical pathology. It may take as long as 2 years to produce the healing that would occur at 6 months in an adolescent. Some clinical tips are mentioned in Table 11.1.

Table 11.1 Some clinical tips

Access	Cleaning and shaping
1. *Coronal*: because of the risk of easy perforations of the floor of the pulp chamber, always try to measure/approximate the depth of pulp chamber from the RVG (or x-ray) or distance from occlusal to the furca and be mindful of the fact that due to increased calcifications/presence of pulp stones in the pulp chamber, the bur doesn't always give the "drop-in" feeling. Always try to remove dentinal shelf 2. *Radicular*: preflare the orifice (try crown-down technique), and an anticurvature filing is recommended (if you work manually)	• Copious irrigation should be done • Use EDTA in gel form (RC-prep) as much as you can • Use a watch-winding motion to negotiate tight canals • Remove overhanging dentine ledges to obtain straight-line access. This reduces total canal curvature

11.19 Success/Failure of Endodontic Therapy

Persistence or the development of the symptoms should not be ignored, and the extent of failure should be closely examined before re-treatment attempt; surgery or extraction is suggested. With vital pulps, repair of periapical tissues is determined by the presence of local and systemic factors. With non-vital pulps and periapical pathology, repair is slow because of arteriosclerotic changes of blood vessels and altered viscosity of connective tissues. Periapical repair is more difficult as the rate of bone formation decreases with age.

Intentional replantation is not a good alternative treatment in geriatric patients in case of failure of any case. If necessary, the simplest surgical alternatives (i.e., incision and drainage) are possible. But if the patient is healthy, endodontic surgery can be planned (if the surgery is only alternative), i.e., very valuable abutment to save if there is no any other alternative or treating and correcting some procedural errors (Fig. 11.5a–h). This is discussed in the surgery chapter. If an implant application is possible, a dental consultation team must decide for this procedure.

Conclusions

In conclusion, geriatric endodontics will gain a more significant role in complete dental care because of the "aging society." Dental services, including root canal procedures, for the elderly population of the future are anticipated to be of two general types (1) services for the relatively healthy elderly who are functionally independent and (2) services for elderly patients with complex conditions and problems who are functionally dependent. The second group will require care from practitioners who have specialized and advanced training in geriatric dentistry. This age group is being targeted in dental education programs and advanced training through improved curriculum research and publications on aging.

11.20 Futuristic Recommendations

Teaching geriatric endodontics as a specialty (and/or as a part of endo programs, specific clinical courses, or subspecialty of endodontics) to handle the new clinical challenges for coming elder generation will be useful. Geriatric consultation teams (gerodontic team) and mobile services (dental mobile units to serve elderly and compromised patients near their place) needed to be established. Government (social services)-university dental health team coordination to create new health policies for geriatric dental patients is necessary and needed to be improved.

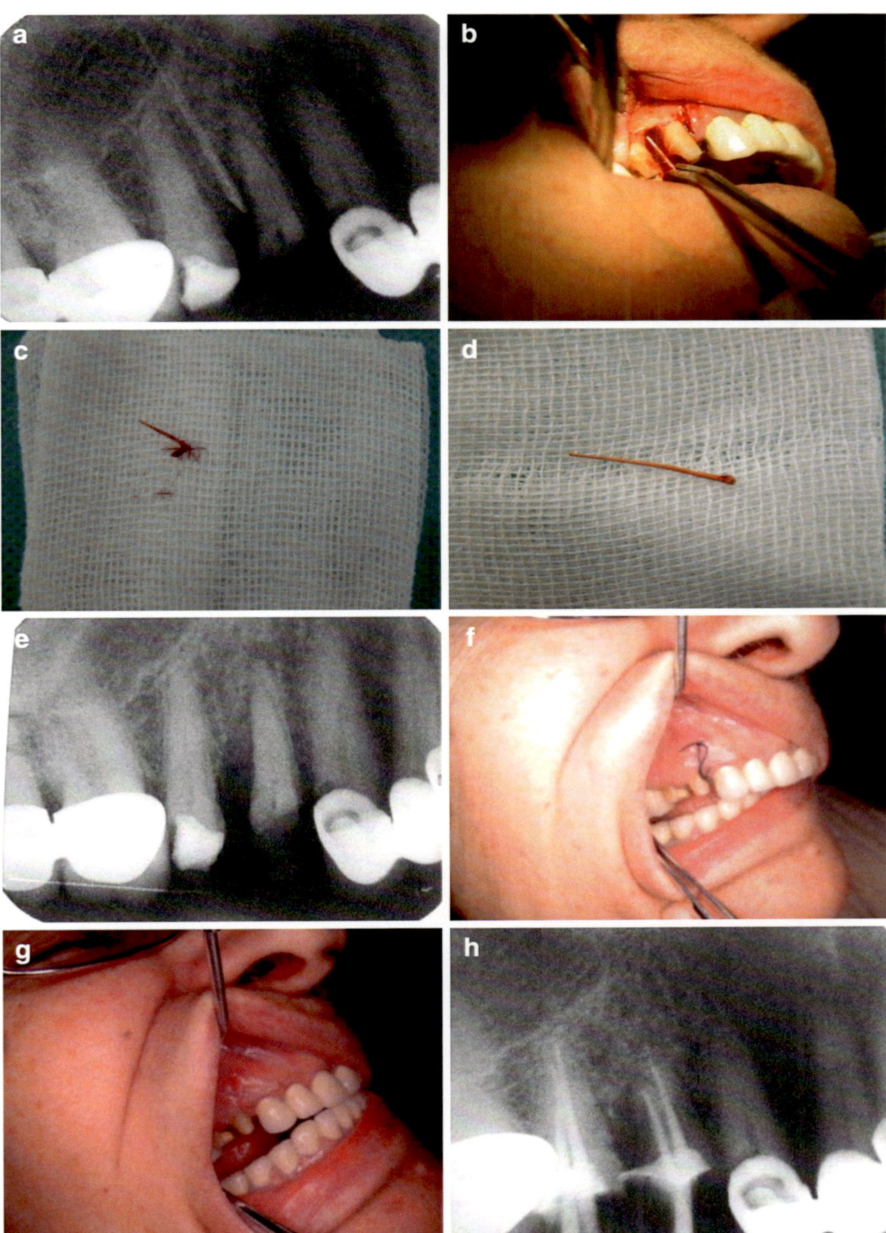

Fig. 11.5 (**a, b, c, d, e, f, g, h**) The serial pictures represent a female patient (72 years old). Medically stable and not compromised. A root canal treatment was attempted on tooth 14, but the procedure ended up with a procedural error and distal perforation. Endodontic surgery was the only alternative. Flap was raised, and the gutta-percha points were removed. The surgical site was properly healed. Tooth 15 was also found to be necrotic. Both teeth were obturated following the root canal treatment. The patient was then referred for prosthetic restorations with crowns. Therefore, even in an elderly patient, the treatment was finalized with endodontic surgical approaches

References

1. Singh SK, Kanaparthy A, Kanaparthy R, Pillai A, Sandhu G. Geriatric endodontic. J Orofac Res. 2013;3(3):191–6.
2. Mulligan R. Geriatrics: contemporary and future concerns. Dent Clin N Am. 2005;49:11–3.
3. Beers H, Berkow MD. Merk manual of geriatrics. Demographics - chapter 2. 2014
4. Government of India. Report of expert committee on population projections for India up to 2001-registrar general of India, Minister of planning and programme implementation. New Delhi; 1998.
5. Persson RE, Persson GG. The elderly at risk for periodontitis and systemic disease. Dent Clin N Am. 2005;49:279–92.
6. Ettinger RL, Beck JD. Geraitric dental curriculum and the needs of the elderly. Spec Care Dentist. 1984;4:207–13.
7. Durso SC. Interaction with other health team members in caring for elderly patients. Dent Clin N Am. 2005;49:377–88.
8. Kendall DM, Bergenstal DM. Comprehensive management of patients with diabetes type-II, establishing priorities of care. Am J Manag Care. 2001;7(Suppl 10):273–83.
9. Williams BR, Kini J. Medication use and prescribing considerations for elderly patients. Dent Clin N Am. 2005;49:411–27.
10. Yellowitz JA. Cognitive function, aging, and ethical decisions: recognizing change. Dent Clin N Am. 2005;49:389–410.
11. Patil MS, Patil SB. Psychological and emotional considerations during dental treatment. Gerodontology. 2009;26:72–7.
12. Murray PE, Stanley HR, Matthews JB, Sloan AJ, Smith AJ. Age related changes odontometric changes of human teeth. Oral Surg Oral Med Oral Pathol Oral Radio Endod. 2002;93:474–82.
13. Bhaskar SN. Orban's oral histology and embryology. 11th ed. St Louis: Mosby; 1990.
14. Jimena ME. Endodontic needs of geriatric patients in private practice. J Philipp Dent Assoc. 1998;49(4):5–21.
15. Goodis HE, Rossall JC, Kahn AJ. Endodontic status in older U.S. adults. Report of a survey. J Am Dent Assoc. 2001;132(11):1525–30.
16. Walton RE. Endodontic considerations in the geriatric patient. Dent Clin N Am. 1997;41(4):795–816.
17. Allen PF, Whitworth JM. Endodontic considerations in the elderly. Gerodontology. 2004;21(4):185–94.
18. Sperber GH, Yu DC. Patient age is no contraindication to endodontic treatment. J Can Dent Assoc. 2003;69(8):494–6.
19. Philippas GG, Applebaum E. Age factor in secondary dentin formation. J Dent Res. 1966;45:778–89.
20. Smith JW. Calcific metamorphosis: a treatment dilemma. Oral Surg Oral Med Oral Pathol. 1982;54:441–4.
21. Solheim T. Amount of secondary dentin as an indicator of age. Scand J Dent Res. 1992;100:193–9.
22. Morse DR, Esposito JV, Schoor RS. A radiographic study of aging changes of the dental pulp and dentin in normal teeth. Quintessence Int. 1993;24:329–33.
23. Kveal S, Kolltveit K, Thomsen I, Solheim T. Age estimation of adults from dental radiographs. Forensic Sci Int. 1995;74:175–85.
24. Nielsen CJ, Bentley JP, Marshall FJ. Age-related changes in reducible crosslinks of human dental pulp collagen. Arch Oral Biol. 1983;28:759–64.
25. Ketterl W. Age-induced changes in the teeth and their attachment apparatus. Int Dent J. 1983;33:262–71.
26. Bernick S. Effect of aging on the nerve supply to human teeth. J Dent Res. 1967;46:694–9.
27. Bernick S. Differences in nerve distribution between erupted and non-erupted human teeth. J Dent Res. 1964;43:406–11.

28. Johnsen DC, Harshbarger J, Rymer HD. Quantitative assessment of neural development in human premolars. Anat Rec. 1983;205:421–9.
29. Fried K. Changes in innervation of dentin and pulp with age. Front Oral Physiol. 1987;6:63.
30. Bennett CG, Kelln EE, Biddington WR. Age changes of the vascular pattern of the human dental pulp. Arch Oral Biol. 1965;10:995–8.
31. Bernick S. Age changes in the blood supply to human teeth. J Dent Res. 1967;46:544–50.
32. Johnsen DC. Innervation of teeth: qualitative, quantitative, and development assessment. J Dent Res. 1985;64 Spec No:555–63.
33. Drusini AG, Toso O, Ranzato C. The coronal pulp cavity index: a biomarker for age determination in human adults. Am J Phys Anthropol. 1997;103:353–63.
34. Fuss Z, Trowbridge H. Assessment of electric and thermal pulp testing agents. J Endod. 1986;12:301–5.
35. Replogle K, Reader A, Nist R. Cardiovascular effects of intra osseous injections of 2 percent lignocaine with 1:100000 epinephrine and 3% mepivacaine. J Am Dent Assoc. 1999;130:169–74.
36. Berbick S, Nedelman C. Effect of ageing on human pulp. J Endod. 1975;3:88–95.
37. Barkhorder R, Linder D. Pulp stones and ageing (abstract 669).
38. Bui D. The ageing mouth. J Dent Res. Special Issue: 1990;192–7.
39. Moreinis SA. Avoiding perforation during endodontic access. J Am Dent Assoc. 1979;98:707–12.
40. MK W, Wesselink P, Walton R. Apical terminus of root canal treatment procedures. Oral Surg Oral Med Oral Pathol Oral Radiol Endod. 2000;89:99–103.
41. Kuyk K, Walton R. Comparison of radiographic appearance of root canal size to its actual diameter. J Endod. 1990;16:528–33.

12 Endodontics in Systemically Compromised Patients

Catherine Wynne

12.1 Introduction

The common medical conditions encountered by the dentist in daily practice that necessitates extra knowledge include cardiac diseases, pulmonary diseases, hypertension, diabetes, bleeding disorders, pregnant patients, multiple drug interactions, infectious diseases, renal complications, diabetes, and patients undergoing radiation therapy [1]. When treatment is carried out in a healthy individual, it is sufficient to concentrate on the technical part of the procedure, but when there is a need to treat patients with systemic illness who are under medical management, it is equally important to avoid any potential medical emergency or complication.
The world is experiencing growth in the number and proportion of older persons in the population, because of this the incidence of a number of pathologies has been increasing and thus is producing an increase in the number of individuals with systemic medical conditions that can affect oral health and subsequent dental treatment. The dental management of medically compromised patients can be sometimes problematic in terms of oral complications, dental therapy, and emergency care. One of the challenges faced by dental specialists today is the assessment and management of these patients. As mentioned in detail in Chap. 11 geriatric patients are much more likely to be at least partially dentulous having a complex medical history and the use of multiple medications.

In order to ascertain a patient's medical status, a thorough history taking is essential. This chapter will focus on guidelines for endodontists to manage such medical conditions in a dental office. It should be noted that this book covers endodontic considerations in commonly occurring medical conditions, a comprehensive list of all medical conditions is exhaustive and beyond the scope of this book.

C. Wynne
American Academy of Cosmetic Surgery Hospital, Dubai, UAE
e-mail: catherinewynne10@gmail.com

P. Jain (ed.), *Common Complications in Endodontics*,
https://doi.org/10.1007/978-3-319-60997-3_12

For information on other medical conditions and more detail on those listed below, the reader is advised to refer to other books and journals and to consult their medical colleagues with respect to specific patient cases.

12.2 Importance of History Taking

Obtaining a thorough medical history is of great importance [2]. It is an information gathering process for assessing a patient's health status and comprises a systematic review of the patient's chief or primary complaint, a detailed history related to the complaint, information about past and present medical conditions, pertinent social and family histories, and a review of symptoms by organ system. Interpretation of this information collected achieves three important objectives: enables the monitoring of medical conditions and the evaluation of underlying systemic conditions of which the patient may or may not be aware, provides a basis for determining whether dental treatment might affect the systemic health of the patient, and provides an initial starting point for assessing the possible influence of the patient's systemic health on the patient's oral health and/or dental treatment [3, 4].

Each identified condition during the process of history taking can affect dental care in a unique manner. For example, medication prescribed for a medical condition might produce a problem during the administration of a local anesthetic, or it could interact with pain medication prescribed posttreatment. Certain medically compromised patients should only be treated in a hospital setting where emergency issues, should they arise, can be immediately addressed and promptly attended to in a controlled manner.

Past dental history (PDH) should also be obtained as a review of systems, especially when the patient presents with complicating dental and medical factors such as restorative and periodontal needs coupled with a systemic disorder such as diabetes. Details of any previous untoward complications of dental treatment must be recorded or must be obtained subsequently if not immediately available from the patient.

Dental treatment causes changes to the patient's homeostasis. A risk assessment should be performed to evaluate and determine the modifications to be required before, during, and after dental treatment. Different modifications may be necessary at each stage of treatment such as antibiotic prophylaxis or steroid replacement may be necessary before treatment, or it may not be possible to place the patient in a supine position during dental procedures, or specific hemostatic agents may need to be employed after extractions. Many different medical conditions are discussed hereby, and protocols for the modification of dental care are suggested.

In the patient with pre-existing disease, preparation for dental treatment should include determination of disease status. The clinician should have an understanding of the nature of the patient's disease and how it can impact their physiology and his/her response to dental management and postdental treatment healing. Knowing how to manage potential complications is also important and is discussed in the following chapter.

12.3 Cardiac Disorders

Cardiovascular disease (CVD) has become increasingly common in modern times; therefore, a dentist must be aware of the modifications and precautions to take while treating a patient suffering from cardiovascular disorders. According to WHO, Global status report on noncommunicable diseases (2014), 17.5 million people die each year from CVD, an estimated 31% of all deaths worldwide.

Patients suffering from cardiovascular disease are vulnerable to physical and emotional stress. If, in addition, the patients have to undergo dental treatment, it will add to their stress. Cardiac patients have a higher risk of collapse, other cardiac emergencies such as angina attacks and/or drug interactions, in the dental clinic.

Cardiovascular problems that require special attention and dental-treatment-plan modification include infective endocarditis, ischemic heart disease, myocardial infarction, cardiac arrhythmias, and congestive heart failure. In patients with cardiovascular disease, the most important considerations during treatment include the maintenance of blood pressure, pulse, cardiac output, and myocardial oxygen and the prevention of bacteremia via prophylactic antibiotic. A comprehensive dental evaluation involving a thorough medical history and premedical evaluation should be carried out including an assessment of vital signs (e.g., pulse, blood pressure, the rate and depth of respiration, and temperature).

12.3.1 Hypertension

Blood pressure is determined by how much blood the heart pumps (i.e., cardiac output) and by the resistance to blood flow in the vascular system. Cardiac output in turn is determined by how often the pump contracts (i.e., heart rate) and by the amount of blood ejected during each beat (i.e., stroke volume) [5]. Hypertensive patients are defined as those receiving treatment for hypertension or those with a mean systolic blood pressure (SBP) of 140 mm Hg or greater and/or mean diastolic blood pressure (DBP) of 90 mm Hg or greater [6] (Table 12.1). The same classification is used in young, middle-aged, and elderly subjects. Patients with prehypertension are at increased risk of developing hypertension, those with blood pressure values 130–139/80–89 mmHg have a two times greater risk of developing hypertension than those with lower values [7].

Patients with untreated or inadequately treated hypertension are at increased risk of developing acute complications like myocardial infarction, stroke, and chronic complications of hypertension. Hypertension is a highly prevalent cardiovascular

Table 12.1 Classification of hypertension [8]

Classification	SBP (mmHg)	DBP (mmHg)
Normal	<120	and <80
Prehypertension	120–139	or 80–89
Stage 1 hypertension	140–159	or 90–99
Stage 2 hypertension	≥160	≥100

SBP systolic blood pressure; *DBP* diastolic blood pressure

Table 12.2 White coat hypertension, the white coat effect, and masked hypertension [9]

Diagnosis	Office blood pressure	Blood pressure outside office	Associated with adverse outcomes
White coat hypertension	Elevated	Normal	Controversial
White coat effect	Elevated	Normal or high	Controversial
Masked hypertension	Normal	Elevated	Yes

disease, which affects over 1 billion people worldwide [8]. Hypertension was called the "silent killer" because it often affects target organs (the kidney, heart, brain, eyes) before the appearance of clinical symptoms.

12.3.1.1 White Coat Hypertension

Office BP is usually higher than BP measured out of the office, which can be attributed to anxiety and/or a conditional response to the unusual situation [1]. *White coat hypertension* (WCH) refers to a persistently elevated office blood pressure in the presence of a normal blood pressure outside of the office [4]. WCH is different from the white coat effect (WCE), which refers to a high office blood pressure but whereby hypertension may or may not be present outside the office setting. *Masked hypertension* refers to when a patient has a normal office blood pressure but has hypertension outside of the office (Table 12.2).

WCH and masked hypertension are important for clinicians to recognize. It is controversial as to whether WCH is associated with increased cardiovascular risk, but patients with masked hypertension are at increased cardiovascular risk.

12.3.2 Ischemic Heart Disease

When coronary atherosclerotic heart disease becomes sufficiently advanced to produce symptoms, it is referred to as ischemic heart disease. It is relatively common in the general population, especially with increasing age, and typically presents as angina or heart failure [10]. Angina is often precipitated by physical activity or stress and may radiate to the arm or jaw or may present as facial or dental pain. Fear and anxiety associated with a dental procedure may be a precipitating factor for angina in some patients [11].

12.3.3 General Considerations in Patients with Cardiovascular Disorders

12.3.3.1 Physician Consent

Consultation with the patient's physician is mandatory before the initiation of dental treatment. A green signal from the patients' physician is crucial when treating medically compromised patients for the safety of the patient from medical complications as well as the safety of the dentist from medicolegal complications. It is important for a physician/cardiologist report before initiating any elective dental surgical procedure in a cardiovascular patient. The proposed treatment plan should be reviewed, and any medical recommendations should be documented [12]. In addition, a careful preoperative dental evaluation is recommended. This helps in reducing the incidence of dental emergencies.

12.3.3.2 Stress Reduction

Dental treatment has the potential to induce stress in patients. It can be either physiological (pain) or psychological (anxiety, fear). The body responds to stress by increased release of catecholamines (epinephrine and norepinephrine) from the adrenal medulla into the cardiovascular system. This, in turn, can increase the workload on the heart (i.e., increased heart rate and strength of myocardial contraction and an increased myocardial oxygen requirement) in patients with hypertension or coronary artery disease [13]. Therefore patients with cardiovascular disease are more vulnerable to physical or emotional stress that may be encountered during dental treatment than a normal patient [12]. Various steps should be taken to minimize stress encountered during dental treatment procedure. These are:

- Patients should be given reassurance to prevent or reduce anxiety.
- Medically compromised patients are better able to tolerate stress when rested. Therefore, appointments should be scheduled in the mornings [13].
- Angina-prone patients who experience greater than normal stress from the thought of dental work benefit from the administration of oral anxiolytics or nitrous oxide [12, 14].
- Patients should be seated comfortably (semi-supine) in the dental chair [14]
- Pain control is critical for lessening the chances of angina in ischemic heart disease patients by producing and maintaining profound local anesthesia in the surgical area via the use of longer-acting anesthetics, such as bupivacaine, or by using an anesthetic containing a vasoconstrictor, after careful aspiration [14, 15].
- Intermittent rest should be provided to the patient thereby reducing fatigue.
- Appointments should not be long [13].

12.3.3.3 The Use of Vasoconstrictors

Incorporation of a vasoconstrictor to local anesthetic provides better pain control, which in turn reduces anxiety and stress usually associated with dental treatment [16].

Control of pain and anxiety is very important in patients with high medical risk. Patients with cardiovascular disease have a high risk of complications due to endogenous catecholamines (adrenaline and noradrenaline) released from pain and stress. These catecholamines may increase dramatically BP and cardiac output. This effect is reduced by controlling dental pain. Local anesthetics with epinephrine produce a longer and more effective anesthesia than simple LA, thus avoiding an exaggerated response to stress [17]. But the commonly used vasoconstrictors such as epinephrine can cause a rise in heart rate [18]. Hence, the use of vasoconstrictor should be limited in individuals with cardiac disease, taking care not to exceed 0.04 mg of adrenaline. In turn, if anesthetic reinforcement is needed, it should be provided without a vasoconstrictor [14]. Aspiration before any injection is mandatory to avoid intravascular administration [15].

The maximum recommended dose of epinephrine in a patient with cardiac risk is 0.04 mg, which is equal to that containing about two cartridges of LA with 1: 100,000 epinephrine or 4 cartridges with 1: 200,000 epinephrine [16].

Vasoconstrictor is an absolute contraindication in patients with unstable angina pectoris or in patients with uncontrolled hypertension, refractory arrhythmias, recent myocardial infarctions (less than 6 months), recent stroke (less than 6 months), recent coronary bypass surgery (less than 3 months), and uncontrolled congestive heart failure [18]. Furthermore, since vasoconstrictors can interact with certain anti-hypertensive medications, they should be used only after consultation with the patient's physician [12].

12.3.4 Endodontic Consideration in Hypertensive Patients

Patients with hypertension are at an increased risk of suffering from angina pectoris, myocardial infarction, stroke, and heart failure. All of these are medical emergencies which can occur during and after dental care [14, 19]. Although clear guidelines for establishing a cutoff point for dental treatment emergency or routine are lacking, it is generally accepted that patients with SBP greater than 180 or DBP greater than 110 should be taken for medical consultation and treatment prior to dental treatment and only emergency management of pain or acute infection should be considered [11].

Routine dental treatment should be deferred until acceptable blood pressure levels are achieved, and the patient should be referred for medical evaluation. Antihypertensive drugs may cause certain oral side effects. Orthostatic hypotension occurs to varying degrees in most of the patients taking antihypertensive medicines [14]. Therefore, dentists should avoid making sudden changes in the patients' body position during treatment [19].

Prolonged use of certain nonsteroidal anti-inflammatory drugs (NSAIDs), such as ibuprofen, indomethacin, or naproxen, is shown to reduce the effectiveness of certain antihypertensive drugs (beta-blockers, diuretics, ACEIs) [14, 18]. Paracetamol can be used to avoid this side effect. Excessive bleeding especially is a possibility in hypertensive patients. Therefore, aggressive dental surgical procedures should be performed with great caution in these patients [19].

Dental treatment should include short morning appointments, good procedural pain control, stress and anxiety reduction that could include preoperative or intraoperative conscious sedation or other non-pharmacologic techniques, and good post-operative follow-up with pain control using appropriate medication.

Although vasoconstrictors may precipitate significant elevations in blood pressure, they lower the risk of endogenous catecholamine release that may result from inadequate pain control.

However, elective dental care should be avoided in the following situations:

- Stage 2 hypertensive patients with blood pressure greater than or equal to 180/110
- Patients who have hypertensive symptoms such as occipital headache, failing vision, ringing in the ears, dizziness, weakness, and tingling of the hands and feet

In these cases, if emergency dental treatment is necessary, medical consultation is required and vasoconstrictor amounts should be limited to one to two cartridges of 1:100,000 solution (0.018–0.036 mg of epinephrine). In patients with Stage 2 hypertension (blood pressure of 160–179/100–109), epinephrine should be limited to three cartridges (0.054 mg). Intraligamentary and intrabony injections should be avoided in these patients [6, 20].

12.3.5 Endodontic Considerations in Patients with Congestive Cardiac Failure

In congestive cardiac failure, there is a mismatch between blood supply and organ demand. A determination must be made via physician consultation on the status of the disease prior to treatment (i.e., is it stable or unstable?). The condition is often confounded by hypertension, a history of MIs, renal failure, thyrotoxicosis, and chronic obstructive pulmonary disease (COPD).

Following a recent MI, patients may have damaged myocardium and be susceptible to reinfarctions, possibly predisposing to heart failures.

The amount of epinephrine delivered can be a critical aspect to the disease. It is advisable to avoid vasoconstrictors in patients receiving digitalis as it can precipitate cardiac arrhythmias [12]. Since aspirin can lead to sodium and fluid retention, it is important to avoid it in patients with heart failure. Medications used by patients with heart failure can be associated with certain side effects of dental significance like xerostomia, lichenoid reaction, and orthostatic hypotension [14].

The clinician should be prepared for potential complications. In the patient with multiple comorbid conditions, only urgent dental needs should be provided, preferably in a hospital setting. For the patient who is considered stable and without significant complications, routine conservative dental care can be performed in an outpatient setting. Prior to treatment, a prothrombin time should be obtained, and, during treatment, the patient should be placed in an upright position to prevent additional pulmonary fluid collection. Placing a patient with poorly compensated heart in supine position can cause shortness of breath and can precipitate pulmonary edema, thus complicating dental treatment procedures [21]. Prothrombin time is measured with the international normalized ratio (INR), and it is used to monitor the effects of anticoagulants on patients. The accepted range of INR to perform elective endodontic procedures is 2–4 [22] and should be checked on the day prior to endodontic therapy.

Important considerations are [23]:

1. Premedication, 2–5 mg diazepam 1 h before procedure to reduce anxiety.
2. Anesthesia without vasoconstrictors can be used for procedures.
3. Short appointments, semi-supine chair position, and availability of sublingual form of nitroglycerine are considered as safety procedures.
4. Patients receiving aspirin can be considered normal, though increased bleeding may be associated.

12.3.6 Endodontic Considerations in Patients with Ischemic Heart Disease (IHD)

When coronary atherosclerotic heart disease becomes sufficiently advanced to produce symptoms, it is referred to as ischemic heart disease. It is relatively common in the general population, especially with increasing age, and typically presents as angina or heart failure [10]. Angina is often precipitated by physical activity or stress and may radiate to the arm or jaw or may present as facial or dental pain. Fear and anxiety associated with a dental procedure may be a precipitating factor for angina in some patients [11].

Angina attacks resulting from cardiac ischemia may be precipitated by dental treatment. This can lead to infarction and cardiac arrest. Dental patients with previous history of angina or a myocardial infarction are approached similarly. Patients who have a history of myocardial infarction less than 6 months prior to dental consultation should be deterred from elective dental care because of their increased susceptibility to repeat infarctions and other cardiovascular complications. Dental treatment should be reserved for emergency situations intended to provide odontogenic pain relief [18]. Patients with angina in the ambulatory setting should not be sedated, as it impairs their ability to report angina. Dentist should regularly check the patient's heart rate and BP during long appointments [15].

These patients benefit from empathy, short morning appointments, oral premedication with anxiolytics or prophylactic nitroglycerin, nitrous oxide-oxygen sedation, and slow delivery of an anesthetic with epinephrine (1:100,000) with aspiration, adequate pain management (during and after dental appointment), and cardiac monitoring [24]. The patient with mild or moderate angina should be reminded to bring with them their nitroglycerin tablets in case of an attack during treatment. If comorbid pulmonary disease (chronic obstructive pulmonary disease) exists, the dose of oxygen provided via cannula or nitrous-oxygen delivery should not exceed 3 L/min. Patients should be placed in a semi-supine position in the dental chair. This helps to prevent potential aspiration of fluid or materials.

It should also be remembered that IHD can rarely be felt as an orofacial pain complaint. Such a referred pain of cardiac origin can lead to a diagnostic dilemma for the clinicians. An improper diagnosis can result in unnecessary dental treatment and more significantly, it can delay the proper treatment of the cardiac problem. Differentiating the site of pain from the source of pain is important so that the treatment will be properly directed toward the source of pain [11].

Anticoagulants and antiplatelet drugs used in the prevention of atherothrombosis in cardiac patients can be associated with increased perioperative bleeding during dental surgical procedures [22]. Since stopping these drugs can result in serious complications, it is advisable not to discontinue these medications when performing minor surgical procedures [15, 22].

If the patient is receiving antiplatelet medication, excessive local bleeding should be controlled 1 [4]. If the patient is receiving anticoagulants, the international normalized ratio (INR) on the day of treatment should be determined. Minor oral surgical procedures can be carried out with an INR of less than 4.0, with additional aid of local hemostasis [18]. Patients with an INR greater than 4.0 should not undergo any dental surgical procedure without being referred to their cardiologist for medication alteration, expert opinion, and consent [14].

Potential adverse reactions need to be taken into account after treatment (e.g., the interaction between NSAIDs, penicillin, tetracyclines, metronidazole, and anticoagulants) because prophylactic antibiotic may need to be considered to prevent infection. Cardiac patients may also be prescribed digitalis (digoxin in some countries), which can increase nausea as well as exacerbate the gag reflex, a consideration if a rubber dam is not used.

12.3.7 Endodontic Considerations in Patients with Valvular Disease

Prosthetic heart valves carry the higher risk of thromboembolism, and valves placed in the aortic region are more risky than the one in mitral position [24].

An infection on or near the heart valves caused by a bacteremia is termed as infective or bacterial endocarditis. Patients with valvular disease present two primary considerations for dental treatment: potential risk for infective endocarditis (IE) and risk of excessive bleeding in patients on anticoagulant therapy [25].

Though IE is not an emergency condition in the dental clinic, the bacteremia associated with dental treatment can contribute to this potentially fatal disease in patients with valvular heart disease [14]. Therefore, patients with pathologic valve disease are to be managed in close consultation with their physicians, especially to determine the need for antibiotic premedication [21].

According to the most recent guidelines, antibiotic prophylaxis is only recommended for dental procedures that involve manipulation of gingival or the periapical tissue. In general, procedures associated with nonsurgical root canal treatment such as local anesthetic injection, placement of the rubber dam, and instrumentation within the canal system do not place the patient at significant risk for infective endocarditis. The incidence and magnitude of bacteremia when canal instrumentation does not extend into the periapical tissues is very low, and therefore, antibiotic prophylaxis is not required [26].

The highest risk of infective endocarditis (IE) is for patients with prosthetic cardiac valves, those with a history of IE or significant congenital heart disease, or cardiac transplant recipients who develop cardiac valvulopathy [10, 27]. The antibiotic regimen as per the guidelines from the *American Heart Association* before a dental procedure in patients with high risk for IE is given in Table 12.3.

Maintaining good oral hygiene and eradicating dental disease is shown to decrease the frequency of bacteremia from routine daily activities. Hence, the importance of oral health should be emphasized especially in patients with valvular diseases. Moreover, all the standard infection control protocols should be followed such as sterilization of instruments, barrier techniques, and disinfecting the dental clinic and the surgical area, in general maintaining the hygiene of the operatory. Antimicrobial mouth rinse (0.2% chlorhexidine) given before any dental treatment is shown to reduce bacteremia of oral origin [14].

Table 12.3 Antibiotic Prophylactic Regimens for Endocarditis, as recommended by the *American Heart Association*

Regimen	Drugs (single dose 30–60 min before procedure)
Standard regimen	Adults: 2.0 g amoxicillin Children: 50 mg/kg amoxicillin
Patients allergic to penicillin (oral)	Adults: 2 g cephalexin or other first- or second-generation cephalosporin Or 600 mg clindamycin Or 500 mg azithromycin or clarithromycin Children: 50 mg/kg cephalexin or other first- or second-generation cephalosporin (or) 20 mg/kg clindamycin Or 15 mg/kg azithromycin or clarithromycin
For patients allergic to penicillin and unable to take oral medications, IM/IV routes of administration is considered	Adults: 1.0 g IM or IV cefazolin or ceftriaxone Or 600 mg IM or IV clindamycin Children: 50 mg/kg IM or IV cefazolin or ceftriaxone Or 20 mg/kg IM or IV clindamycin within 30 min before the procedure

12.3.8 Endodontic Considerations in Patients with Cardiac Arrhythmias

Patients with cardiac arrhythmias are at greater risk for more serious cardiac complications including cardiac arrest. Most patients presenting for dental treatment will know they have an arrhythmia and will be taking controlling medication such as procainamide, quinidine, or propranolol. If the patient's cardiac status is unclear, treating in a more controlled hospital environment may be best. Best practice also includes the avoidance of excessive anesthetic with epinephrine. The excessive delivery of anesthetic with epinephrine by intraligamentary injection is contraindicated because it has been reported to act in a similar manner to intravenous epinephrine injection.

The general considerations during dental treatment of a cardiac patient (physician consultation, patient monitoring, stress reduction, and limited use of vasoconstrictors) should be strictly adhered to. Patients with dysrhythmias are sometimes managed with electronic devices such as pacemakers that emit electrical signals. These devices have been shown to be sensitive to electromagnetic signals produced by certain dental instruments like electrosurgical unit, electric pulp tester, electronic apex locator, etc. Although the newer models (bipolar devices with electromagnetic shielding) are generally not affected by the small electromagnetic fields generated by dental equipment, care and precaution should be taken when operating ultrasonic scalers and ultrasonic cleaning systems, and selecting composite curing lights in the vicinity of individuals who have pacemakers or implantable cardioverter-defibrillators [14, 28].

12.4 Diabetes

Diabetes affects blood glucose metabolism and vessel pathology. The condition may be the result of absolute insulin deficiency (type 1 diabetes), a problem with insulin function (termed relative or type 2 diabetes), or both conditions. Other types of diabetes include gestational diabetes and diabetes occurring secondary to other diseases.

According to *International Diabetes Foundation* (2015), diabetes mellitus is now an epidemic with 415 million people affected globally. This number is projected to rise to 642 million in 2040. It is estimated that one in two adults with diabetes is undiagnosed. Diabetes is reported to have been responsible for 5 million deaths worldwide in 2015.

It is characterized by hyperglycemia (increased blood glucose level) with or without glycosuria resulting from an absolute or conditional deficiency of insulin [26, 27]. Hyperglycemia leads to an increase in the urinary volume of glucose and fluid loss, which then produces dehydration and electrolyte imbalance. It is the inability of the diabetic patient to metabolize and use glucose, the subsequent metabolism of body fat, and the fluid loss and electrolyte imbalance that causes metabolic acidosis. Complications in the diabetic patient that can occur during and after dental treatment include hypoglycemia, coma, or infection and delayed healing.

Diabetes mellitus is diagnosed as a fasting blood glucose level greater than 125 mg/dL, and the normal fasting blood glucose level is considered to be less than 110 mg/dL. Patients with fasting plasma glucose levels greater than 110 mg/dL but less than 126 mg/dL represent a transitional condition between normal and DM and are considered to have impaired glucose tolerance [29, 30].

In poorly controlled diabetes, gingivitis, periodontitis, and periodontal bone loss are common oral manifestations. In uncontrolled diabetes, there are chances of infection and poor wound healing [31, 32].

12.4.1 Endodontic Considerations

In patients with controlled diabetes, no special treatment is required for routine dentistry including prophylaxis and dental restorative care. The patient should be told to continue with their normal eating and injection regimen. Morning appointments are recommended because cortisol levels are highest at this time and will provide the best blood glucose level. The morning meal should not be skipped [33]. If an appointment is likely to lead to a delayed or missed meal, the diabetic regimen may have to be modified with the assistance of the patient's physician. For patients receiving insulin therapy, appointments should be scheduled so that they do not coincide with peaks of insulin activity, since this is the period of maximal risk of developing hypoglycemia [34]. Before the procedure, it has to be ensured that the patient has eaten normally and taken medication as usual [3]. Emotional and physical stress increases the amount of cortisol and epinephrine secretion that induces hyperglycemia. Therefore, if the patient is very apprehensive, pretreatment sedation should be contemplated [34].

The type 1 patient should not be scheduled immediately after an insulin injection because this may result in a hypoglycemic episode. No more than two carpules of lidocaine 1:100,000, prilocaine HCL (1:200,000) or bupivacaine with 1:200,000 epinephrine should be delivered for anesthesia. In the moderately controlled diabetic patient, a maximum of two carpules of bupivacaine or prilocaine should be used. In the uncontrolled or brittle diabetic patient, only acute dental infection should be treated on an outpatient basis. Delivered anesthetic should not include epinephrine.

Non-insulin-controlled patients may require insulin, or the insulin dose for some insulin-dependent patients may have to be increased. Acute infections in diabetic patients should be managed using incision and drainage, pulpectomy, antibiotics, and warm rinses [35].

Prophylactic antibiotics are not indicated for endodontic surgery in well-controlled diabetics as they are at no greater risk of postoperative infection than the nondiabetics [36]. Whereas when endodontic surgery is required in a poorly controlled diabetic, prophylactic antibiotic should be considered due to altered function of neutrophils.

Lengthy appointments should be avoided. If a lengthy, especially surgical, procedure is to be undertaken, the patient's physician should be consulted. Blood glucose level should be constantly monitored during a lengthy surgical procedure. Hypoglycemia is a common complication during dental treatment in diabetic patients. Symptoms of hypoglycemia may range from mild, such as anxiety, sweating, and tachycardia, to severe, such as mental status changes, seizure, and coma. The patient usually senses that they are becoming hypoglycemic and requests any form sugar such as orange juice. Severe hypoglycemic episodes are medical emergencies and should be treated promptly with 15 g of oral carbohydrate such as 6 oz orange juice or 3–4 teaspoons of table sugar. If the patient is unable to cooperate or swallow, 1 mg of glucagon may be administered by subcutaneous or intramuscular injection [37].

If hypoglycemia appears to be developing, dental treatment should be terminated and glucose administered. Loss of consciousness is the most serious complication of hypoglycemia. Medical assistance should be quickly sought. Posttreatment problems can include delayed healing and infection. In uncontrolled diabetics, electrolyte imbalance can also present a problem following dental treatment.

12.5 Endodontic Considerations in Patients with Bleeding Disorders

Many dental procedures are associated with postoperative bleeding, which in most cases, is self-limiting and non-problematic. However, some people are at an increased risk of bleeding due to inherited bleeding disorders, in which even relatively minor invasive procedures can precipitate a prolonged bleeding episode [38, 39]. Although patients with congenital bleeding disorders have an increased risk of significant bleeding from invasive dental and oral surgery procedures [40, 41], the majority of routine nonsurgical dental treatment can be provided in a general dental practice [42, 43].

Some of the bleeding disorders are hemophilia (type A and B), von Willebrand's disease, platelet function disorders, thrombocytopenia, and hypofibrinogenemia and dysfibrinogenemia.

12.5.1 Hemophilia

Individuals with hemophilia (inherited bleeding disorder) do not bleed more profusely than an individual with normal coagulation but may bleed for a longer period of time [44] and may experience delayed bleeding due to clot instability. There are two main types of hemophilia: hemophilia A is the commonest, accounting for approximately 85% of all cases of hemophilia, and characterized by a deficiency of factor VIII. Hemophilia B is characterized by a deficiency of factor IX. Both types of hemophilia are inherited as X-linked recessive conditions and share identical clinical manifestations [45].

Patients with congenital bleeding disorders require formulation of a comprehensive treatment plan with an overall goal of achieving satisfactory hemostasis. It is essential to prevent accidental damage to the oral mucosa when carrying out any procedure in the mouth by implementing general measures such as careful use of saliva ejectors and care in the placement of radiographic films [40, 46].

Local anesthetic infiltration using a slow injection technique and modern fine gauge single-use needles can usually be used without the need for factor replacement therapy [40, 46–48] (Table 12.4). There are no restrictions regarding the type of local anesthetic used, although those with vasoconstrictors may provide additional local hemostasis [49]. Articaine has been described for infiltration as an alternative to inferior dental block in the restoration of mandibular molars, removing the need for preoperative factor cover [50]. A buccal infiltration can be used without any factor replacement. It will anesthetize all the upper teeth and lower anterior and premolar teeth. The intraligamentary technique or interosseous technique should be considered instead of the mandibular block.

Endodontic treatment is generally low risk for patients with bleeding disorders. Nonsurgical endodontic procedure can be performed without any modification in anticoagulant therapy, although it is important to ascertain that patient's international normalized ratio (INR) value is in the therapeutic range of (2–3.5) especially if a nerve block injection is required [51]. Periapical surgery may pose a greater challenge for hemostasis even for patients well maintained within the therapeutic

Table 12.4 Dental anesthetic techniques and factor replacement therapy [47]

No hemostatic cover required	Hemostatic cover required
Buccal infiltration	Inferior dental block
Intrapapillary injections	Lingual infiltrations
Intraligamentary injections	

range; therefore, a consultation with the patient's hematologist is required in developing an appropriate treatment plan.

It is important that the procedure be carried out carefully with the working length of the root canal calculated to ensure that the instruments do not pass through the apex of the root canal. Sodium hypochlorite should be used for irrigation in all cases, followed by the use of calcium hydroxide paste to control the bleeding.

Dental pain can usually be controlled with a minor analgesic such as paracetamol (acetaminophen) and codeine-based preparations. Aspirin should not be used due to its inhibitory effect on platelet aggregation. The use of any nonsteroidal anti-inflammatory drug (NSAID) must be discussed beforehand with the patient's hematologist because of their effect on platelet aggregation. Antibiotics should only be prescribed if there is local spread or signs of systemic infection. There are no contraindications to any of the antibiotics for patients with congenital bleeding disorders.

12.6 Infectious Diseases

Infectious conditions that are problematic in terms of dental management include hepatitis B (HBV), hepatitis C (HCV), HIV, and tuberculosis. Less likely to cause a problem but of additional concern are viral infections such as that seen in severe acute respiratory syndrome (SARS) or healthcare-associated infections such as methicillin-resistant *Staphylococcus aureus* (MRSA). Several potential complications can occur during dental treatment such as the risk of transmission, medication interactions in patients being treated for active disease.

HIV is a blood-borne retrovirus infection transmitted primarily by blood and bodily fluids by intimate sexual contact and parenteral route. After infection, enzyme reverse transcriptase allows the virus to integrate its own DNA into the genome of an infected cell and replicate using the infected cell's ribosomes and protein synthesis. Initially, immune seroconversion with antiviral antibody production occurs followed by a significant decrease in CD4+ lymphocytes over a period of years.

The most effective management in the progression of HIV infection and AIDS is a combination of antiviral agents known as highly active antiretroviral therapies (HAART), which has significantly increased the lifespan and the quality of life of individuals infected with HIV [52, 53].

12.6.1 HIV and Endodontics

In general, endodontic treatment of patients with apical periodontitis would have a poorer prognosis in immunocompromised patients such as HIV-infected patients. This is due to the fact that T cells play an important role in the pathogenesis as well as healing of apical periodontitis.

One of the challenges faced by HIV-positive patients and their dentist is the potential for adverse drug interactions. Because HIV-positive patients usually take an antiretroviral regimen of three or more drugs from at least two different classes, there exists a potential for unwanted side effects and toxicities [54].

Many of the medications dentists commonly administer or prescribe may interfere with the metabolism of the antiretroviral medications [55, 56]. Statistically, the chances of treating a HIV-positive patient in a dental practice have increased because of a steady state of new HIV infections annually and increasing longevity from highly active antiretroviral therapy. Thus, HIV-positive patients are seeking routine dental care rather than episodic treatment for the oral manifestations of HIV/AIDS, and dental clinicians should know how to appropriately care for them.

The dental clinician should know the medications that their HIV-positive patients are taking, understand the potential drug interactions with medications they prescribe, and be prepared to prescribe medications from a different class when interactions are possible.

Controversy exists in the literature regarding the need for antibiotic coverage before performing dentistry. A small subgroup of patients with advanced HIV disease may require customized modification, such as antibiotic prophylaxis or transfusion of blood products for their care [57]. If the granulocytes count ranges above 500 cells/μL of blood, endodontic treatment should be performed under prophylactic antibiotic cover. Patients with CD4 cell counts below 200 cells/μL might suffer from a disorder of blood coagulation. If the thrombocyte count is more than 60,000 cells/mm^3, routine dental treatment is possible without the risk of hemorrhage.

Infiltration and/or intraligamentary anesthesia is preferred to avoid any complications of block anesthesia. Antibiotic mouth rinses (chlorhexidine) can be prescribed 2–3 days before the treatment to achieve reduction in oral microorganisms and to avoid any postoperative complications.

Endodontic treatment for an HIV-infected patient is seen on an outpatient basis. These patients have the same prognosis with nonsurgical root canal treatment as medically healthy patients [53]. Finally, the practitioner should be aware of occupational risks in treating these patients, should familiarize himself / herself with the CDC's postexposure prophylactic guidelines, implement preventive measures to prevent occupational exposures, and provide occupational risk training for their staff.

Wounds and needle stick injury following dental procedures resulting in bleeding and subsequent instrument or materials contamination represent the biggest problem with respect to potential viral transmission to clinical staff. The risk of seroconversion after a needle stick injury with HIV-infected blood is approx. 0.03% [58, 59]. In case of deep penetrating injury with accidental exposure to HIV-infected blood and body fluids, a prophylactic administration of a triple antiretroviral therapy along with immediate referral to a specialist is recommended.

Precautions such as not putting the used injection needle back into the sheath and wearing gloves and goggles during the treatment are considered as adequate infection control precautions [60].

It is important to inform all staff members of the patient's infection before starting the treatment to ensure vigilance. Since HIV can be found in both pulpal tissues and apical granuloma, the use of rubber dam is considered mandatory [61]. With using rotary instruments, not only should the used instruments but also the handpiece must be disinfected and sterilized after every treatment.

A dentist may not ethically refuse to provide treatment purely because of the patients HIV status.

12.6.2 Hepatitis B and C and Endodontics

Hepatitis B virus (HBV) is a DNA virus and was originally known as "serum hepatitis" [62]. Hepatitis C is a hepatotropic viral infection caused by hepatitis C virus (HCV), which is a major cause of acute hepatitis and chronic liver disease. It is characterized by inflammation of the liver and in many cases permanent damage to liver tissue. The most common types of hepatitis are hepatitis A, B, C, D, E, and G. Hepatitis B and C can lead to permanent liver damage and in many cases, death [62].

Physicians, dentists, nurses, laboratory staff, and dialysis center personnel are at high risk of acquiring infection. HCV prevalence varies widely among countries, with the highest being in several African and eastern Mediterranean countries [63]. The frequency of exposure to HBV was the highest among dental healthcare workers according to a study conducted in Japan [64]. Even after the introduction of many programs and strategies, hepatitis infection continues to remain a health problem in dental settings.

The most significant problems associated with hepatitis B and C in dental settings include the risk of viral contagion on the part of the dental professionals and patients (cross infection), the risk of bleeding in patients with serious liver disease, and alterations in the metabolism of certain drug substances that increase the risk of toxicity [65]. It has been found that HBV and HCV exist on various surfaces in the dental operatory even many days after treating patient's positive with hepatitis B and C [66]. HCV can remain stable at room temperature for over 5 days [67]. Therefore, standard precautions, i.e., the use of barrier methods, with correct sterilization and disinfection measures, must be followed [65]. The conventional sterilization techniques usually eliminate specific proteins and nucleic acids (HBV DNA and HCV RNA) from dental instruments previously infected with HBV and HCV.

Elective treatment is postponed in an unfavorable state. However, in case treatment is carried out, the dentist must have local hemostatic agents such as oxidized and regenerated cellulose, as well as antifibrinolytic agents (tranexamic acid), platelets, and vitamin K [65]. If antibiotic prophylaxis is suggested, the physician treating the patient therefore should be consulted to establish which drugs are used, their doses, and their possible interactions [68].

Endodontic treatment can be provided for these patients with adequate sterilization care and infection control protocol. The most important factor is in choosing which of the medications and drugs metabolized in the liver should be avoided. Drugs such as erythromycin, metronidazole, or tetracyclines must be avoided entirely [69]. Ampicillin is the choice of antibiotic, while acetaminophen may be used for pain relieving [70]. Nonsteroidal anti-inflammatory drugs should be used with caution or avoided, due to the risk of gastrointestinal bleeding and gastritis usually associated with liver disease. Local anesthetics are generally safe, provided the total dosage does not exceed 7 mg/kg, combined with epinephrine.

In case there is an accidental exposure:

1. Carefully wash the wound without rubbing, as this may inoculate the virus into deeper tissues, for several minutes with soap and water or using a disinfectant of established efficacy against the virus (iodine solutions or chlorine formulations). The rationale behind these measures is to reduce the number of viral units to below the threshold count required to cause infection (the infectious dose).
2. A complete detailed medical and clinical history of the patient must be recorded to rule out possible risks.

All staff should be vaccinated appropriately. Infection control recommendations are mentioned in Appendix 12.1.

12.6.3 Endodontic Treatment in a Pregnant Patient

Pregnancy does not classify as being medically compromised; therefore, dental treatment should not be denied simply because a woman is pregnant. But the pregnant woman who presents for dental care may require special considerations.

Usually, pregnant patients are not immunocompromised; however, in pregnancy, there is suppression of the maternal immune system in response to the fetus [71] subsequently causing a decrease in cell-mediated immunity, as well as natural killer cell activity [72]. The odontogenic infections have the potential to progress rapidly to deep-space infections eventually compromising the oropharyngeal airway. In addition, pregnant women may also require a prescription and/or over-the-counter analgesics to control serious pulpal pain. Some of these drugs rather than benefitting effects may have deleterious effects on the fetus and the pregnant mother. Therefore, it is imperative that odontogenic infections should be treated promptly at any time during pregnancy. An understanding of the patient's physiologic changes, the effects of chronic infection, and the risks or benefits of medications is necessary to advise a patient on her options regarding medical care.

Fortunately, most of the drugs prescribed/used by a dentist are considered to be safe for both pregnant patients and their unborn child. However, if in any doubt, about either dental medication choices or the risk factors for pregnant patients, he or she should refer to the patient's obstetrician (Tables 12.5 and 12.6).

12.6.3.1 Local Anesthesia

Local anesthetics are most commonly used medications by dentists. Lidocaine and prilocaine are FDA category B rating when given in a therapeutic range and should be the first-line choices for local anesthesia for pregnant women who do not have any contraindications, such as allergy [73, 74]. Bupivacaine, mepivacaine, and articaine are FDA category C ratings.

Table 12.5 FDA drug categories during pregnancy [74, 75]

Category	US Food and Drug Administration risk stratification of drugs
A	Controlled studies in humans have failed to demonstrate a risk to the fetus, and the possibility of fetal harm appears remote
B	Animal studies have not been indicated fetal risk, and human studies have not been conducted, or animal studies have shown a risk, but controlled human studies have not
C	Animal studies have shown a risk, but controlled human studies have not been conducted, or studies are not available in humans or animals
D	Positive evidence of human fetal risk exists but in certain situations that drug may be used despite its risk
X	Evidence of fetal abnormalities and the fetal risk exists based on human experience, and the risk outweighs any possible benefit of use during pregnancy

Table 12.6 Common drugs used in pregnancy in dental treatment

Drug	Use in pregnancy	FDA category
Antibacterial		
Amoxicillin Metronidazole Erythromycin Penicillin Cephalosporins	Yes	B
Tetracycline Gentamicin	No • Discoloration of teeth with tetracycline • Fetal ototoxicity with gentamicin	D
Analgesics		
Oxycodone	With caution	B
Aspirin Ibuprofen Naproxen	Not in 3rd trimester • Postpartum hemorrhage with aspirin	B (D in 3rd trimester)
Acetaminophen Morphine Meperidine	Yes • Respiratory depression with morphine	B
Codeine		C (D in 3rd trimester)
Local anesthetics		
Lidocaine Prilocaine	Yes	B
Mepivacaine Bupivacaine	With caution • Fetal bradycardia with mepivacaine and bupivacaine	C
Sedatives/hypnotics		
Nitrous oxide	Not in 1st trimester • Spontaneous abortions with nitrous oxide	Avoid
Barbiturates and benzodiazepines	No • Cleft lip/palate with benzodiazepines	D

None of the above-listed local anesthetic agents are considered unsafe when given in dental therapeutic dose ranges [73, 75]. Additionally, the use of vasoconstrictors such as epinephrine or levonordefrin is not contraindicated when they are a part of the commercially available local anesthetics. Though they are FDA category C rating, these vasoconstrictors, when used in low concentrations in prepackaged local anesthetic cartridges, cause no fetal harm as long as normal precautions are taken. These precautions include avoiding injection within the blood vessels and maintaining total dosages at or below therapeutic ranges such as 0.04 mg for epinephrine and 0.2 mg for levonordefrin [73, 75].

12.6.3.2 Antibiotics

There are situations when antibiotics may be a necessary course of action. Most of the antibiotics used in dental care are FDA category B for pregnancy risk. These include the penicillin family, the erythromycins (except for the estolate form), azithromycin, clindamycin, metronidazole, and the cephalosporins [18]. However, tetracycline, minocycline, and doxycycline are given D ratings due to their likelihood of chelating in bones and teeth. Thus, tetracycline, minocycline, and doxycycline should be normally avoided [74].

12.6.3.3 Analgesics

Not all NSAIDs are considered safe for the fetus. Neither aspirin nor diflunisal is recommended for a pregnant woman. Both these drugs have both been associated with prolonged gestation and labor, anemia, increased bleeding potential, and premature closure of the ductus arteriosus of the heart [75]. Ibuprofen, ketoprofen, and naproxen are also contraindicated in the third trimester of pregnancy, as they are considered FDA category D choices, due to their risks of prolonged labor, hemorrhage risk during delivery, and premature closure of the ductus arteriosus.

The first-line choice of a NSAID should be acetaminophen which is considered to be FDA B rating for all three trimesters of pregnancy [18]. If stronger pain medication is necessary, most narcotic combinations are relatively safe for short durations, despite their risks for fetal growth retardation or fetal dependency if prescribed for long periods.

12.6.3.4 Anxiolytics

When treating anxiety in the dental setting, non-pharmaceutical methods are preferred because they reduce the fetus's exposure to medication. Most benzodiazepines for anxiolytic relief are classified in categories C or D for pregnancy risk [75, 76]. Intranasal nitrous oxide use is very controversial because there is risk of reduced uterine blood flow or teratogenic effects when it is used in high concentrations [76]. Short-term (i.e., %30 min) use of nitrous oxide, when used in combination with 50% oxygen for nonelective dental procedures, may be warranted if patient management is not possible without anxiolytic management.

12.6.4 Endodontic Management

Endodontic treatment in pregnancy is directed toward controlling disease, maintaining a healthy oral environment, and preventing potential problems that could occur later in the pregnancy or during the postpartum period and has been certified safe in pregnancy [77]. Nevertheless, it has been recommended that elective procedures be avoided until the end of pregnancy and only emergency treatment to be given or if possible, be delayed until the second trimester [78].

The initial 3 months of pregnancy are considered vital to the growth of the fetus. It has been recommended that any avoidable treatment in the first trimester should be moved to the next trimester to prevent any threat of untoward effects of dental treatment [72]. By the end of the first trimester, the uterine size is not large enough to make sitting on the dental chair uncomfortable, and nausea has generally waned. These make the second trimester an ideal period to undertake endodontic treatment. However, extensive elective endodontic procedures should be postponed until after delivery.

During the first trimester (conception to 14th week), there is a great risk of susceptibility to stress and teratogens, and 50–75% of all spontaneous abortions occur during this period [79]. Avoid routine radiographs. Use selectively and when needed.

During the second trimester (14–28th week), organogenesis is completed and therefore the risk to the fetus is low. Some elective and emergent dentoalveolar procedures are more safely accomplished during the second trimester. During the third trimester (29th week until childbirth), although there is no risk to the fetus during this trimester, the pregnant mother may experience an increasing level of discomfort. Short dental appointments should be scheduled with appropriate positioning while in the chair to prevent supine hypotension. The supine position poses an increased risk of developing DVT, by compression of the inferior vena cava, leading to venous stasis and clot formation. The ideal position in the dental chair is the left lateral decubitus position with the right buttock and hip elevated by 15°. Put a ref.

It has been researched that neither the cleansing irrigant, hypochlorite, nor root canal filling materials used in endodontic treatment is detrimental to the fetus [80]. Intraoral radiographs are considered safe for pregnant patients as the X-rays are directed to the mouth and not the abdomen, along with the use of protective measures such as high-speed film, collimation, filtration, lead apron, and a thyroid collar [81]. It has been proposed that *the As Low As Reasonably Achievable (ALARA)* principle should always be practiced, and only radiographs necessary for diagnosis and treatment should be obtained [82].

Local anesthetics are relatively safe when administered properly and in the correct amount during pregnancy [72]. For a healthy pregnant patient, the 1:100,000 epinephrine concentration used in dentistry, administered by proper aspiration technique and limited to the minimal dose required, is safe [77].

Feelings of joy, anxiety, or fear can be common during pregnancy. When combined with dental fears or phobia, pregnant patients may delay or avoid dental care. Anxiety may lead to transient increases in blood pressure, hyperventilation, or uterine cramping. It is important to remember that treatment is being given to two patients: mother and child. All treatment should be done only after consultation with the patient's gynecologist. It is best to avoid drugs and therapy that would put a fetus at risk in all women of child-bearing age or for whom a negative pregnancy test has not been ensured.

12.7 Endodontic Considerations for Patients Undergoing Chemo/Radiation Therapy and on Bisphosphonates

Cancers that are amenable to surgery and do not affect the oral cavity require few treatment plan modifications. Patients who previously had or are undergoing radiation therapy, chemotherapy, and others taking bisphosphonate medications require special consideration regarding their dental treatment. Prior to the beginning of cancer treatment, the patient should always be carefully evaluated by a dentist. The main goals of preventive dental measures are to remove any oral infection, pathology, or risk factors in order to obtain a stable oral health situation, preventing the necessity for invasive dental procedures in the near or intermediate future [83].

Whenever possible, non-restorable teeth and those with poor long-term periodontal prognosis should be extracted more than 2 weeks prior to radiation therapy. Symptomatic non-vital teeth can be endodontically treated at least 1 week before initiation of chemotherapy. Conservative endodontic and prosthodontic therapies of teeth with good prognosis should be completed. American Heart Association (AHA) has recommended antibiotic prophylaxis (refer to Table 12.2) as cancer patients may have catheters which may be susceptible to infection. This is controversial in literature [84].

For a patient receiving chemotherapy, WBC count and platelet status should be carefully monitored before commencement of dental procedure. Endodontic procedures can be performed if the neutrophil count is greater than 2000 cells per cubic mm and platelets are greater than 50,000 per cubic mm. Postradiation osteonecrosis (PRON) results from radiation-induced changes in the jaws, may arise in bones exposed to high radiation, and is characterized by asymptomatic or painful bone exposure.

Preventive measures and protocols used to reduce radionecrosis include selection of endodontic therapy over extraction, atraumatic surgical procedures, use of non-lidocaine local anesthetics that contain no or low concentrations of epinephrine and prophylactic antibiotics plus antibiotics during the week of healing [85]. Although nonsurgical endodontic treatment is a relatively safe procedure, caution is essential.

12.7.1 Patients Taking Antiresorptive and Anti-angiogenic Medication

Bisphosphonates are used to treat patients with metastatic breast cancer, multiple myeloma,

Paget's disease of the bone, hypercalcemia of malignancy, and for patients with documented bone metastases from any solid tumor (prostate cancer, lung cancer, and renal cell carcinomas).

Bisphosphonates are inhibitors of bone resorption. Bone remodeling is a normal physiologic function. It removes and replaces the damaged bone with new elastic osseous tissue [86]. Bisphosphonates inhibit osteoclast function, prevent bone turnover, and have anti-angiogenic properties [87, 88].

The management of bisphosphonate-associated osteonecrosis of the jaws represents an additional challenge to professionals. In 2014, the American Association of Oral and Maxillofacial Surgeons (AAOMSs) suggested to change the nomenclature from bisphosphonate-related osteonecrosis of the jaw (BRONJ) to MRONJ to accommodate the growing number of osteonecrosis cases involving the maxilla and mandible associated with other antiresorptive (denosumab) and anti-angiogenic therapies [89]. MRONJ or medication-related osteonecrosis of the jaw is a severe adverse drug reaction, manifesting as a progressive bone destruction in the maxillofacial region of patients. The dental treatment of patients receiving oral or intravenous bisphosphonate therapy is principally preventive in nature.

Intravenous (IV) bisphosphonates are utilized to treat conditions associated with cancer as well as hypercalcemia of malignancy, skeletal-related events connected with bone metastases from solid tumor, and for the management of lytic lesion related to multiple myeloma. Patients taking IV bisphosphonates are at higher risk for developing bisphosphonate-associated ONJ than those taking oral BPs. Oral BPs are used to treat osteoporosis, osteopenia, or other less common conditions such as Paget's disease and osteogenesis imperfecta. RANK ligand inhibitor (denosumab) is an antiresorptive medication that inhibits osteoclast function, decreases bone resorption, and increases bone density [90, 91]. It is used in patients affected by osteoporosis or metastatic bone diseases. Anti-angiogenic medications hinder the development of novel blood vessels, blocking the angiogenesis-signaling cascade [92].

Osteoporotic patients starting oral BP therapy should be instructed to the risk of developing MRONJ. Informative and educational documents about the current knowledge of MRONJ as well as the instruction to quickly report every signs and symptoms should be given to patients. Periodic clinical-radiological follow-ups are recommended. The importance of oral hygiene and dental health should be underlined [89]. Data are limited, so an informed consent for a non-quantifiable risk of long-term developing of MRONJ should be obtained. The risk of developing MRONJ associated with oral BPs is very low, and it increases when the duration of therapy exceeded 4 years [93].

Nonsurgical endodontics instead of tooth extraction should be performed whenever possible, even if the tooth is non-restorable. Endodontic surgical procedures and every invasive procedure that involves bone injury are not recommended. Consider BONJ when developing a differential diagnosis of non-odontogenic pain.

Endodontic procedures should be performed with care to avoid trauma to the surrounding periodontal tissues. Rubber dam placement with clamps should avoid impinging gingival tissue, or a modified isolation technique (split dam technique) should be considered.

Procedural errors resulting in periodontal tissue damage (perforation or apical foramen damage) should be prevented. Improved knowledge of root canal anatomy, careful instrumentation, correct working length measurement, and using an operating microscope and electronic apex locater are all helpful tools. A subgingival matrix band placement should be avoided. A decoronation procedure should be considered and endodontic treatment of the remaining roots for teeth with extensive coronal destruction, subgingival margin, or if not restorable. The tooth can be left with a permanent seal or prepared as an over-denture abutment.

Utilize the entire healthcare team, including the patient's general dentist, oncologist, and oral surgeon, when developing treatment plan for these patients. Be aware that the knowledge base for MRONJ is rapidly increasing and it is likely that these recommendations may change over time. The prudent practitioner is encouraged to continually review publications for new developments and treatments in antiresorptive therapy [94].

12.8 Patients with Chronic Kidney Disease

Chronic kidney disease is associated with progressive deterioration of renal function resulting in reduced glomerular filtration rate. Drugs used for its management tend to alter the common oral manifestations associated with the disease. The patients require special considerations for endodontic management because of increased tendency toward bleeding episodes, odontogenic infections, and drug interactions.

For renal disease patients with conservative medical management, the frequent episodes of hypertension require to constantly monitor the blood pressure during the procedure. Nephrotoxic drugs such as tetracyclines and aminoglycosides must be strictly avoided. Antibiotics such as amoxicillin/clavulanate, erythromycin, azithromycin, and analgesics such as paracetamol and ibuprofen do not require any dose alteration for these patients [95].

12.8.1 For Patients on Hemodialysis

These patients have bleeding tendencies due to uremia and hemodialysis [96]. During hemodialysis, the patient's blood is anticoagulated with heparin to assist blood transportation [97]. For this reason, endodontic procedures with a risk of bleeding should not be executed on the day of hemodialysis. Dental treatment should commence on a day after dialysis, to ensure the absence of circulating heparin [98].

Local anesthetics like lidocaine are generally safe and can be administered in their usual dose, and anesthesia can be achieved through infiltration, while nerve block is generally not advised unless deemed necessary because of bleeding tendencies. These patients should undergo complete blood count and coagulation profile tests before initiating the surgical endodontics and nerve blocks in nonsurgical root canal therapy.

These patients are highly prone to the risk of infection and of transmission possibility of hepatitis B virus, hepatitis C virus, and HIV. Appropriate diagnostic tests must be carried out to confirm the negative results for these infections.

12.8.2 For Patients with Renal Transplant

It is important that in the first 6 months after transplantation, any elective dental treatment should be avoided [99]. Treatment with corticosteroids, calcineurin inhibitors (Cs, tacrolimus), and inhibitors of lymphocyte proliferation (azathioprine and mycophenolate mofetil) is common in renal patients, and hence, they will be in an immunosuppressed state. Antibiotic prophylaxis, as per nephrologist's guidelines, is mandatory prior to endodontic procedure.

12.9 Patients on Corticosteroid Therapy

For these patients, it is necessary to assess whether patient is currently on steroid therapy or if there is a history of steroid intake for 2 weeks or longer within the past 2 years. In such condition, the patient's physician should be consulted if any extra dosage of steroid will be needed and confirm the pre- and post-procedural steroid dosages to avoid the risk of adrenal crisis [100]. Increased dose shift is not compulsory if the prednisolone dose is <7.5 mg/day. Morning appointments should be preferred for these patients.

12.10 Respiratory Disorders

12.10.1 Asthma

Asthma is a respiratory disease that affects the respiratory system characterized by inflammation and bronchoconstriction. A distinction should be made between allergic and non-allergic asthma [3].

Clinicians should be aware of the potential for dental materials and products to exacerbate asthma. These include dentifrices, fissure sealants, tooth enamel dust, and methyl methacrylate. Before starting the endodontic procedure, it is essential to understand about the type (mild, moderate, and severe), frequency of attack, and precipitating factors for avoiding the stimulators, and we should follow the emergency protocols [77]. Patients' immune status depends on the level of immunosuppressive medications they are taking. Only the most severely affected asthmatic patients who are taking large doses of systemic corticosteroids fall into this category. For severe conditions, procedures should be carried out with the physician's consent.

If the patient uses a bronchodilator inhaler, it is essential to advise him/her to bring the inhaler during each dental visit. Anxiety is a trigger and dental treatments often trigger an acute asthmatic attack. A well-planned and uncomplaining approach of the dentist and dental team members may help to lessen the anxiety.

When antibiotic therapy is indicated, macrolides (i.e., erythromycin, azithromycin, and clarithromycin), ciprofloxacin, and clindamycin should be avoided in patients taking theophylline because of the potential adverse effect of methylxanthine toxicity. NSAID group of medicines, barbiturates, and narcotics should be avoided for all asthmatic patients. Acetaminophen and Cox-2 inhibitors can be used as anti-inflammatory drugs for these patients since they do not precipitate bronchospasm. However, recent studies have suggested that long-term daily or weekly acetaminophen use is associated with a more severe asthma. Although there is reason for caution, acetaminophen still is the preferred analgesic for asthmatic patients [101].

LA-containing epinephrine should be avoided as their sulfite preservative component may induce acute asthmatic attacks and allergic reactions. Improper positioning of suction tips or the use of cotton rolls could trigger a hyper reactive airway response in sensitive subjects. Rubber dams should be used judiciously to avoid possible respiratory compromise or aggravation. Prolonged supine positioning can also trigger an asthmatic attack in the dental setting. In the event of an acute asthmatic attack during dental treatment, the clinician should stop the procedure, remove all intraoral implements and rule out foreign body aspiration, and initiate the emergency protocol for managing acute asthmatic exacerbation.

12.10.2 COPD

Chronic obstructive pulmonary disorder (COPD) is a collective term for lung diseases including chronic bronchitis, emphysema, and chronic obstructive airway diseases [74]. COPD patients have breathing problems primarily due to their constricted airways. Medical treatment is directed toward managing the acute and chronic symptoms because COPD cannot be cured completely Endodontic considerations are the same as in asthma.

Conclusion

The potential always exists for development of a medical emergency in a medically compromised patient. Enough emphasis cannot be given to the importance of a detailed history taking. All dentists and dental office staff must be prepared to recognize and treat adverse responses using appropriate current guidelines. Although there is a huge range of systemic illnesses, this chapter focussed on only selected conditions that need utmost care. Endodontic therapy rather than extraction, maybe the treatment of choice for medically compromised patients due to their health condition as well as psychological status. Today, endodontists are very well informed regarding systemic diseases and can deliver a high standard of endodontic treatment, while at the same time minimizing the potential problem related to general health of the patient.

Appendix 12.1: Infection Prevention Recommendations (Modified and Adapted from CDC, US Department of Health and Human Resources, 2016)

Administrative measures

1. Develop and maintain written infection prevention policies and procedures specific for the dental setting based on evidence-based guidelines (e.g., CDC/Healthcare Infection Control Practices Advisory Committee [HICPAC]), regulations, or standards.
2. Infection prevention policies and procedures should be reassessed at least annually.
3. At least one individual trained in infection prevention is assigned responsibility for coordinating the program.

Dental healthcare personnel safety (DHCP)

1. All staff should be immunized according to the current CDC recommendations for immunizations, evaluation, and follow-up. There is a written policy regarding immunizing DHCP, including a list of all required and recommended immunizations for DHCP (e.g., hepatitis B, MMR (measles, mumps, rubella), varicella (chicken pox), Tdap (tetanus, diphtheria, pertussis)).
2. A log of needlesticks, sharps injuries, and other employee exposure events should be maintained.
3. Referral arrangements should be in place to qualified healthcare professionals (e.g., occupational health program of a hospital) to ensure prompt and appropriate provision of preventive services, occupationally related medical services, and postexposure management with medical follow-up.
4. Establish routine evaluation of the infection prevention program

Sharps safety

1. Sharp items (needles, burs, scalers, etc.) that are contaminated with patient blood and saliva should be considered as potentially infective.
2. Do not recap used needles by using both hands or any other technique that involves directing the point of a needle toward any part of the body.
3. Place used disposable syringes and needles and any other sharp items in appropriate puncture-resistant containers located as close as possible to the area where the items are used.

Sterilization and disinfection of patient care devices

1. Written policies and procedures should be available to ensure reusable patient care instruments, and devices are cleaned and reprocessed appropriately before use on another patient.
2. Clean and disinfect/sterilize reusable dental equipment appropriately before use on any other patient, according to the manufacturer's instructions. If the manufacturer does not provide such instructions, the device may not be suitable for multi-use.
3. Wear appropriate PPE (personal protective equipment) when handling contaminated patient equipment (e.g., examination or heavy duty utility gloves, protective clothing, masks, eye protection) to prevent exposure to infectious agents or chemicals.
4. Routine maintenance for sterilization equipment should be performed according to manufacturer instructions and documented by written maintenance records.

References

1. Peacock ME, Carson ME. Frequency of self-reported medical conditions in periodontal patients. J Periodontol. 1995;66:1004–7.
2. Jain kittivong A, Yeh CK, Guest IF, Cottone JA. Evaluation of medical consultations in a predoctoral dental clinic. Oral Surg Oral Med Oral Pathol Oral Radiol Endod. 1995;80:409–13.

3. Little JW, Falace DA, Miller CS, Rhodus NL. Dental management of the medically compromised patient. 6th ed. St. Louis, MO: Mosby; 2002.
4. Smeets EC, de Jong KJ, Abraham-Inpijn L. Detecting the medically compromised patient in dentistry by means of the medical risk-related history. A survey of 29,424 dental patients in The Netherlands. Prev Med. 1998;27:530–5.
5. Segura-Egea JJ, Jimenez-Moreno E, Calvo-Monroy C. Hypertension and dental periapical condition. J Endod. 2010;36:1800–4.
6. Lessard E, Click M, Ahmed A, Saric M. The patient with a heart murmur: evaluation, assessment and dental considerations. J Am Dent Assoc. 2005;136:347–56.
7. Vasan RS, Larson MG, Leip EP, et al. Impact of high normal blood pressure on the risk of cardiovascular disease. N Engl J Med. 2001;345(18):1291–7.
8. Chobanian AV, Bakris GL, Black HR, et al. The seventh report of the joint national committee on prevention, detection, evaluation and treatment of high blood pressure: the JNC 7 report. JAMA. 2003;289(19):2560–72.
9. Hogan J, Radhakrishnan J. The assessment and importance of hypertension in the dental setting. Dent Clin N Am. 2012;56:731–45.
10. Wilson W, Taubert KA, Gewitz M, Lockhart PB, Baddour LM, Levison M, et al. Guidelines from the American Heart Association for the quality of care and outcomes from Research Interdisciplinary Working Group. J Am Dent Assoc. 2007;138:739–60.
11. Herman WW, Konzelman JL, Prisant LM. New national guidelines on hypertension: a summary for dentistry. J Am Dent Assoc. 2004;135:576–84.
12. Hargreaves KM, Cohen S, Berman LH. Case selection and treatment planning. In: Rosenberg PA, Frisbie JC, Hargreaves KM, Cohen S, editors. Cohen's Pathways of the pulp. 10th ed. St. Louis, MO: Mosby Elsevier; 2011. p. 71–87.
13. Malamed SF. Knowing your patients. J Am Dent Assoc. 2010;141:S3–7.
14. Cruz-Pamplona M, Jimenez-Soriano Y, Sarrión-Pérez MG. Dental considerations in patients with heart disease. J Clin Exp Dentist. 2011;3:97–105.
15. Hupp JR. Ischemic heart disease: dental management considerations. Dent Clin N Am. 2006;50:483–91.
16. Margaix-Muñoz M, Jiménez-Soriano Y, Poveda-Roda R, Sarrión G. Cardiovascular diseases in dental practice. Practical considerations. Med Oral Patol Oral Cir Bucal. 2008;13:296–302.
17. Malamed SF. Handbook of dental anesthesia. 5th ed. St Louis, MO: Elsevier Mosby; 2004.
18. Pérusse R, Goulet JP, Turcotte JY. Contraindications to vasoconstrictors in dentistry: part I. Cardiovascular diseases. Oral Surg Oral Med Oral Pathol. 1992;74:679–86.
19. Bavitz JB. Dental management of patients with hypertension. Dent Clin N Am. 2006;50:547–62.
20. Connolly HM, Crary JL, McGoon MD, Hensrud DD, Edwards BS, Edwards WD, et al. Valvular heart disease associated with fenfluramine—phentermine. N Eng J Med. 1997;337:581–8.
21. Warburton G, Caccamese JF Jr. Valvular heart disease and heart failure: dental management considerations. Dent Clin N Am. 2006;50:493–512.
22. Pototski M, Amenábar JM. Dental management of patients receiving anticoagulation or antiplatelet treatment. J Oral Sci. 2007;49:253–8.
23. Bonow RO, Carabello BA, Kanu C, de Leon AC Jr, Faxon DP, et al. American College of Cardiology/American Heart Association Task Force on Practice Guidelines; Society of Cardiovascular Anesthesiologists; Society for Cardiovascular Angiography and Interventions; Society of Thoracic Surgeons. ACC/AHA 2006 guidelines for the management of patients with valvular heart disease: A report of the American College of Cardiology/American Heart Association Task Force on Practice Guidelines (writing committee to revise the 1998 guidelines for the management of patients with valvular heart disease): Developed in collaboration with the society of cardiovascular anesthesiologists: Endorsed by the society for cardiovascular angiography and interventions and the society of thoracic surgeons. Circulation. 2006;114:e84–231.
24. Lockhart PB, Loven B, Brennan MT, Fox PC. The evidence base for the efficacy of antibiotic prophylaxis in dental practice. J Am Dent Assoc. 2007;138:458–74.
25. Brennan MT, Wynn RL, Miller CS. Aspirin and bleeding in dentistry: an update and recommendations. Oral Surg Oral Med Oral Pathol Oral Radiol Endod. 2007;104:316–23.

26. Little JW Falace DA, Miller CS, Rhodus NL. Management of the hypertensive patient in dentistry. 5th ed. St Louis, MO: Mosby; 1997. p. 176–92.
27. Beck DE. New guidelines for prevention of infective endocarditis. Ochsner J. 2007;7:106.
28. Roedig JJ, Shah J, Elayi CS, Miller CS. Interference of cardiac pacemaker and implantable cardioverter-defibrillator activity during electronic dental device use. J Am Dent Assoc. 2010;141:521–6.
29. Larsen ML, Hørder M, Mogensen EF. Effect of long-term monitoring of glycosylated haemoglobin levels in insulin-dependent diabetes mellitus. N Engl J Med. 1990;323:1021–5.
30. Firrilio J. Endodontic management of patient with diabetes. Dent Clin N Am. 2007;50:561–606.
31. Montoya-Carralero JM, Saura-Pérez M, Canteras-Jordana M, Morata-Murcia IM. Reduction of HbA1c levels following nonsurgical treatment of periodontal disease in type 2 diabetics. Med Oral Patol Oral Cir Bucal. 2010;15:808–12.
32. Wang CH, Chueh LH, Chen SC, Feng YC, Hsiao CK, Chiang CP. Impact of diabetes mellitus, hypertension, and coronary artery disease on tooth extraction after nonsurgical endodontic treatment. J Endod. 2011;37:1–5.
33. Living with diabetes. http://www.diabetes.org/living-with-diabetes/treatment-and-care/oral-health-and-hygiene/. Accessed 19 Feb 2017. Last Edited: January 22, 2014.
34. Azodo CC. Current trends in the management of diabetes mellitus: the dentist's perspective. J Postgrad Med. 2009;11:113–29.
35. Cohen S, Hargreaves KM. Pathways of the pulp. 9th ed. St. Louis, MO: Mosby; 2006. p. 85.
36. Mc Kenna SJ. Dental management of patients with diabetes. Dent Clin N Am. 2006;50: 591–606.
37. Ingle JI, Bakland LK, Baumgartner JC. Ingle's endodontics. 6th ed. Hamilton: BC Decker Inc.; 2008. p. 763.
38. Scully C, Wolff A. Oral surgery in patients on anticoagulant therapy. Oral Surg Oral Med Oral Pathol Oral Radiol Endod. 2002;94:37–64.
39. Cannon PD, Dharmar VT. Minor oral surgical procedures in patients on oral anticoagulants—a controlled studies. Aust Dent J. 2003;48:115–8.
40. Hewson ID, Daly J, Hallett KB, et al. Consensus statement by hospital based dentists providing dental treatment for patients with inherited bleeding disorders. Aust Dent J. 2011;56:221–6.
41. Heiland M, Weber M, Schmelzle R. Life-threatening bleeding after dental extraction in a haemophilia A patient with inhibitors to factor VIII: a case report. J Oral Maxillofac Surg. 2003;61:1350–3.
42. Dougall A, Fiske J. Access to special care dentistry, part 5. Safety. Br Dent J. 2008;205: 177–90.
43. Dougall A, O'Mahoney B. Evaluation of a collaborative model of shared care designed to increase access to preventive and restorative dentistry for patients with haemophilia. Haemophilia. 2010;16(Suppl 4):50. (Abs no 11FP04).
44. Berry E, Hilgartner M, Mariani G, Sultan Y. Members of the Medical Advisory Board, World Federation of Haemophilia. In: Jones P, editor. Haemophilia: facts for health care professionals. Geneva: World Health Organization; 1996.
45. Bolton-Maggs PH, Pasi KJ. Haemophilias A and B. Lancet. 2003;361:1801–9.
46. Brewer A, Correa ME. Guidelines for dental treatment of patients with inherited bleeding disorders. Montréal: World Federation of Haemophilia; 2006. (Treatment of Haemophilia monograph, no 40).
47. Brewer AK, Roebuck EM, Donachie M, et al. The dental management of adult patients with haemophilia and other congenital bleeding disorders. Haemophilia. 2003;9:673–7.
48. Freedman M, Dougall A, White B. An audit of a protocol for the management of patients with hereditary bleeding disorders undergoing dental treatment. J Disabil. Oral Health. 2009;10:151–5.
49. Richter S, Stratigos GT. Management of a hemophiliac with a dental abcess and subsequent root canal therapy and apicoectomy. N Y State Dent J. 1973;39:11–4.
50. Robertson D, Nusstein J, Reader A, Beck M, McCartney M. The anaesthetic efficacy of articaine in buccal infiltration of mandibular posterior teeth. J Am Dent Assoc. 2007;138:1104–12.
51. Jafri SM. Periprocedural thromboprophylaxis in patients receiving chronic anticoagulation therapy. Am Heart. 2004;147:3–15.

52. Suchina JA, Levine D, Flaitz CM. Retrospective clinical and radiologic evaluation of nonsurgical endodontic treatment in human immunodeficiency virus (HIV) infection. J Contemp Dent Ract. 2006;7:1–8.
53. Quesnell BT, Alves M, Hawkinson RW Jr. The effect of human immunodeficiency virus on endodontic treatment outcome. J Endod. 2005;31:633.
54. Hastreiter RJ, Jiang P. Do regular dental visits affect the oral health care provided to people with HIV. J Am Dent Assoc. 2002;133:1343–50.
55. Williams M. The HIV positive dentist in the United Kingdom the decline of the undiagnosed clinician. J Am Med Dent Assoc. 1999;130:509–20.
56. Bonito AJ, Patton LL, Shugars DA, et al. Management of dental patients who are HIV-positive. Evidence Report/Technology Assessment No. 37 (Contract 290-97-0011 to the Research Triangle Institute-University of North Carolina at Chapel Hill Evidencebased Practice Center). AHRQ Publication No. 01-E042. Rockville, MD: Agency for Healthcare Research and Quality; 2002.
57. Goldman M, Cloud GA, Wade KD, Reboli AC, Fichtenbaum CJ, Hafner R, et al. A randomized study of the use of fluconazole in continuous versus episodic therapy in patients with advanced HIV infection and a history of oropharyngeal candidiasis: AIDS Clinical Trials Group Study 323/Mycoses Study Group Study 40. Clin Infect Dis. 2005;41:1473–80.
58. Petereit G, Kirch W. Arzneimittelkommission: Beryfliche HIV- exposition und medikamentose Postexpositionsprophylaxe. Zahnartl Mitt. 1997;87:72–3.
59. Marcus U. Risiken und Wege der HIV- Ubertragung. Auswirkungen auf Epidemiologie und Pravention der HIV- Infektion. Bundesgesundheitsblatt Gesundheitsforschung Gesundheitsschutz. 2001;44:554–61.
60. Guidelines of the DGZMK. Virusinfektionen in der Zahnarztpraxis. Dtsch Zahnarztl Z. 2000;55:298–9.
61. Gerner NW, Hurlen B, Dobloug G, Brandtzag P. Endodontic treatment and immunopathology of periapical granuloma in an AIDS patient. Endod Dent Traumatol. 1988;4:127–31.
62. Ramsay DB, Friedman M, Borum ML. Does the race or gender of hepatitis C infected patients influence physicians' assessment of hepatitis A and hepatitis B serologic status? South Med J. 2007;100:683–5.
63. Papatheodoridis G, Hatzakis A. Public health issues of hepatitis C virus infection. Best Pract Res Clin Gastroenterol. 2012;26:371–80.
64. Nagao Y, Matsuoka H, Kawaguchi T, Ide T, Sata M. HBV and HCV infection in Japanese dental care workers. Int J Mol Med. 2008;21:791–9.
65. Grau-García-Moreno DM. Dental management of patients with liver disease. Med Oral. 2003;8:23.
66. Younai FS, Murphy DC, Kotelchuck D. Occupational exposures to blood in a dental teaching environment: results of a ten-year surveillance study. J Dent Educ. 2001;65:436–48.
67. Lodi G, Porter SR, Scully C. Hepatitis C virus infection: review and implications for the dentist. Oral Surg Oral Med Oral Pathol Oral Radiol Endod. 1998;86:8–22.
68. Centers for Disease Control and Prevention (CDC). Updated CDC recommendations for the management of hepatitis B virus-infected health-care providers and students. MMWR Recomm Rep. 2012;61:1–40.
69. Golla K, Epstein JB, Cabay RJ. Liver disease: current perspectives on medical and dental management. Oral Surg Oral Med Oral Pathol Oral Radiol Endod. 2004;98:516–21.
70. Krasteva A, Panov VE, Garoval M, Velikova R, Kisselova A, Krastev Z. Hepatitis B and C in dentistry. JMAB. 2008;14:38–40.
71. Gordon MC. Maternal physiology in pregnancy. In: Gabbe SG, Niebyl JR, Simpson J, editors. Obstetrics: normal and problem pregnancies. 4th ed. New York: Churchill Livingstone; 2002. p. 63–91.
72. Giglio JA, Lanni SM, Laskin DM, Giglio NW. Oral health care for the pregnant patient. J Can Dent Assoc. 2009;75:43–8.
73. Haas DA. An update on local anesthetics in dentistry. J Can Dent Assoc. 2002;68(9):546–51.
74. Wynn RL, Meiller TF, Crossley HL. Drug information handbook for dentistry. 10th ed. Hudson, OH: Lexi-Comp; 2005. p. 47–50. 145–8, 174–7, 294–6, 348–50, 369–71, 471–4, 562–3, 594–6, 603–5, 702–4, 783–5, 823–6, 870–2, 917–20, 931–4, 1003–4, 1027–8.

75. Haas DA, Pynn BR, Sands TD. Drug use for the pregnant and lactating patient. Gen Dent. 2000;48(1):54–60.
76. Alexander RE. Eleven myths of dentoalveolar surgery. J Am Dent Assoc. 1998;129(9):1271–9.
77. Little JW, Falace DA, Miller CS, Rhodus NL. Dental management of the medically compromised patient. 7th ed. St. Louis, MO: C.V. Mosby; 2008. p. 268–78. (456).
78. Garg N, Garg A. Pregnancy considerations in dentistry. Indian J Res Dent. 2014;1:8–11.
79. Yuan K, Wing LY, Lin MT. Pathogenetic roles of angiogenic factors in pyogenic granulomas in pregnancy are modulated by female sex hormones. J Periodontol. 2002;73:701–8.
80. Risks Associated and Best Strategy for Root Canal Treatment During Pregnancy. 2017. http://www.monashdentalgroup.com.au/endodontic/risks-associatedandbest-strategy-for-root-canal-treatment-duringpregnancy/.
81. Richards AG, Colquitt WN. Reduction in dental X-ray exposures during the past 60 years. J Am Dent Assoc. 1981;103:713–8.
82. Katz VL. Prenatal care. In: Scott JR, Gibbs RS, Karlan BY, Haney AF, editors. Danforth's obstetrics and gynecology. 9th ed. Philadelphia: Lippincott, Williams & Wilkins; 2003. p. 43–8.
83. Hellstein JW, Adler RA, Edwards B, Jacobsen PL, Kalmar JR, Koka S, et al. Managing the care of patients receiving antiresorptive therapy for prevention and treatment of osteoporosis: Executive summary of recommendations from the American Dental Association Council on Scientific Affairs. J Am Dent Assoc. 2011;142:1243–51.
84. American Association of Oral and Maxillofacial Surgeons position paper on medication-related osteonecrosis of the jaw. 2014.
85. Delmas PD. Clinical potential of RANKL inhibition for the management of postmenopausal osteoporosis and other metabolic bone diseases. J Clin Densitom. 2008;11:325–38.
86. Fizazi K, Carducci M, Smith M, Damião R, Brown J, Karsh L, et al. Denosumab versus zoledronic acid for treatment of bone metastases in men with castration-resistant prostate cancer: A randomised, double-blind study. Lancet. 2011;377:813–22.
87. Tenore G, Palaia G, Gaimari G, Brugnoletti O, Bove L, Lo Giudice R, et al. Medication-related osteonecrosis of the jaws (MRONJ): etiological update. Senses Sci. 2014;1:147–52.
88. Lo JC, O'Ryan FS, Gordon NP, Yang J, Hui RL, Martin D, et al. Prevalence of osteonecrosis of the jaw in patients with oral bisphosphonate exposure. J Oral Maxillofac Surg. 2010;68:243–53.
89. American Association of Endodontics, Colleagues for Excellence, Fall 2012. Bisphosphonate-associated Osteonecrosis of the Jaw.
90. Thomson PJ, Greenwood M, Meekan JG. General medicine and surgery for dental practitioners. Part-6 cancer, radiotherapy and chemotherapy. Br Dent J. 2010;2:65–8.
91. Main JHP. Dental care for cancer patients. Can Med Assoc J. 1983;128:1062–3.
92. Ott SM. Long-term safety of bisphosphonates. J Clin Endocrinol Metab. 2005;90:1897–9.
93. Rogers MJ, Watts DJ, Russell RG. Overview of bisphosphonates. Cancer. 1997;80:1652–60.
94. Fleisch H. Development of bisphosphonates. Breast Cancer Res. 2002;4:30–4.
95. de la Rosa García E, Mondragón Padilla A, Aranda Romo S, Bustamante Ramírez MA. Oral mucosa symptoms, signs and lesions, in end stage renal disease and non-end stage renal disease diabetic patients. Med Oral Patol Oral Cir Bucal. 2006;11:E467–73.
96. Hedges SJ, Dehoney SB, Hooper JS, Amanzadeh J, Anthony J. Evidence-based treatment recommendations for uremic bleeding. Nat Clin Pract Nephrol. 2007;3:138–53.
97. Sharma DC, Pradeep AR. End stage renal disease and its dental management. N Y State Dent J. 2007;73:43–7.
98. Klassen JT, Krasko BM. The dental health status of dialysis patients. J Can Dent Assoc. 2002;68:34–8.
99. Gudapati A, Ahmed P, Rada R. Dental management of patients with renal failure. Gen Dent. 2002;50:508–10.
100. Little JW, Falace DA, Miller CS, Rhodus NL. Little and Falace's dental management of the medically compromised patient. 8th ed. St. Louis, MO: Mosby; 2012. p. 240–50.
101. Hunt LW, Frigas E, Butterfield JH, Kita H, Blomgren J, Dunnette SL, et al. Treatment of asthma with nebulized lidocaine: a randomized, placebo-controlled study. J Allergy Clin Immunol. 2004;113:853–9.

Erratum to: Strategies to Reduce the Risk of Reinfection in Endodontics

Federico Foschi

Erratum to:
Chapter 8 in: P. Jain (ed.), *Common Complications in Endodontics,*
https://doi.org/10.1007/978-3-319-60997-3_8

The spelling of the author was inadvertently published as Federico Foshi in the table of contents and chapter 8.
This has now been amended throughout the book as Federico Foschi

The updated online version of the original chapter can be found at
https://doi.org/10.1007/978-3-319-60997-3_8

F. Foschi, BDS, MSc, PhD, FHEA, FDS RCS
Department of Endodontics, King's College London, Guy's Hospital, Tower Wing,
Fl 22, Great Maze Pond, London, SE1 9RT, UK
e-mail: federico.foschi@kcl.ac.uk

P. Jain (ed.), *Common Complications in Endodontics*,
https://doi.org/10.1007/978-3-319-60997-3_13

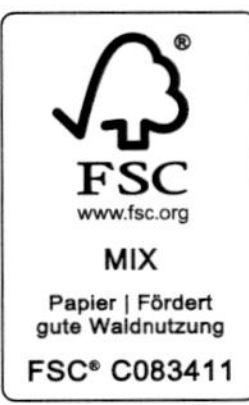

Zeitfracht Medien GmbH
Ferdinand-Jühlke-Straße 7
99095 Erfurt, Deutschland
produktsicherheit@kolibri360.de